FAST FOOD
GENOCIDE

Also by Joel Fuhrman, M.D.

The End of Heart Disease
The End of Dieting
Eat to Live Cookbook
The End of Diabetes
Super Immunity
Eat for Health
Disease-Proof Your Child
Fasting and Eating for Health
Eat to Live
Eat to Live Quick & Easy Cookbook

FAST FOOD GENOCIDE

How Processed Food Is Killing Us and What We Can Do About It

Joel Fuhrman, M.D.

WITH RESEARCH AND CONTRIBUTIONS BY ROBERT B. PHILLIPS

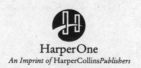

HarperOne
An Imprint of HarperCollinsPublishers

HarperOne

FAST FOOD GENOCIDE. Copyright © 2017 by Joel Fuhrman, M.D. All rights reserved. Printed in the United States of America. No part of this book may be used or reproduced in any manner whatsoever without written permission except in the case of brief quotations embodied in critical articles and reviews. For information, address HarperCollins Publishers, 195 Broadway, New York, NY 10007.

HarperCollins books may be purchased for educational, business, or sales promotional use. For information, please email the Special Markets Department at SPsales@harpercollins.com.

FIRST HARPERCOLLINS PAPERBACK EDITION PUBLISHED IN 2018

Designed by Kris Tobiassen of Matchbook Digital
Illustrations by Colin Goh

Library of Congress Cataloging-in-Publication Data is available upon request.

ISBN 978-0-06-257122-9

18 19 20 21 22   LSC   10 9 8 7 6 5 4 3 2 1

This book is dedicated to the thousands of people that "give back" to others across the globe; people who encourage compassion for others in their work, sacrifice their own comforts, and even take personal risks to aid others. This country was founded and built on people fighting for every person's rights, dignity, and pursuit of happiness.

CONTENTS

PARTICIPANTS IN OUR OWN DESTRUCTION

It isn't that they can't see the solution. It's that they can't see the problem.

—G. K. CHESTERTON

We are facing a tragic and unprecedented destruction of human lives in the United States and much of the developed world. Processed, fake, and fast foods have become the primary source of calories in this country, and they're on track to become the same in other countries. This attachment to fast food over natural foods and fresh produce is moving us toward widespread chronic disease, mental illness, and shortened life spans. I believe that the growing fast food addiction in this country and abroad is a genocide, as these foods destroy life with frightening efficiency and this damage is worsening. The food industry has evolved to effectively feed the majority of our citizens with mass-marketed, factory-produced foods that do not have the biological and chemical properties of natural produce. The result is the destruction of human potential, along with an explosion of chronic illness, human suffering, and the premature death of millions.

The American Heritage Dictionary defines genocide as "the deliberate destruction of an entire race or nation."

On the surface it may seem that we are in control of our food choices and therefore "genocide" does not apply here. We typically think of genocide as a crime that one group commits against another. But that is not always the case; sometimes we are participants in our own destruction. Multiple factors combine to remove choice from the equation, leaving all of us in peril.

In an effort to improve efficiency and cost-effectiveness, food companies have developed ways to feed a great many people with highly processed, highly addictive foods. These foods are designed to hook us and impair our taste buds in the process. Despite the wealth of the nation, many people live in parts of the country where fresh ingredients are difficult to get. When healthy foods are simply out of reach, individuals have no opportunity to make informed choices about what they eat. Furthermore, the medical establishment offers quick-fix surgery or a lifetime supply of pills in place of a simple dietary regimen that can reverse and prevent disease and save millions of lives from medical tragedy and premature death. The harm of these medical interventions is glossed over, and the benefits are exaggerated, while this food-induced health care crisis continues to grow. Last but not least, the idea that unhealthy food leads only to weight gain and not unhappiness, disease, and death remains a permanent myth that permeates society. We need to make clear that the issues are far more than just about waistlines; they are about lifelines.

Despite the tremendous evidence coming from the worlds of nutritional and social sciences, these "Frankenfoods"—or unnatural, human-made, processed fast foods—continue to destroy the fiber of our society, creating new social problems and damaging the health and happiness of a large proportion of our population. Modern science reveals that this pervasive and serious damage to our health can even damage our genes, resulting in severe harm being passed on to future generations. This is information that everyone must know.

Most health problems facing Americans today are the direct consequence of Frankenfoods. Heart attacks, strokes, adult and childhood cancers, our growing epidemic of attention deficit hyperactivity disorder (ADHD), autism, allergies, and autoimmune diseases all have their basis in the common dietary practices that are ubiquitous across the United States. According to studies, our diet, not just during pregnancy but even before conception, has profound effects in determining the health, intelligence, and immune systems of our children.[1] The problem is deeper, more serious, and more pervasive than anyone imagined, and no one is safe. It is widely accepted that mental illness, antisocial behavior, reduced intelligence, and most life-altering chronic diseases are primarily genetic; that is, they are not the result of dangerous foods. But this assumption is dead wrong. Further, this false belief perpetuates bigotry, contempt, and a growing, but generally ignored atrocity occurring right under our noses in urban communities.

By itself, a single pebble is harmless. However, put enough small pebbles together and start them rolling down the side of a mountain, and suddenly you have an avalanche. An avalanche doesn't just move earth and rocks from one place to another; it destroys everything in its path. We are already experiencing an expanding crisis of physical and mental health deterioration from an avalanche of commercially prepared convenience food. There is compelling evidence that the modern epidemic of learning disabilities, poor school performance, depression, aggressive behavior, and despair are all influenced by the avalanche of fake food that has invaded our nation and taken over our cities.

Malnutrition caused by the lack of natural food and fresh produce has troubled humanity for eons. Today, malnutrition is no longer the exclusive problem of underdeveloped nations that have poor economies and inadequate food distribution networks. It is increasingly being experienced throughout the entire modern world as people eat foods that lack the micronutrients humans need for good health. In other words, "excess-calorie malnutrition" is spreading disease to all parts of the globe.

However, this new widespread malnutrition—what I call "fast food malnutrition"—is not as obvious as it would be without the influence of conventional medicine. Fast food malnutrition creates chronic inflammation and causes weight gain, but subtle micronutrient deficiencies disproportionately target the brain. Fast food malnutrition goes largely undetected because conventional medicine has developed its quick-fix solutions that allow us to destroy our bodies with fast food even as we appear perfectly healthy. Prescriptions and pills have created a new normal; our blood vessels and organs are routinely damaged by our chemical- and calorie-dense diets, but the medical establishment persuades us that our health is beyond our control and we need its pharmacologic solutions in order to thrive.

But the truth is this: Our diets are the primary driver of our health and longevity, and the medical community is doing us a disservice when it entices us to pop pills in answer to all that ails us. Disease is not inevitable. People are now enslaved to their illnesses and food addictions, accompanied by years of chronic suffering and medical dependence before a premature death, and this problem has become ubiquitous. The wrong food damages the brain, too, and is destroying lives and the American dreams of liberty and success.

Fast food malnutrition is resulting in fast food genocide.

America's future is being threatened by pebbles.

The choice to eat unhealthy foods may seem inconsequential. Yet this choice doesn't just make us fatter; it also contributes to an avalanche of health and social problems, including chronic disease, diminished intelligence, attention deficits, reduced educational and occupational opportunities, and even increased drug addiction, violence, and crime. In the following pages, I share the details of how unhealthy food has affected our nation and the devastating consequences that have followed. Escalating health tragedies are worsening in all demographics and regions of the country, and more so in younger people and in impoverished communities with poor access to fresh produce.

Robert Phillips, my collaborator, and I want to shine a light on the challenges of these impoverished communities and specifically the African American urban community now and in the past. However, as you read the data, the studies, and the history presented throughout this book, remember that this damage is occurring today all over our country, to all ethnic and racial groups where fast food consumption is high.

But without question, it is clear from the evidence that the African American urban community has suffered greatly. Compared with white Americans, if you are African American and live in an urban area in the United States:

- You are less likely to complete high school.[2]

- You have a 47 percent greater chance of having high blood pressure.[3]

- You have an 80 percent greater risk of experiencing a fatal stroke.[4]

- You have a 50 percent greater risk of dying from heart disease.[5]

- You are twice as likely to have diabetes.[6]

- You are more than four times more likely to have severe kidney disease.[7]

- You are more likely to get cancer and die of it.[8]

- You are more than twice as likely to get Alzheimer's disease.[9]

Studies show again and again that in every health and social category, African Americans generally fare worse than whites. A primary reason is that systemic racism has led to disenfranchisement, decreased school funding, and decreased economic opportunity that perpetuate poverty and ill health. This is certainly a multifactorial and complicated issue, but I would like to propose and prove to you an additional reason for these dismal statistics that may change the way that you see the world. Mounting scientific evidence suggests that each and every point listed above is directly linked to diet and to social forces that perpetuate unhealthful eating.

This does not mean that there aren't many other contributors to the persistent poor health we see in certain communities, or that people bear no responsibility for their own circumstances. Still, the evidence is unmistakable: An unhealthy diet conspires to unfavorably transform our DNA. Fake food alters us, both mentally and physically. It affects the way we act, and it undermines our health. None of us is immune to the destructive impact of this devastating problem.

Even though African Americans are disproportionately affected, fast food addiction, fast food malnutrition, and fast food genocide are not just an African American problem. Millions of Americans of all skin colors and economic strata are eating a dangerous diet loaded with soda, sweets, toxic additives, and junk food. And the more harmful foods you consume, the higher your risk of developing the physical, intellectual, and emotional problems they cause.

Our love for and acceptance of fast food as part of an everyday diet and our obsession with unhealthy foods (like bacon, cheese, white bread, and ice cream) blind us to other, even bigger problems. Diminished concentration and intelligence are consequences that we don't currently associate with an unhealthy diet, but we should. Sadly, we live in a world where the vast majority of people have been conditioned to believe that what we put into our mouths simply doesn't matter. However, whether one is considering serious disease, premature death, or functional intelligence, dietary influence—not heredity—is the major factor governing every outcome. The idea that individuals or ethnic groups have inferior genes is demonstrably false.

Furthermore, current science indicates that diet and lifestyle behaviors play a larger role in overall health and function, and genetics a smaller role, than was widely believed in the past. This means that health, brain function, and chronic diseases are primarily the result of environment and diet exposure, with a relatively small component of genetic predisposition. Nutrition overpowers genetics. For example, even in certain more genetically homogenous populations, such as American Indian tribes with an enhanced proclivity to develop obesity and diabetes, these conditions will only develop given a low-nutrient, high-calorie diet.

Lives are being destroyed daily by food choices. If we accept the untruth that people are just "born with" these problems, then we don't have to face the truth that food is the real cause. The role of genetics has been grossly overemphasized in the study of disease. Genetics plays a role in a person's susceptibility to a toxic nutritional insult, but that role is a relatively small one. This misplaced emphasis on genetics has led us to a larger cultural ignorance about environmental influences that can be modified. For example, the amount you smoke, and the number of years you smoke—not your genetics—are the major determinant of your risk of getting lung cancer.

We have the daily ability to positively affect our lives and overall health. And yet the importance we place on something we can't control—our genes—absolves us from taking responsibility, personally and collectively.

Humans were designed to eat specific natural substances in a balanced way, but we now eat a wide array of unnatural substances in an unbalanced way. And we have done so to such a degree that most people have lost their taste and desire for life-giving, whole foods.

As a result, most Americans now prefer to eat foods that we know shorten our lives and damage our brains. This damage also alters our genetic structure. Changes to our DNA accumulate from eating commercially designed foods that are incompatible with our genetic design. These gene defects have devastating consequences for us, but also can be passed on to our children and grandchildren. If nothing is done, the harmful effects of our fast food diet style today will continue through future generations, creating a decline in population intelligence and an increase in autism, learning difficulties, childhood cancers, diabetes, and other serious metabolic abnormalities as people mature, further weakening the delicate fabric of our society.

This fast food genocide is fueled by a vicious cycle in which the food industry, the medical establishment, and society at large turn a blind eye to the real cause and effect of our nation's dietary patterns. The food companies profit from producing low-cost, low-nutrition Frankenfoods designed to be addictive. The medical establishment profits from treating disease on a cause-by-cause basis, refusing to acknowledge, prescribe, or enforce effective lifestyle changes that actually prevent and reverse symptoms and diseases. And last, as a culture we continue to embrace unhealthy foods as if the data on how these foods are destroying lives do not exist or do not apply to us.

We have been in similar situations before. It took us decades to combat cigarette addiction, despite ample evidence that smoking caused heart disease and cancer. The fight against corporate greed, lies, and apathy is an uphill one. We may be the victims here, but we have the power to change this dangerous reality.

If we are to survive in good health, enjoy economic prosperity, and live in peace and harmony with each other, we have to consider the damage that poor food choices inflict on our society. We have to learn from our past mistakes and cultivate a nutritionally adequate diet for all, to enable people to live up to their potential for productivity, kindness, and happiness. Food can destroy the world, but food can also heal it.

This book addresses the many different issues that are influenced by our food choices: health, education, productivity, intelligence, economics, crime, and even drug addiction. To change society in a positive fashion, we have to explore from whence we came—and we have to stop fast food genocide.

My books have reached millions of people over the years with this simple message:

The secret to achieving your ideal weight, reversing disease, and delaying aging is consuming a diet that has the full spectrum of nutrients humans need, without consuming excess calories.

I offer a no-nonsense approach to eating and health that eliminates toxic substances and loads your diet with a variety of high-nutrient foods. I'm proud to say that many people who have read my books have lost the weight they needed to lose and, more importantly, regained their health.

However, most people are looking for an easier, almost magical approach that does not involve eating so healthfully. They prefer to maintain their current food behaviors and falsely believe that they are fine. To attract this audience, most "health" and diet books have catchy titles that feature weight-loss programs, gimmicks, and promises. Not many people are as interested in books about maintaining and earning health through excellent nutrition; instead, they seek short-term fixes and expect doctors to prescribe their long-term medical difficulties away. This just complicates the problem, adding the toxic insults from medications, while the poor dietary exposure continues—an approach that accelerates the deterioration of mental and physical health.

This book looks at the foundation of our nutritional beliefs, how these beliefs developed, and their broad effect on society. By understanding the concepts presented here, and the widespread benefits to society of those concepts, you can improve your personal health and achieve a healthy weight. This will happen despite the fact that the main focus of the book is not weight loss or dieting. We need to see how and why we have come to the place where we are today, and where we are headed. This is necessary if we are to change.

According to my standards of ideal weight (a body mass index of 23 or less), more than 80 percent of people in the United States are overweight, not just two-thirds, as is commonly claimed.[10] This statistic demonstrates the ubiquitous nature of unhealthy eating across our country. However, this epidemic weight gain now sweeping across the globe is only a single consequence of unhealthy eating. It overshadows a constellation of more serious problems: the widespread occurrence of chronic degenerative diseases, including intellectual and mental disorders associated with these foods. The impact on society caused by this human suffering is incalculable. Fundamentally, we have eaten our nation into a medical and social crisis. And much of this crisis is neither understood nor appreciated.

We look for magical cures for mental illness, breast cancer, autism, and autoimmune diseases, yet the cure has been under our noses all along. Take lung cancer, for instance. No matter how many billions of dollars we throw at searching for a cure for lung cancer, it is highly unlikely that we will develop a medicine that can enable us to smoke three packs of cigarettes a day for forty years and not develop the disease; nor can we undo the cancer once it appears because of smoking. Likewise, it is highly unlikely that we can develop an easy solution for breast or other common cancers, no matter how many research dollars are allocated, while we continue to ingest the standard American diet (SAD) (which I also call the deadly American diet [DAD]).

Our food choices not only shape our bodies and our futures; they also shape our intelligence and our behavior because food profoundly affects our brains. But perhaps most interesting of all, our choice of food is not our own. Humans are social animals, and as such, we are subject to invisible social forces. Our brain reasons that if everyone else is eating a certain way, it must be okay. Our choice of food is one of the most important decisions that we make, and it is a decision that we unconsciously allow invisible social forces to govern. These forces have the power to compel dangerous eating behavior that can alter us on a genetic level, and this in turn leads people to become self-destructive and to make even worse choices as time goes on. This cycle, supported by the addictive nature of highly processed food, is insidious, pervasive, and powerful.

Americans have abandoned natural foods such as vegetables, fresh fruits, and other plant foods in favor of a dizzying array of chemically altered, nutrient-deficient Frankenfood substitutes. We are paying for this exchange with an unaffordable, bloated, and unsustainable health care system. Chronic diseases—a direct result of not eating enough natural foods—affect record numbers of Americans. But this is only a part of the problem. Commercial food substitutes contribute to people being more depressed, more violent, less intelligent, and less forgiving. I explain the biological reasons for these effects in the chapters that follow. For now, suffice it to say that a biological problem caused by the way foods are made today is creating enormous social consequences that we presently don't associate with our modern radically altered diets.

Many crimes occur in places where people must survive on unhealthy food substitutes because they don't have access to real foods; such areas are sometimes called "food deserts." What if we could prevent a significant number of violent crimes by eliminating food deserts and changing how people eat? What if we could similarly improve school performance? And what if we could reduce or even eradicate poverty by fundamentally changing how everyone thinks about food? This is a matter of justice.

Most Americans are free to choose what types of foods they eat. But within the borders of this great nation are vulnerable people who have almost no choice other than to eat a brain-damaging, disease-promoting diet consisting of commercial food substitutes. And worst of all, the people who live outside the food deserts are doing only slightly better—they are so addicted to the same dietary style that they can't see the problem.

We are victims of a status quo based on a fundamentally flawed way of thinking. At one time, people believed that the Earth was the center of the universe. Then, in 1543, Nicolaus Copernicus published *On the Revolutions of the Heavenly Spheres,* in which he proposed that the Earth and the other planets revolved around the sun. Copernicus was talking about the revolution of the planets, but in a broader sense, he launched a revolution that fundamentally altered and forever changed the way people thought about and saw the world.

The idea that the Earth is the center of the universe became entwined with religious dogma and was the generally accepted worldview for a long time. Challenging this idea was dangerous. Copernicus didn't live to see the change that he ushered in; he waited nearly thirty years to publish his work. (It is said that he saw the first copy of his published book on the day that he died.) He experienced the backlash that came from challenging such orthodoxy: His book was banned by the Catholic Church.

Copernicus launched a scientific revolution that paved the way for the likes of Galileo, René Descartes, and Sir Isaac Newton. He challenged twelve hundred years of entrenched thought. But this did not happen all at once; the questions Copernicus raised were not settled for another 150 years. Today, the idea that the Earth revolves around the sun is self-evident. We take it for granted, but it is a relatively recent insight and was such a groundbreaking change that it became known as the Copernican Revolution.

We need another Copernican Revolution today. The simple premise of this book is that all humans are created equal, but all calories are not. **The lower the nutrients in the food that you eat, the more calories you crave.**

Many people think the problem is that Americans are overeating. But the real problem is that Americans are eating the *wrong things.* Unhealthy foods alter our brains in ways that make us emotionally attached to the very foods that are doing us the most harm. The way we eat affects our brains in ways that prevent us from seeing the problem with the way we are eating.

This message might be hard to swallow, but many people have already heeded the call and have changed the way that they eat. As a result, they have resolved their desire to overeat and, with time, have retrained their palates to prefer the flavors of healthy food choices. The outcome is not just weight loss, but recovery from high blood pressure, high cholesterol, diabetes, headaches, acne, fatigue, and excessive menstrual bleeding and cramps. They have also tremendously improved their emotional outlook on life. Thousands have reported that the "fog" clouding their thoughts has lifted; they are no longer depressed and feel newly excited about life and their future.

These concepts gleaned from scientific studies are still ignored or contested. With all the research data available, you would expect that achieving an adequate amount of food-based antioxidants and phyto-chemicals for optimal health and brain function should be an accepted norm and known by everyone. The idea that heart disease, diabetes, dementia, stroke, and most cancers are preventable and are largely the result of poor nutrition is still not fully accepted, either by authorities or by society at large. Powerful social and economic interests support the status quo. Massive societal awareness and change are desperately needed, but we can expect these concepts to be contested and denied for years to come—Copernicus was not the only one whose revolutionary, but correct, idea was opposed.

These pages show that there is a direct and clear connection between the foods that you eat and the way that you behave and live. It is to be expected that interested parties will attempt to discredit the science and fight back.

The diet industry is a big business. There is no shortage of diet advice: eat more, eat less, eat more frequently, eat less frequently, use herbs or natural stimulants to speed up your metabolism, eliminate carbs, eat less fat, or eat more fat—it doesn't really matter anymore. All of these recommendations have some basis in fact. And yet, our nation's dieting mentality and dieting efforts have not put even the slightest dent in the problem of obesity.

Despite a $40 billion-a-year diet industry, people are fatter now than ever. In the end, the advice and products offer virtually no long-term return on investment—measured, of course, in pounds permanently

lost. According to a review of seventeen studies on long-term maintenance of weight loss, ranging from three to fourteen years in duration,
85 percent of dieters fail to keep the weight off.[11] *And always keep in
mind that no health benefits occur from temporary weight loss.* It is necessary to
understand the addictive nature of commercial food, and its connection
to our failures, in order to achieve a new chance at success. We need to
move the needle of social behavior into a favorable range—and that can
happen only when we are properly educated about the power of the
food we put on our plates and the power of these laboratory-designed
foods to control us.

This book challenges some fundamental beliefs, but many of these
commonly held beliefs are simply wrong. However, being wrong, by
itself, is not a problem unless it causes us to act in harmful ways. The real
problem is that the untrue beliefs that are tackled here are toxic. These
untrue beliefs have cost the lives of millions of people and continue to
have a negative health influence on billions of others across the globe.
Unless something is done, it will get worse, much worse.

The ideas in this book have been distilled from years of scientific
research, and this critical information calls for widespread awareness and
action. Turn these pages and study this problem carefully, because greater
knowledge can lead to a solution: a solution to your personal health
issues and a solution for our society. It has to start with you.

CHAPTER ONE

FAST FOOD AND DISEASE

Of all the preposterous assumptions of humanity over humanity, nothing exceeds most of the criticisms made on the habits of the poor by the well-housed, well-warmed, and well-fed.

—HERMAN MELVILLE

Let's start with the basics: "Fast food" is, literally, fast food. That means you can get it fast, eat it fast, digest it fast, and assimilate it into your fat cells fast—all with minimal effort.

Addiction to fast food is likely the most far-reaching and destructive influence on our population today. As I show in the following pages, this addiction has had an increasingly and dramatically negative effect on our society. Certainly, given what we know about the health effects of cigarettes, you have to be insane to smoke, but in this book I explain why the health effects of regularly consuming fast food may be even more severe than smoking.

I define fast food in two ways: First, it is the food served at commercial chain restaurants, where processed meats, pizza, burgers, French fries, pretzels, soft drinks, and rich desserts are made in an assembly-line process, with commercial ingredients that are duplicated and dispersed all over the world. Second, it is any commercially made food that includes artificial ingredients, processed grains, sweeteners, salt, and oil, with minimal nutrient content.

Most of us are aware that many chain restaurants aren't serving up healthy foods, but the second definition of fast food is often confusing to many and just as lethal. These "fake" foods—the frozen waffle, the deli sandwich, the frozen pizza, the bag of chips, and much more—are easily available at our local supermarkets and convenience stores. Processing foods removes and destroys the fragile micronutrients and phytochemicals we need for cellular normalcy, and also adds toxins.

Toxins added to fast foods and processed foods include artificial colors, artificial flavors, preservatives, pesticides, antifoaming agents, emulsifiers, stabilizers, and thickeners. These ingredients give foods the texture and consistency that consumers expect. Added toxins also include cleaning chemicals, whitening chemicals, and packaging components. Fast foods are toxic; they accelerate death through these added toxins but also by supplying concentrated calories without substantial fiber or the micronutrients humans need to sustain a normal life.

This book is not an exposé about fast food restaurants. Fast food includes all types of junk food too, regardless of where it is purchased. These human-created fakes are not only served at fast food restaurants, but in almost every food store across the country. After all, fast food restaurants could decide now, or in the future, to serve healthy (or healthier) foods. Instead, this book is a condemnation of the fast food style of eating—the consumption of mass-processed convenience foods in general. These foods include commercial and preserved (deli) meats and cheeses, cold breakfast cereals, sandwiches that use bread and rolls made from white flour, burgers, pizza, soft drinks, ice cream, doughnuts, cookies, marshmallows, and candies. These, and other "recreational" foods, have drug-like effects that are damaging the emotional fabric of our country and creating an immense and growing burden of human health tragedies. When I use the terms "fast food" or "junk food" throughout this book, I refer to this broad definition—not merely the foods served at quick-serve, take-out restaurants.

FAST FOOD IS SUICIDE ON THE INSTALLMENT PLAN

Obesity affects approximately 35 percent of Americans. This means that a staggering 100 million people are obese in the United States, and 100 million more are significantly and dangerously overweight, but not yet obese.[1] This is not just a cosmetic issue; fat on the body is indicative of heart disease, diabetes, and cancer lurking within, if not now, then in a few years. Fast food causes disease: The more you eat of it, the fatter and sicker you become, and the faster you age. **Eating fast food kills more people prematurely than smoking cigarettes.**[2]

Gallup polls have shown that today in the United States, 19 percent of adults smoke, which pales in comparison with the 45 percent of adults who smoked in the 1950s.[3] Compare this 19 percent of Americans who smoke to the proportion of Americans who eat fast food: 16 percent eat fast food several times a week; 28 percent eat fast food about once a week; and 80 percent eat fast food at least once a month. Only 4 percent say they never eat fast food.[4] But this is only the tip of the iceberg because they are using the narrow definition of "fast food," considering only food purchased in fast food restaurants when over half the American diet is nutrient-barren processed foods not purchased at fast food establishments.

A person who eats fried foods, fast food, and processed foods has at least ten times the heart attack risk of someone who eats reasonably healthy food.[5] This link between unhealthy foods and heart disease was confirmed in the Harvard Health Professionals Follow-up Study, which showed that if we follow men over time, those making healthier lifestyle choices are associated with a 90 percent drop in heart disease risk, while women making healthier lifestyle choices had a 92 percent drop.[6] This huge drop in heart attacks underestimates the benefits of healthy eating, because although the diets evaluated were better than average, they were far from ideal. Based on epidemiologic studies, survey studies, and clinical evidence, a person following a Nutritarian diet style (which I will describe in detail in Chapters 3 and 7) has at least a hundredfold less risk of developing heart disease than one eating the SAD.

Heart disease is the leading cause of death in the United States.[7] Researchers at the University of Minnesota School of Public Health evaluated the frequency of more than fifty thousand individuals eating Western-style fast food and their risk of dying of heart disease. They found the following:

- Eating fast food two to three times per week increased the risk of dying from coronary artery disease more than 50 percent.

- The greatest risk was found when subjects ate fast food four or more times weekly; the risk of dying from coronary artery disease rose to 80 percent under those conditions.

- Even eating fast food just once a week increased heart disease risk by 20 percent.[8]

These heart disease deaths, and the risks reported, were also greatly underestimated, as the participants were followed for only about fifteen years. Plus, all the unhealthy, processed food eaten outside of fast food restaurant settings were not included in the analysis. The participants were not eating anything resembling an ideal cardioprotective diet, which could have offered dramatic protection against heart disease.

FAST FOOD HAS SIX CHARACTERISTICS:

- It is digested and absorbed rapidly.
- It contains multiple synthetic ingredients.
- It is calorically dense.
- It is nutritionally barren.
- It is highly flavored.
- It contains excess salt and sugar.

The faster the calories of a food enter the bloodstream, the higher the release of fat storage hormones and the greater the increase in dopamine

Speed of Absorption of Calories in Fast Food Versus Slow Food

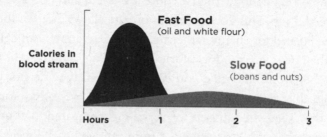

(a driver of addiction in the brain). Because of these hormonal effects, fast foods initiate and perpetuate food addiction and cravings. The chief fat storage hormone is insulin, and the excessive insulin response to fast food leads to the promotion of fat storage, weight gain, cellular replication, and eventually cancer.

The *glycemic index,* or glycemic load, considers the rate at which glucose builds up in the bloodstream over time. The more rapid and concentrated the elevation of glucose in the blood, the more significant the risk of life-threatening disease developing. The more quickly the brain can sense that rush of sugar into the bloodstream, the more its pleasure center gets stimulated and trained to direct more sugar-seeking behavior. Eating sweets and high-glycemic carbohydrates enhances the desire and craving for these foods. This influences decision-making and makes stimulating, addictive behaviors desirable. Despite the known dangers of these foods, the American public has demonstrated that they will fight to maintain their favorite addictive substances—sugar and white flour—and ignore the undeniable amount of accumulated evidence revealing the dangers of these substances.

In contrast, the more subtle levels of sugar in natural foods, in conjunction with the fiber and phytochemicals that slow the entry of sugar into the bloodstream, make for a very different biological and neurological experience that does not feed addictive behavior and addictive eating.

Similar dangers are associated with fat entering the blood quickly. The oils and concentrated fats from animal products can enter the blood-stream rapidly; in contrast, the fat content of seeds and nuts is absorbed over several hours. This slower absorption rate allows more of the calories to be burned for energy, rather than stored as fat, and can delay and reduce the body signaling for calories (the feeling of hunger).

In other words, oils give you calories fast, so they do not trigger satiety signals to stop eating—they actually induce overeating—and neither do they keep you satisfied for very long, compared to consuming a similar number of calories ingested from eating nuts and seeds. When you use nuts and seeds, which are a whole, natural food, as the major source of fat in your diet, you get anti-hunger and weight-favorable benefits. In addition, when you eat nuts and seeds, all the fat calories consumed are bound to plant fibers and not fully absorbed, resulting in a significant percentage of calories that are removed from the body via the stool and deposited in the toilet.[9] A hallmark of the fast food diet style, which promotes obesity, is a high amount of fat calories coming from oil and very little from natural nuts and seeds.

CRAZY FOR WHITE BREAD?

Processed fats and oils are certainly bad for you, but sugar and white flour take the cake as the most dangerous fast food ingredients. According to accumulating evidence, these high-glycemic carbohydrates, with their huge glycemic load, are the most powerful obesity-causing, diabetes-causing, heart disease–causing, and even depression-causing components of fast food.

Let's be perfectly clear: Commercial baked goods containing white flour are devoid of nutrients and have almost the same glycemic load as pure white sugar.[10] Eating breads, rolls, pizza, and pastries is not much different from sucking on a cube of sugar or eating candy. These foods not only promote obesity, heart disease, and diabetes—they also promote cancer.[11]

A HIGH-GLYCEMIC DIET IS LINKED TO

Colon cancer

Breast cancer

Endometrial cancer

Lung cancer

Pancreatic cancer

Prostate cancer

Fast food is not just loaded with sugar, sweetening agents, and chemicals; it also contains high-fructose corn syrup and other products made from white potato and white flour. To make things even worse, fast food is usually fried in oil, which increases its glycemic rush, obesity-promoting potential, and toxicity. Fry white flour, sugar, and artificial flavorings and colorings in oil, and you have a doughnut—a Frankenfood linked to a high risk of death.[12]

According to the American Heart Association, the maximum amount of *added* sugar (other than what is contained in fruit and other natural plants) that you should have in a day is 25 grams or 100 calories. According to me, you should have none. Nevertheless, a 64-ounce soda, which equates to a large size at many fast food restaurants, can contain as much as 200 grams of sugar. That is mass addiction in action—and it's legal. Even worse, many sugar-addicted parents give these harmful substances to their children.

Addiction can be a powerful drive and difficult to resist, but food addiction is particularly insidious—it destroys people's health, leads to medical dependence, and splits families apart. There is an epidemic of junk food addiction in many of our inner cities, where lack of access to fresh produce keeps segments of society sickly, sluggish, and mentally burdened—and thwarts their chances for educational and economic opportunities.

FAST FOOD IS ADDICTIVE

Consuming fast food is legal and socially acceptable. But these foods, rich in added sweeteners, salt, oils, and artificial flavoring (called "highly palatable foods" by scientists) have addictive properties. Eating a little makes you want more. Overeating and substance/drug abuse share important common characteristics, including tolerance (needing greater amounts over time to reach the same "high"), unsuccessful efforts to cut back on consumption, and use of the substance despite negative consequences.[13]

Sugar-izing all foods to reach the "bliss point" that maximizes pleasure (and purchases), leads to a gradual deadening of the taste buds. Over time, this has two negative consequences: First, you crave more and more sugar; and second, the level of sweetness in natural foods (such as berries and carrots) no longer has any appeal. Children raised on fast food meals, soda, and frequent junk food treats do not like fruits and vegetables. Why? Because they can hardly taste these foods. Their taste buds have been shut down by excess salt and sugar and simply can't register the nuances of flavors in real food.

Fast food prevents you from tasting the naturally delicious flavors of fruits and vegetables; therefore, the very foods that provide the body with the necessary nutrients to thrive and live a long, healthy life are made less desirable by human-made processed foods designed to cultivate addictive consumption.

Feeding sweetened soda, doughnuts, cake, and junk food to children is practically the same as handing them a shot of whiskey or lighting up a cigarette for them. There is just a small degree of difference between one addictive, dangerous substance and another. The same brain centers are stimulated by cocaine, narcotics, and super-sweetened foods. It is debatable which is more deadly, as so many people eat super-sweetened foods multiple times a day, every day.

Drugs and food can have similar effects in the brain.[14] We don't eat solely because we're hungry; we crave the pleasurable feelings we derive from food. *Dopamine* is a neurochemical that regulates motivation, pleasure, and reinforcement related to certain stimuli, such as food. The amount of pleasure we derive from eating a food correlates with the amount of dopamine released in the brain.[15]

In the long-ago past, the dopamine reward system was a survival advantage, driving early humans to consume calorie-rich foods so they could store up energy for times when food was scarce. However, the effect of today's processed, Frankenfood environment on these drives is a dangerous experiment thrust upon our species. Not only do these fast food calories shorten life span, but they slowly destroy the brain (see Chapter 2). Fast food calories affect intellectual function and judgment and can contribute to depression, aggression, and memory loss. Fast food intake also promotes drug addiction. Since fast food consumption can depress mood, decrease intelligence, and affect judgment it makes it more difficult to break free from food addiction. People become caught in a vicious cycle of brain stimulation with dangerous foods, which makes them more susceptible to all kinds of addiction, including dependence on prescription drugs.

When someone abuses a substance—whether it's alcohol, a drug, or addictive food—the brain reduces the number of dopamine D2 receptors, which is thought to result in a diminished reward response and a higher tolerance to the substance. In the case of overeating and obesity, for example, frequent consumption of ice cream has been shown to

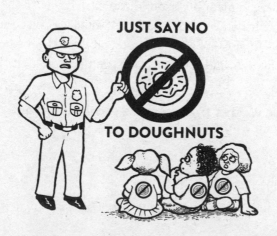

reduce the reward response. This means that over time, lesser amounts are no longer satisfying, and the consumption of more sweetened calories is needed to elicit the same amount of pleasure.[16] The more fast foods people eat, the more they lose dopamine receptor function. This enhances the drive for more and more fast food and contributes to other addictive behaviors. The desire for fast food actually becomes more intense the more often it is eaten, because it excites impulse pathways in the brain. This drives the deadly cycle of overeating, weight gain, and more overeating.

FAST FOOD: PLEASURE AND PAIN

In addition to the effects on the brain, withdrawal symptoms from toxins that accumulate in the body because of fast food also contribute to overeating and food addiction. *Toxic metabolites* are waste products produced by the body that can cause inflammation and disease if allowed to accumulate. Consuming a diet low in micronutrients and phytochemicals results in inflammation, oxidative stress, and the accumulation of these toxic metabolites, including free radicals.[17] The more fast food eaten, the higher the amount of toxic waste products in the body. The toxic load to the body and the simultaneous lack of micronutrients and antioxidants inhibit repair and removal of waste, leading to chronic inflammation and the inevitable development of serious diseases.

Fast foods contribute to a constellation of substances that can congest our cells and lead to disease. Some are wastes produced by the body from consuming such foods, and some are toxins in the food itself.[18]

CELLULAR TOXIC WASTES THAT INCREASE FROM FAST FOOD CONSUMPTION

Advanced glycation end products (AGEs)

Free radicals

Lipofuscin and A2E (a component of cell lipofuscin)

Lipid peroxides

Malondialdehyde

Heavy metals

Petrochemicals

Phthalates (DEHP and DINP)

Bisphenol-A (BPA)

FOOD ADDITIVES CAN BE TOXIC

- **Potassium bromate** is used in bromated flour and sold to commercial bakers to make dough more flexible and allow for higher rising. Bromine interferes with the body's ability to metabolize iodine, promoting thyroid disease. It also induces tumors and cancers in rats.[19] Bromated flour is considered a class 2B carcinogen by the International Agency for Research on Cancer and has been shown to cause malignant tumors and to damage human DNA. It is banned in most of the world, including the United Kingdom, Europe, India, and China. Even though many fast food chains have stopped using it, bromated flour is still one of General Mills's best sellers; the company supplies it to bakeries, supermarkets, and commercial food manufacturers within the United States.

- **Sodium phosphate** or **phosphoric acid** is added to most fast foods and processed foods for leavening and to add moisture, color, and flavor. The least expensive processed foods, fast foods, and baked goods contain the most added phosphorus.[20] In other words, the food purchased at convenience stores and fast food establishments are loaded with phosphorus. High levels of phosphorus in the blood are not just linked to the development of kidney disease in the future and death in kidney disease patients; high normal serum phosphate levels have been a predictor of cardiovascular death. This additive is associated with intravascular inflammation and calcifications as well, weakening bones.

- **Artificial coloring agents,** such as Yellow No. 5, Yellow No. 6, and Red No. 40, are added to just about every fast food menu item. The yellow colorings supply a golden hue to sauces, cheese, puddings, and soft drinks, while the red color is added to meats, shakes, and desserts that contain fruit.

These toxic food additives mix with the metabolic toxins that accumulate in the body from eating a low micronutrient diet, leading to immune system dysfunction, autoimmune disease, and chronic degenerative diseases. The amount of toxins in the body rises with fast food consumption in proportion to the amount of fast food consumed. These toxins are linked to lower IQ, fibroids, endometriosis, thyroid disease, and the development of serious autoimmune disease.[21] Unfortunately, not many people recognize the link between the accumulation of cellular toxins and poor health, serious autoimmune disease, premature aging, and excess weight and obesity.

TOXIC HUNGER

When digestion is complete after eating a meal, the body attempts to mobilize and eliminate accumulated waste products. This causes uncomfortable symptoms such as headaches, light-headedness, irritability, and fatigue. I call these withdrawal symptoms from an inadequate diet *toxic hunger*. Since eating halts this detoxification and removes the symptoms, people mistakenly believe that these uncomfortable withdrawal sensations indicate hunger.

I have been researching this phenomenon for the past thirty years. During this time, I have observed that my patients' perceptions of hunger change as they improve their diets. Their feelings of hunger become less frequent, less uncomfortable, and morph to be mainly felt in the mouth and throat, rather than in the head or stomach.

My observations and conclusions have been documented in a study of 764 individuals published in a 2010 issue of *Nutrition Journal*. In the study, we showed that enhancing the micronutrient quality of a person's diet, and removing processed foods, led to changes in the experience of hunger and a reduction in uncomfortable symptoms associated with hunger, despite a lower caloric intake.[22] A diet of healthy food does not produce withdrawal symptoms; when the body is fed mostly vegetables, fruits, beans, nuts, and seeds, there is nothing to detoxify. With natural healthful foods, toxic metabolites are minimized, and people no longer feel the need to overconsume calories to keep their energy up. When you eat healthfully, with adequate colorful produce, you don't feel hungry between meals. When hunger eventually does kick in, it is because your body has a real biological need for calories.

True hunger does not cause fatigue; it is not painful, and it is not uncomfortable. True hunger is a signal that directs the body to the appropriate amount of food it needs to maintain a healthy weight. True hunger does not drive overeating behavior; only toxic hunger does that. Responding to, and satisfying, true hunger cannot cause obesity. True hunger symptoms, felt mainly in the throat, only occur to maintain muscle mass, not to store fat. Improving the nutritional quality of your diet is the most effective and sustainable way to achieve—and maintain—a normal body weight.

RESOLVING FOOD ADDICTION

The only way to break an addiction is to abstain from the addictive substance, and that can be difficult at first. The period of discomfort associated with breaking your ties to addictive foods usually lasts two to three days, and then the discomfort lessens considerably. Two to three days of discomfort is a small price to pay for breaking away from food addiction.

Trying to eat fast foods or sweets in moderation almost always fails, because your toxic hunger symptoms and addictive drive kick in. This is evident in the fact that most randomized controlled trials on weight loss have reported only a 6- to 13-pound sustained weight loss after two years.[23] Compare that to the average 50-pound weight loss after two years reported by individuals who started out obese and switched to a high-nutrient diet.[24]

To achieve sustainable weight loss, you need to pay attention to nutritional quality and eat a sufficient amount and variety of nutrient-rich, natural plant foods. If you continue to eat fast foods and try to lose weight by attempting to reduce calories, you are highly likely to fail. Eating unhealthful foods that cause toxic hunger will leave you forever fighting against powerful addictive drives that urge you to eat more, and to eat more frequently.

Natural plant foods are not as intensely sweet and salty and as fatty as the processed fast foods that are purposely engineered to excite your bodily reward systems. When you consistently base your diet on healthful foods, in time your tastes change and the addictive desire for junk food fades away. Plus, as you continue to take care of your body and know that you are taking care of your future health, your self-esteem rises. *Eating right is self-care, not deprivation.*

People should be aware that withdrawal symptoms from unhealthy foods, especially excess sugar and salt, can sometimes be severe. Fatigue, headaches, itching, low-grade fever, sore throat, and mild anxiety are common. Because people initially feel so ill when they try to eat healthfully, many are deterred from sticking with it. But as I've said, these symptoms rarely last longer than three days.

The slow poisoning of the body from fast food does not merely occur from the toxins within the food. As a higher and higher percentage of our caloric pie is taken up by foods with empty calories—that is, calories that provide energy but very little nutrition—it becomes impossible to meet our requirements for micronutrients. Plus, for the body to digest and assimilate those empty-calorie foods, is uses micronutrients that are then subtracted from the body's stores of nutrients. Modest micronutrient insufficiency is ubiquitous in the United States and is a major cause of immune system malfunction and chronic disease.[25]

SWEETENERS AND THE KISS OF DEATH

Fast food restaurants add high amounts of high-fructose corn syrup (HFCS) to everything. It is not just in milk shakes and sweet desserts;

HFCS is also hidden in breads, pizza crust, tomato sauce, and salad dressing, and even in the chopped meat used for burgers.

HFCS is much sweeter than simple cane sugar, and it's also cheaper. In addition, it acts as a preservative, extending the shelf life of foods. Fructose is highly soluble and does not crystalize, so it can remain effective in processed foods forever and not cause the food to harden. This allows products like cookies and candy to stay soft. HFCS is cheaper than sugar because of government corn subsidies, so the average soda size has ballooned from being 8 ounces to 20 ounces at little financial cost to manufacturers. But the human cost—increased obesity, diabetes, and chronic disease—is great.

Any type of sugar causes obesity, diabetes, and heart disease; sugar is also a major cancer promoter when used in excessive amounts. The person who regularly eats fast food and processed foods can be exposed to the equivalent of 100 teaspoons of sugar a day or more. Just one large soft drink or milk shake may contain the equivalent of 50 teaspoons of sugar. That is more sugar than our ancestors would have been exposed to in a month of eating natural fruits.

Interestingly, for more than fifty years, the soft drink industry and the sugar industry have provided millions of dollars of research funding to academic and governmental researchers to influence and cover up the health risks associated with consuming sugar. A recent medical investigation published in *JAMA Internal Medicine* and reported in the *New York Times* revealed that five decades of research into the role of nutrition and heart disease, including many of today's dietary recommendations, have been largely shaped by the financial influence of the sugar industry. "They were able to derail the discussion about sugar for decades," said Stanton Glantz, a professor of medicine at the University of California, San Francisco, and an author of the *JAMA* paper.[26] Information regarding the dangers of modern processed foods is effectively suppressed by powerful economic interests that spend lots of money to influence public perception.

Biochemically, HFCS is only slightly different from white cane sugar, and the dangerous effects on your health are the same. Regular table sugar (sucrose) is 50 percent fructose and 50 percent glucose, and

HFCS contains up to 55 percent fructose and 45 percent glucose. Fructose is a naturally occurring substance, but it never occurs naturally in the concentrated and isolated way that it does in soft drinks and other processed foods. In whole foods, most of the fructose and glucose are usually bound together as sucrose and are always balanced with micronutrients and fiber, which reduce the glycemic effects of sucrose and the insulin response by the pancreas.[27]

Although consuming fructose by itself doesn't excite insulin secretion, consuming concentrated fructose, in foods containing HFCS such as soft drinks, baked goods, breakfast cereals, and snack foods, is dangerous. That's because instead of being taken up by muscle cells all over the body, the fructose goes right to the liver and triggers the production of fats such as triglycerides and cholesterol. This is called *lipogenesis*. This is why the major cause of liver damage in this country, which affects 70 million people, is "fatty liver."[28] The liver was not designed to metabolize the large quantities of fructose found in artificial commercial foods.

HFCS has been shown to increase insulin resistance. This means that it interferes with the removal of other sugars from the blood, requiring the pancreas to produce more insulin to do so.[29] The explosion in the occurrence of obesity and type 2 diabetes in the past fifty years was caused (partially) by this high exposure to sugar and HFCS in fast foods and soft drinks.[30] Excess HFCS—and fructose in particular—also contributes to high blood pressure, not only by its promotion of plaque buildup (atherogenesis), but also by inhibiting a key enzyme called endothelial nitric oxide synthase, which is important for maintaining normal vascular elasticity.[31]

Exposure to HFCS has created a nation of metabolically challenged individuals who are overweight, diabetic or prediabetic, and have high levels of cholesterol and triglycerides. This is called *metabolic syndrome* and is a condition that has led to a health crisis of unprecedented proportions. Fructose-induced insulin resistance is linked to both diabetes and Alzheimer's disease.[32]

HFCS and other fast food ingredients increase advanced glycation end products, or AGEs, which age tissues, destroy the insides of the eyeball, and create nerve damage, kidney damage, and other complications of diabetes. If this weren't bad enough, HFCS is manufactured using chemicals that are commonly contaminated with mercury, and mercury residue has been found in significant amounts in such products. This is especially concerning for long-term problems developing in children exposed to these products.[33]

AGEs Age Us Rapidly

Advanced glycation end products, also known as *glycotoxins*, are a diverse group of highly oxidant compounds that cause cumulative pathogenic damage and are a significant factor in chronic disease development, premature aging, and death. AGEs form within the body as metabolic toxins when we eat sweets and have higher blood glucose levels, but we also consume them from dry-cooked fast foods, particularly commercially baked products. Dry heat in cooking promotes new AGE formation by tenfold to one-hundred-fold above the uncooked state across food categories. Animal-derived foods contain the most AGEs and produce high additional amounts of AGEs during dry cooking, especially broiling, frying, and roasting. In contrast, high-water-content fruits and vegetables or water-based cooking such as steaming or cooking in soups or stews prevents AGE formation.

When AGE formation occurs from the darkening of food, the reaction is known as the "Maillard" or "browning" reaction. The disease-causing effects are not only related to the ability of AGEs to promote oxidation and inflammation; AGEs also bind with cell surface receptors or cross-link with body proteins, altering their structure and function.

The types of foods and cooking methods that fast food restaurants favor promote the production of AGEs. In particular, grilling, broiling, roasting, searing, and frying propagate and accelerate new AGE formation. When these foods are infused with HFCS before cooking, they become even more potent in their disease-promoting effects.[34]

HEALTH-DAMAGING EFFECTS OF HFCS

Obesity

High blood pressure

Diabetes

Blindness

Liver disease

Kidney disease

Premature aging

High triglycerides

High cholesterol

Heart attacks

Dementia

Strokes

Cancer

This constellation of risk from HFCS, AGEs, heterocyclic amines (see below), chemical colorings, and nutrient deficiency from fast food leads to an accumulated toxic burden, resulting in "brain fog." This is characterized by difficulty in concentrating, loss of the ability to work a full day, and loss of memory, and it will likely lead to eventual dementia.[35] More and more people with dementia are flooding nursing homes, and many require round-the-clock care.

Processed foods are also linked to the incidence of strokes.[36] The epidemic of stokes, occurring at younger and younger ages[37] has sparked an entire industry of health care facilities that cater to impaired young people who have destroyed large sections of their brains with fast food. The incidence of strokes before the age of forty-five is five times more common in black populations, likely due to the increased consumption of fast food.[38]

The combined effect of the fast food and processed food industries has resulted in an explosive epidemic of obesity and diabetes, with its resultant kidney failure, limb amputations, and heart problems. Medical bills to treat diseases associated with obesity alone are more than $185 billion annually.[39]

SIX FOODS WITH THE HIGHEST AMOUNT OF AGEs AGE/KU	PER 100 GRAM	PER SERVING
1. Beef frankfurter, broiled 5 minutes	11,270	10,143
2. Beef steak, pan fried in olive oil	10,058	9,052
3. Chicken back or thigh (no skin), roasted and barbecued	8,802	7,922
4. Chicken breast, breaded and then oven fried	9,961	8,965
5. Chicken back or thigh with skin, roasted and barbecued	18,520	16,668
6. Bacon, fried 5 minutes	91,577	11,905

GRILLING UP SOME CANCER

Long-term studies with hundreds of thousands of participants have established that diets rich in animal products are associated with a higher incidence of heart attacks and cancers.[40] Animal products also do not contain antioxidants and phytochemicals that offer protection against disease and protect the brain.

But there's worse news about animal products. The processed meats (and other meat) available and prepared at fast food restaurants present a different level of danger because of the way they are processed, the chemicals and flavorings added to them, and then the way they are prepared. These processed meats often contain sodium nitrite, a known carcinogen, and also contain heterocyclic amines, which are linked to colon cancer. Heterocyclic amines, polycyclic aromatic hydrocarbons, and lipid peroxides are chemicals formed when muscle meat, including beef, pork, fish, and poultry, is cooked using high-temperature methods, such as pan frying, grilling, and barbecuing. These compounds have been found to be *mutagenic*—that is, they cause changes in DNA that increase the risk of cancer.[41]

Substances that enter the body along with cooked red meat also include N-nitroso compounds, which have been shown to damage genetic material, leading to cancer. The heme iron in red meat promotes lipid peroxidation and the formation of reactive oxygen species and N-nitroso compounds, all of which contribute to the development of cancer.[42] Increased consumption of processed meat, and meats cooked with typical fast food cooking techniques, correlates positively with the likelihood of developing breast cancer as well as colorectal, pancreatic, and prostate cancers.[43]

If you choose to eat a small amount of animal products in your diet, it should never be breaded, deep fried, pan fried, barbecued, or grilled. These are the ways that animal products are traditionally prepared by fast food restaurants and street vendors—and these are the most dangerous way to incorporate animal products into your diet. Fast food–style animal

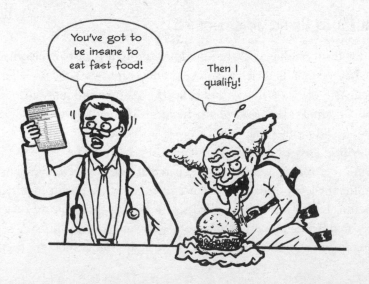

products also lack eicosapentaenoic acid (EPA) and (docosahexaenoic acid) DHA, the two omega-3 fatty acids found in seafood and small wild animals.

The problem is clear: The American food industry has succeeded in its quest to "hook" Americans—especially populations in the inner city, where healthy foods are not as available—on the most dangerous and destructive foods ever devised. It has taken the most disease-causing foods and found a way to make them even worse.

SALT IN FAST FOOD

The processed food and fast food industries are also responsible for increasing salt intake. The excessive level of sodium in the modern diet has caused an epidemic of high blood pressure. Living in the United States, your lifetime probability of developing high blood pressure is higher than 90 percent, with accompanying increased risks of heart attack, heart failure, and stroke.[44] High salt intake causes scarring of the heart, called *coronary fibrosis,* which further increases the risk of developing a dangerous cardiac arrhythmia or irregular heartbeat.[45]

The important issue is that your lifetime salt intake correlates best with your risk of having a heart attack or stroke in later life. This means that feeding kids, teenagers, and young adults salty foods is not without risk, even though their blood pressures have not elevated yet. All the salt they consume when they are young cumulatively adds up and results in damage to the body's vascular system.[46] People pay a steep price for the high salt fast food they eat when they are young, with years of suffering and chronic diseases down the road. Excessive salt intake also increases the risk of developing asthma, autoimmune disease, stomach cancer, osteoporosis, and kidney failure.[47]

Shockingly, salt is added to almost every fast food. Even soda, ice cream, milk shakes, and other desserts contain added salt. Salt is a natural preservative, but the real benefit to fast food vendors is salt's effect on their customers' thirst. The more salt hidden in a fast food meal, the more the customer will drink. And drinks are the most profitable item on a junk food menu, selling for five times the price of gasoline, even though they are mostly water, chemicals, and sweetening agents, and they put salt in them too.

The highest amounts of salt are found in fast food fried potatoes, which can hardly be called potatoes anymore, as fast food French fries have as many as twenty-three ingredients in them, including sweeteners, salt, antifoaming agents, preservatives, and colorings. They are more a potato-chemical slurry, with extra HFCS and salt mixed into the batter—and after they're fried, they're coated with even more salt.

The burgers aren't just meat; HFCS and salt are mixed into the meat before it is fried or grilled. One fast food meal gives you such a dangerous amount of salt, that even if you were to eat nothing else and drink only water for the rest of the day, you would still be in the salt danger zone. For example, a Big Mac from McDonald's, with no salted fries or soda, already supplies 950 milligrams of sodium.[48] A typical meal from Kentucky Fried Chicken (KFC) supplies more than 3,000 milligrams of sodium—and that's just one meal.[49] One box of popcorn at a movie or ballgame has so much salt in it that you'll find yourself waiting in long lines to buy drinks to satisfy your increased thirst.

Salt is also just like the other "white stuff"—sugar: When you eat salted foods regularly, you deaden the taste for salt, you like salty foods, and you crave more and more salt. People like lots of salt because when they were young, they routinely ate lots of hidden salt in all their foods.

Manufacturers also add salt to their foods because it makes people eat more food; scientific studies confirm that salted foods increase appetite and caloric intake. The results of careful investigations indicate that salt intake shuts down the cues to stop eating when full.[50] Salting food prevents people from knowing when they have eaten enough food and induces overeating and obesity.[51]

The "Processed Food Era" started about two to three generations ago, right after World War I. Soon, heart attacks and stroke rates skyrocketed. Yet there are still areas of the world where people eat a more natural diet, and salt intake is comparatively very low. Pockets of people live on diets without added salt in New Guinea, the Amazon Basin, and the highlands of Malaysia—and high blood pressure is unheard of in these regions.[52]

According to the National Institutes of Health (NIH), consuming less sodium is one of the most important ways to prevent cardiovascular disease.

Salt reduction to 1,200 milligrams a day is estimated to prevent fifty-four thousand to ninety-nine thousand heart attacks each year in the United States.[53]

MANY SCHOOL LUNCHES SERVE FAST FOOD

Our addiction to fast food has invaded college campuses, high schools, and even elementary schools. Chicken nuggets, pizza and hamburgers (with bromated flour), soda, and French fries are common fare on school lunch menus. For example, a California statewide sample found these fast foods at 71 percent of schools, and more than half even served brand name products from chains such as Taco Bell and Domino's Pizza.[54]

Furthermore, your child's public school lunch may be held to a lower quality standard than even fast food restaurants. Millions of pounds of meat judged unfit to serve in fast food restaurants makes its way into our school cafeterias. Meat that is only fit for pet food or compost is being served at schools, according to a *USA Today* investigation. The newspaper reported that the Agricultural Marketing Service, which purchases meats for schools, bought meats with levels of *E. coli* and other bacteria that exceeded acceptable levels for fast food outlets.[55]

Hidden dangers lurk in foods commonly served in school lunch programs around the country. For example, look at these ingredients for a hotdog bun marketed to school lunch programs:

INGREDIENTS: ENRICHED BLEACHED WHEAT FLOUR (WHEAT, NIACIN, REDUCED IRON, THIAMINE MONONITRATE, RIBOFLAVIN, FOLIC ACID, **POTASSIUM BROMATE**), WATER, SUGAR, WHEY, DEXTROSE, VEGETABLE SHORTENING (PARTIALLY HYDROGENATED SOYBEAN & COTTONSEED OIL), SOY FLOUR, SALT, MONO & DIGLYCERIDES, EGG, YEAST, SOYBEAN OIL.

MAY CONTAIN 2% OR LESS OF: SODIUM STEAROYLE LACTOLAYTE, WHEAT
GLUTEN, FOOD STARCH, AMMONIUM, DATEM, L-CYSTEIN, VINEGAR,
CALCIUM PROPIONATE, (PRESERVATIVES), MONOCALCIUM PHOSPHATE,
CALCIUM SULFATE ASCORBIC ACID, AZODICARBONAMIDE, ENZYMES.
CONTAINS: WHEAT.

Note that these buns contain partially hydrogenated soybean and
cottonseed oils. Many countries have banned these *trans* fats because
they have been demonstrated to be dangerous and to greatly increase the
risk of heart disease. The Food and Drug Administration (FDA) ruled in
2015 that partially hydrogenated oils are not "Generally Recognized as
Safe" (GRAS) and will require these oils to be phased out from processed
foods by 2018.[56] But in the meantime, since nobody is looking, trans fats
are fed to our kids. Heart disease and increased aggressiveness are both
associated with consumption of trans fats.

The bun ingredients also contain potassium bromate, which is not
only a carcinogen, as we have seen, but is known to impair iodine metabolism, which can lead to iodine deficiency and potential brain damage.[57]
The World Health Organization (WHO) estimates that iodine deficiency
causes an 8- to 10-point drop in the global IQ.[58] Even though potassium
bromate is banned in other countries, and even by most fast food restaurants doing business abroad, we here in the United States somehow see
it as permissible to serve it to young children in our schools.

Corn dogs are another popular menu item in public school lunch
programs. According to a company that manufactures corn dogs for
school lunches, their "100% Whole Grain Chicken Corn Dogs on a
Stick" are "Smart Snack Approved," with portions and nutrition levels
that meet school standards. The nutrition label, and the ingredients on
the company's website, tells a different story. It's a pretty low standard of
excellence, if you ask me.

CHICKEN FRANK: MECHANICALLY SEPARATED CHICKEN, WATER, *CORN
SYRUP SOLIDS*, CONTAINS LESS THAN 2% OF SPICES, SALT, POTASSIUM
LACTATE, POTASSIUM ACETATE, SODIUM PHOSPHATE, POTASSIUM
CHLORIDE, FLAVORINGS, SODIUM DIACETATE, SODIUM ERYTHORBATE,
SODIUM NITRITE.

BATTER: WATER, WHOLE WHEAT FLOUR, WHOLE GRAIN CORN, SUGAR, LEAVENING (SODIUM ACID PYROPHOSPHATE, SODIUM BICARBONATE), SOY FLOUR, SOYBEAN OIL, SALT, EGG YOLK WITH SODIUM SILICOALUMINATE, ASCORBIC ACID, EGG WHITE, DRIED HONEY, ARTIFICIAL FLAVOR. **FRIED IN VEGETABLE OIL.** CONTAINS: WHEAT, SOY, EGG, AND GLUTEN.

Here's a great idea: Feed kids a chicken frank made with corn syrup and sodium nitrite, and then make believe it's a health food! It's really a Frankenfood. And after all, nobody will know that eating more sodium nitrite–preserved meats increases heart disease and diabetes risk,[59] or that sodium nitrite and N-nitroso compounds, when fed to animals, increase low-density lipoprotein (LDL) cholesterol and harm pancreatic beta-cells that produce insulin.[60] Aluminum additives are linked to the development of Alzheimer's disease.[61] This artificially flavored concoction is then deep-fat-fried to make sure it's a cancer promoter. And we thought schools were intended to build brains, not destroy them!

It's crazy that almost half of all entrees served in elementary schools include processed meats (such as hot dogs, ham, sausage, luncheon meats, corned beef, and canned meats), yet *WHO has declared that processed meats are a class 1 carcinogen in humans,* placing them in the same category as asbestos and cigarette smoking.

We need a revolution in information about food. We need our population to educate themselves about food, nutrition, and health. We can have the healthiest population in the history of the world if we take advantage of the recent advances in nutrition and food science. Modern scientific advances in health care and longevity all point to the fact that colorful natural foods, eaten as they were grown or picked from gardens, farms, and trees, contain complex factors that protect human health. Eating fruits, vegetables, beans, nuts, and seeds—the "anti–fast foods"—is the secret to improving our nation's health.

But even more than that: If we feed our most at-risk and economically sensitive populations healthful produce, we will increase their opportunity to reach their intellectual and economic potential. Instead, the fast food, soft drink, and processed food industries have used modern food science and technology to devise the most effective setup to create widespread addiction to their products—magnifying and creating human tragedies. These industries have conditioned humans to prefer, crave, and eat their products instead of real natural foods. This process has engulfed American cities and is spreading throughout the world. It is creating overweight, sickly, and emotionally scarred humans and burdening our societies with spiraling health care problems and overwhelming health care costs.

Certainly, we have the capacity and basic human dignity to put an end to tragic suffering and needless death. But to do this, we must work together to stop the self-destructive human behaviors that hijack human cravings and drives, such as drug addiction and food addiction.

Today, ignorance about fast foods and nutrition is a major killer of humans, both in our country and across the globe. It is a steadily worsening problem that is emotionally maiming our population and creating economic chaos. The next chapter explains this in more depth as we consider "The Brain on Fast Food."

CHAPTER TWO

THE BRAIN ON FAST FOOD

Wherever there is a human being there is an opportunity for kindness.

—SENECA

We are failing to make the connection between food and brain development and behavior. Both criminal propensity and learning capacity are commonly thought to be innate; however, a review of the available evidence suggests that brain function and human potential are undermined by external factors lurking on American dinner plates. The majority of individuals in some areas of the country where healthy foods are hard to find face insidious brain damage; but this is a problem not limited to urban inner cities. These devastating health problems, which affect the health of the brain, affect all races and transcend socioeconomic demographics, occurring wherever processed and fast food consumption is high.

According to research data, poor glucose control has been linked with aggression and poor self-control, and the crime rate in a given area of the country is highly correlated with the rate of diabetes.[1] This correlation remains significant even when controlled for income, meaning that crime is more closely associated with disease than economics. This alone does not necessarily imply causation; however, human studies reveal that study participants became less able to forgive others as their diabetic symptoms worsened.[2]

In 2014, 8.5 percent of New Jersey residents had diabetes.[3] In one crime-ridden Camden zip code the rate of diabetes was almost twice that.[4] In 2012, Camden had a murder rate of 60.6 per 100,000 people, or nearly twelve times the national average; it was the deadliest year in Camden's history.[5] Not surprisingly, in the same year Camden had the highest crime rate in the United States. Low academic achievement, another persistent problem, also afflicts this city. The most recent U.S. Census shows that only 8 percent of people 25 years old and older have a four-year college degree or more, compared with 49 percent for nearby Cherry Hill. The lack of education makes it hard for individuals to escape the cycle of poverty. Thirty-nine percent live at or below the poverty line compared with 6 percent in Cherry Hill.[6] Can it be, despite complex variables and societal factors, that unhealthful food is a major contributor to this conundrum of disease, lower achievement, and even crime?

The human brain, the most complex structure known to humanity, is under attack. We are a long way away from fully understanding this biological engineering marvel; nevertheless, advances in science reveal an inescapable truth: The brain is a living organ that is exquisitely dependent on nutrients, and even small amounts of unnatural foods early in life can wreak havoc on this nutrient-sensitive organ. That damage becomes incrementally worse as we consume these foods in greater amounts.

The evidence indicates that your emotional well-being, willpower, determination, work ethic, patience, concentration, creativity, memory, and intelligence all depend on exposure to sufficient nutrients and healthy food throughout life. It is impossible to have normal brain function and a healthy emotional life when the majority of your food calories come from fast food. Not only are these processed foods leading to premature disease and death, they are negatively affecting our ability to function in everyday life. Fast foods and processed foods simply do not contain the diverse array of nutrients—nutrients that the body and brain desperately needs—that are found in natural unprocessed or minimally processed plant foods. And unfortunately, the majority of Americans today get more than half of their calories from fast food and processed food.

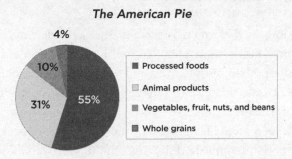

The American Pie

This pie graph represents total food consumption throughout the United States.[7] People in some areas may not eat this poorly, but there are lots of areas of the country where people eat much worse. Keep in mind that the "Vegetables, fruit, nuts, and beans" segment includes white potatoes (even French fries) and ketchup. Most Americans get less than 5 percent of their calories from colorful produce. The combination of lack of micronutrients and phytochemicals, imbalances in fatty acids (see more on page 50), and exposure to fast food–derived toxins damages not just our bodies, but our fragile, nutrient-demanding brains.

Ordinarily, an inadequate diet would be quickly evident and detected because of accompanying severe physical symptoms. However, modern fast foods are specifically designed to deceive human metabolism by limiting these outward symptoms. Commercial foods are fortified with vitamins and enriched just enough to keep us from displaying or dying from an acute deficiency, but they do not have the vast array of nutrients and phytochemicals that are needed to enable our brains to develop and function normally.

Chronic anger, chronic mild depression, and mental inflexibility are symptoms of subclinical nutritional deficiencies that are extremely common and difficult to diagnose. A CNN poll carried out in December 2015 revealed that 69 percent of Americans are angry.[8] This kind of widespread chronic anger, irrational thoughts, and diminished intelligence are red flags telling us that poor nutrition is epidemic. These subtle symptoms worsen significantly as diets get less healthy.

THE BRAIN UTILIZES HUNDREDS OF MICRONUTRIENTS AND PHYTOCHEMICALS

Natural foods such as green vegetables, seeds, berries, and mushrooms contain thousands of nutrients that fuel human health and normality. We need more than just vitamins and minerals; we also need a diverse spectrum of antioxidants and phytochemicals that enable our cells to function normally.

The brain is incredibly resilient; it can recover from occasional traumatic injury or micronutrient shortage. But this recovery process doesn't work in people who consistently consume a diet lacking life-supporting plant compounds. Our brains cannot function normally with a continual and unrelenting buildup of free radicals, other metabolic wastes, and

---

What Is a Phytochemical?

Phytochemicals (also known as phytonutrients) are noncaloric compounds present in plants that have health-promoting and disease-preventing properties. They are not vitamins and minerals, but they augment and sustain human cell function and support the immune system. They act as fuel for cell repair processes on human DNA; therefore, they have powerful anticancer effects. There are more than a thousand known phytochemicals. Some of the well-known phytochemicals are *lycopene* in tomatoes, *isoflavones* in soy, and *flavonoids* in fruits.

Phytochemicals do not merely have anticancer and longevity-promoting effects; they also affect the brain. The central nervous system includes the brain and spinal cord. The brain is composed of more than 100 billion nerve cells called *neurons*. Phytochemicals exert neuroprotective effects in experimental models of psychiatric disorders.[9] As a natural part of the human diet, they are necessary for cell signaling pathways within the brain; that is, *the presence or absence of phytochemicals affects brain development, brain function, and brain pathology.*

toxic irritants that arise from consuming processed foods. *Metabolic wastes* are toxins produced by our body that normally would be removed if phytonutrient exposure were adequate. And let's not forget the unhealthful toxic substances and additives in processed foods.

The average American consumes an extravagant high-calorie, low-nutrient diet that stresses the brain with metabolic wastes while systematically depriving it of the micronutrients necessary to self-cleanse and undo the damage. A healthy and happy brain requires a steady stream of vitamins, minerals, and phytochemical plant compounds—ingredients that are missing from modern commercial foods.

Although many Americans eat a deficient diet by choice, they rarely consider the addictive nature of Frankenfoods and how that affects their "choice." In many areas of the United States where healthy foods are hard to come by, such as Camden, New Jersey, residents have little to no choice of what to eat. They live in communities where natural produce is simply not available, so they are routinely deprived of foods that enable optimal brain function. People from impoverished communities around the country become "hooked" on commercial foods from a very young age, causing them to then reject fruits and vegetables even when available. Once this addictive pattern of craving is established, creative self-delusional rationalizations often justify the self-destructive food behavior that causes so much harm. The thinking pattern and end result is not much different from drug addiction.

An unhealthy diet destroys us from the inside out. It is an invisible threat that goes largely unnoticed until diseases like diabetes, heart disease, and cancer crop up. But way before these diseases become easy to recognize, subtle brain difficulties arise, hinting of these dramatic diseases to come later. Learning difficulties and depression may start fairly young; the statistics are alarming. As many as one in eight adolescents is diagnosed as clinically depressed, and many more have milder forms of mood disorders and learning difficulties. Clinical depression is the top cause of disability for children age 5 and older.

FAST FOOD AND DEPRESSION

Depression doesn't have one specific cause, but one of the major causative factors is an unhealthy diet. Studies have shown fast food as an important factor for many years, yet nutrition is hardly mentioned as part of the cause or treatment for mental health difficulties. A dietary pattern that includes fried food, sweetened desserts, processed meat, and refined grains has been associated with depression, and the consumption of whole natural foods has been shown to be strongly protective.[10]

The relationship between risk of depression and some components of our diet, such as omega-3 fatty acids and B vitamins, has been studied and confirmed,[11] whereas the role of fast food and white bread products has received little attention until recently. Today the evidence is overwhelming. A scientific study published in 2011 evaluated the consumption of fast food (hamburgers, sausages, and pizza) and processed pastries (muffins, doughnuts, and croissants) with a median follow-up of 6.2 years. The researchers found that these fast food and commercial baked goods were linked to depression in a dose-dependent manner.[12] The results revealed that people who eat fast food, compared with those who eat little or none, are 51 percent more likely to develop depression. And the more you consume, the greater the risk.

This depression-inducing dietary pattern is not solely due to sugar and white flour, although the dangerous effects on the brain of these high-glycemic carbohydrates is now well-established. A 2015 study showed a dose-dependent relationship between high-glycemic-load foods (white flour and sweetening agents) and depression.[13] Many people have noted a link between eating sugary foods and feeling "down" the next day, but now we know that the effects are cumulative and long-lasting and can be severe.

The data was collected from roughly seventy thousand women in the Women's Health Initiative Observational Study, none of whom suffered from depression at the study's start. Baseline measurements were taken between 1994 and 1998 and then again after a three-year follow-up. Diets with higher glycemic loads, typically rich in refined

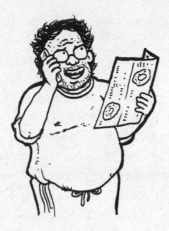

"Hi, I'd like to order the pepperoni doughnut pizza, with Prozac sprinkles."

grains and added sugar, were associated with greater odds of developing depression, while researchers found that eating high-fiber foods such as whole grains, whole fruits, and vegetables lowered the odds.

In addition to being typically overweight and prone to diabetes, the fast food–consuming public is suffering from depressed moods and clinical depression, as well as difficulties in concentration and learning that accompany their depressed moods. Throughout the body, excess sugar is harmful; even a single instance of elevated glucose in the bloodstream can harm the brain, resulting in slowed cognitive function and deficits in memory and attention.[14] In healthy young people, a brain imaging study demonstrated that the ability to process emotion is compromised by elevated blood glucose levels.[15] Increasing stimulation of the brain with calorically concentrated processed foods can lead to sadness and anxiety, and this is not restricted to people who have diabetes.

FAST FOOD DESTROYS THE BRAIN

Excess sugar impairs both our cognitive skills and our self-control (that is, having a little sugar stimulates a hard-to-resist craving for more). The mixture of sugar, salt, and oil derails the ability of the body to control calories or be satisfied with normal amounts of food. Fast foods create human eating machines, that is, individuals with no caloric turn-off switch. This lack of self-control over eating food is like turning on an obesity driving switch that leads to diabetes and other life-altering diseases. Of course, the health complications that follow as a result of eating commercially baked goods and fast food magnify the emotional problems. Let me explain how this works.

Elevated blood glucose levels harm blood vessels, and blood vessel damage is the major cause of the vascular complications of diabetes. This in turn leads to damage to blood vessels in the brain and eyes, causing retinopathy, a disease of the retina that can result in blindness. Studies of long-term diabetics show progressive brain damage leading to deficits in learning, memory, motor speed, and other cognitive functions.[16] This evidence not only shows that frequent exposure to high glucose levels diminishes mental capacity, but that higher glycated hemoglobin (HbA1c) levels have been associated with an increasing degree of brain shrinkage. Even in people who don't have diabetes, higher sugar consumption is associated with lower scores on tests of cognitive function.

Continual exposure to sweets has been shown to impair clear thinking and negatively affect behavior. One study found an increase in behavior and attention problems in 5-year-olds with increased consumption of soda.[17] The researchers adjusted their findings to accommodate potential confounding factors that might affect behavior, such as hours of television watched and a stressful home environment, and they still found that the strongest association was between soda consumption and

Glycated hemoglobin, or hemoglobin A1c (HbA1c), is a marker in the blood that indicates the average blood sugar readings over the previous few months. For people with diabetes, higher HbA1c readings are associated with a higher risk of serious diabetes complications.

aggression, withdrawn behavior, and poor attention. And soda is not the only problem; any junk food eaten during the formative preschool years is associated with hyperactivity and attention issues.[18]

Any sugar added in our food is dangerous. We can avoid these dangers by satisfying our sweet tooth with fresh fruit instead of refined sugars. Other concentrated sweeteners such as agave, honey, and maple syrup are equally dangerous and place the same glycation stress on the body. All of these sweeteners contain excessive amounts of the same basic compounds: fructose, glucose, and sucrose (fructose and glucose bound together). By eating real fresh fruit we get the satisfying sweetness and the added bonus of the fruit's fiber, antioxidants, and phytochemicals that curtail the surge of sugar in the bloodstream and thereby block its negative effects.

Fear not!—you can make delicious desserts and even treats such as brownies and ice creams with fruits, nuts, and dried fruits that are only a little less sweet than conventional desserts (see Chapter 8).

COMPOSITION OF SWEETENERS

	FRUCTOSE (%)	GLUCOSE (%)	SUCROSE (%)	OTHERS (%)
White sugar, granulated			100	
Maple syrup	1	3	96	
Honey	50	45	1	4
Molasses	24	22	54	
Agave nectar	82	18		
Corn syrup, light	7	93		
High-fructose corn syrup	42	53		5
Brown rice syrup		100		

THE OILING OF THE BRAIN

Of course, just because fast food and baked goods contribute to mood disorders and depression doesn't mean that other nutritional inadequacies don't do the same. Deficiencies in EPA and DHA fatty acids are one of the other strong nutritional promoters of depression.[19] These long-chain omega-3 fatty acids are commonly found in fish oil, though vegan EPA and DHA are now available from algae.

But deficiency isn't the only problem; these two fatty acids can also be imbalanced. The commercial meats, dairy, and oils that predominate in the SAD worsen the ratio of omega-6 to omega-3 fatty acids, which negatively affects brain health and function. Heated vegetable oils are almost all omega-6 fats, the "bad cop." Green vegetables, walnuts, flaxseeds, chia seeds, and seafood contain omega-3 fatty acids, the "good cop." As you consume more fried foods and cooked foods made with oil, you pump up the omega-6 content in your body. This doesn't just make you fat; it also increases your requirement for omega-3 fatty acids.

Fast food provides excessive amounts of omega-6 fats, but much of this fat is overheated and oxidized. *Oxidation* means the oils have been degraded by heat and have become rancid, producing numerous volatile, toxic compounds. Oxidation is not one single reaction but a series of complex reactions. Oxidized oils damage brain cells.[20] The brain is particularly sensitive to oxidized oils because it has limited antioxidant activity. These oil-generated compounds are so dangerous that even working near a deep fat fryer and inhaling the fumes is harmful. The toxic compounds produced are linked to birth defects, autoimmune disease, and cancer.[21]

Furthermore, fast food is deficient in the omega-3 fats, specifically— alpha-linolenic acid (ALA), EPA, and DHA—one more added element to the dangerous fast food pattern that primes brain disease. Omega-6 excess and omega-3 deficiency alter the composition and function of the brain and make people more prone to violence by preventing serotonin from passing between neurons.[22]

The Fatty Facts

Omega-6 and omega-3 polyunsaturated fatty acids (PUFAs) are essential for normal functioning of all the tissues of the body. Fatty acid deficiencies can cause dry skin, depression, and serious disease such as dementia with aging.[23]

Omega-3 fatty acids are the fats that are more difficult to find in the SAD. They are found in leafy green vegetables, flaxseeds, chia seeds, hemp seeds, walnuts, and seafood. **Alpha-linolenic acid (ALA),** a short-chain omega-3 fat, is the building block for the body to make **EPA** and **DHA,** which are commonly found in seafood. EPA and DHA are the longer-chain omega-3 fats that have anti-inflammatory effects and are necessary for brain growth and repair. Optimal brain function requires adequate DHA, which makes up 8 percent of the total volume of a healthy brain.

Omega-6 fatty acids are another family of PUFAs that are considered essential for the body, yet they are harmful in excess. The shortest of this class of fats (the building block) is **linoleic acid (LA).** Examples of oils that contain omega-6 fat are corn oil, soybean oil, and canola oil. It is generally recognized that excess omega-6 fat (in relation to omega-3 fat) is pro-inflammatory and accelerates common diseases, such as heart disease and cancer.[24]

The SAD has way too much omega-6 fat and too little omega-3 fat, mainly because of the oils used in cooking. The average American consumes more than 400 calories a day of omega-6–rich oils. It is estimated that the modern diet has a ratio of omega-6 to omega-3 fatty acids of approximately 15 to 1, but for people who eat fast food regularly, the ratio can be as dangerous as 25 to 1. Our cells, and particularly brain cells, need omega-3 fats impregnated in the cell membranes for normal function. The more omega-6 PUFAs you consume, the heavier you become and the more omega-3 PUFAs you need to consume for cell membranes to be healthy and tissue levels to be adequate.

SATURATED FATS IN ANIMAL PRODUCTS ARE NOT HARMLESS

An extremely powerful recent study showed that the saturated fat found in meat and cheese is likely the most dangerous type of fat to eat (excluding, of course, trans fats, which will be outlawed by 2018).[25] The researchers followed 125,000 male and female health professionals for more than thirty years, recording more than 33,000 deaths during this period. Replacing 5 percent of calories from saturated fat with polyunsaturated oils was associated with a 27 percent decrease in deaths, clearly demonstrating that saturated fat intake is more harmful than getting fats from vegetable and seed oils.

In recent years, certain studies have been publicized which concluded that greater intake of saturated fat was not associated with the risk of heart disease. However, these studies did not take into account what people were eating instead of food rich in saturated fats—often equally dangerous, high-glycemic refined carbohydrates.[26] These recent findings have been tremendously misinterpreted, and a huge push to deny the effect of diet on health and longevity has resulted. This misinformation is widespread and dangerous. Far too many doctors, programs, websites, and other information outlets are emphasizing these dangerous high-fat diets. Even the acclaimed cookbook author and former *New York Times* op-ed writer Mark Bittman declared, "Butter Is Back," and the June 23, 2014, issue of *Time* magazine had "Eat Butter" on its cover.[27] Poor scientific studies and irresponsible media continue to propagate this dangerous myth and in turn are contributing to thousands of needless deaths.

Adding to this confusion are recent scientific studies that indicate it is not merely the saturated fats in meat and cheese that promote heart disease, but also excess omega-6 fats in oils.[28] When researchers investigated findings of numerous randomized controlled trials that replaced saturated fats (butter, lard, cream, etc.) with vegetable oils, they found little difference in age of death. This large and detailed analysis of earlier data demonstrated that corn oil, safflower oil, soybean oil, canola oil, sunflower oil, and even olive oil damage the arteries and increase risk of death from heart disease and lead to earlier deaths. Some people have interpreted such data to mean that saturated fats such as butter are not as bad as we thought, but the science demonstrates otherwise: Both saturated fats and excess consumption of oils high in omega-6 fatty acids are harmful. And when any of these fats or oils is consumed in conjunction with sugar (or other high-glycemic carbohydrates), the dangerous effects are multiplied dramatically.

The point is that neither saturated fats nor vegetable oils have passed the test for safety. This is even partially true for olive oil, the linchpin of the supposedly healthy Mediterranean diet. For example, the findings of a study looking at the health of blood vessel linings (the endothelium) after a meal high in olive oil had surprising results demonstrating a decline in blood flow and increase in inflammation. The lead researcher, Dr. Robert Vogel, a cardiologist at the University of Maryland Hospital, concluded from the data "that it is not the olive oil that is the vaso-protective part of the Mediterranean diet [the part that helps keep blood vessels healthy]. It is the natural antioxidants [*in fruits and vegetables*] and the omega-3 fatty acids."[29]

In contrast, consuming one's fat mostly in the form of nuts and seeds protects the heart. When fats come from whole foods such as whole grains and nuts and seeds, instead of oils extracted from those foods, the presence of fat-binding fibers slows the absorption of the fat calories, enabling them to be burned for energy rather than stored as fat. Plus, because of the magnetic effect between the fiber and the fat in nuts and seeds, a significant amount of calories passes through the body into the toilet with that fiber and therefore is lost.[30]

OILS AND DEATH

The health benefits of nuts and seeds disappear when the nuts and seeds are processed and reduced to oils, which changes a weight-favorable food (the nuts and seeds) to an obesity-promoting food (the oils). Oils are not natural foods; they are highly processed foods. This change from consuming the whole foods to consuming the processed oils derived from those foods fundamentally affects behavior on a global scale. The increase in worldwide consumption of high-omega-6 oils over the past century is a large uncontrolled experiment that has shown increased societal burdens of aggression, depression, and cardiovascular mortality.

The danger of all this oil is seen best in the U.S. South, where oil consumption and fried foods are at their worst. People there regularly eat a traditional "Southern" diet that is known for its many deep-fried foods (such as fried chicken), processed meats (like bacon and ham), sugary beverages, and biscuits and gravy. With this diet, Southerners have earned the highest rates of stroke and heart disease in the world.

The large REGARDS (Reasons for Geographic and Racial Differences in Stroke) study addressed this issue by following more than twenty thousand study participants. Researchers found that, compared with other parts of the United States, the area of the country encompassing Alabama, Arkansas, Georgia, Indiana, Kentucky, Louisiana, Mississippi, North Carolina, South Carolina, Tennessee, and Virginia had a whopping 41 percent increased risk of stroke and 56 percent increased risk of heart

---

Common cooking oils are very high in omega-6 fats and very low in omega-3 fats. Humans can make some beneficial EPA and DHA fat (a long-chain omega-3, needed for brain cell membranes) from the short-chain omega-3 found in walnuts and seeds, such as flaxseeds and chia seeds. However, omega-6 oils compete for the same conversion enzymes, so the more omega-6 consumed, the less DHA is produced by the body, and the worse the ratio of omega-6 to omega-3 becomes in cell membranes.

More omega-6 intake → More inflammation
Less omega-6 intake → Less inflammation

Lower DHA levels also impair synthesis of serotonin, increasing the risk of depression as well as cognitive decline in the elderly.[31] In the Framingham Heart Study, the top quartile of blood DHA level was associated with a 47 percent reduction in the risk of developing dementia.[32] It is important to assure adequate amounts of DHA with a dietary source of DHA, such as fish, or a supplement for those who do not consume fish regularly.

attacks, and fried foods are highly implicated. And African Americans in these Southern states have the highest risk—an incredible 63 percent higher incidence of acute cardiovascular events compared with people who abstain from fried foods.[33]

The bottom line is this: When you fry a vegetable in oil, it doesn't count as a vegetable anymore; it's junk food.

The consumption of unhealthy oils that are high in omega-6 fats leads to inflammation, obesity, and heart disease, yet the average American consumes more than 400 calories a day from (fiberless) oil—up 67 percent since the 1950s.[34] And people who eat fast foods consume considerably more oil. We also know that clinical intervention trials and animal studies indicate that increasing dietary intake of long-chain omega-3 fatty acids as well as reducing the intake of omega-6 fatty acids reduces aggressive and violent behaviors. A large study of eight hundred active military personnel who committed suicide also found that the likelihood of suicide was 62 percent higher in those with low levels of DHA.[35]

Since 1909, per capita consumption of soybean oil has increased a thousandfold.[36] The homicide rate in the United States and the United Kingdom tripled between 1961 and 2000, while the percentage consumption of omega-6 oil grew by a similar amount during this period. The NIH compared homicide rates against oil consumption between 1961 and 2000 in Argentina, Australia, Canada, the United Kingdom, and the United States.[37] They collected data for twelve types of oils, including soybean, corn, and canola oils, which are the most popular. A direct correlation was found between the level of oil consumption and the rate of homicide in each population.

Clearly, this link between high consumption of omega-6 oil and violence, suicide, and murder is something that should not be quickly dismissed by claiming that association does not mean causation. The evidence continues to grow showing that chronic exposure to bad food influences bad behaviors. Food plays a huge role in how we think and act, affecting brain fog, depression, mood swings, anxiety, aggression, and even the propensity for violence. There is also much evidence today demonstrating that high consumption of omega-6 oils (and sweeteners) works synergistically to damage the body and the brain.[38] Think of French fries or doughnuts, for example, which are just high-glycemic carbohydrates fried in oil. That's suicide on a plate. Such foods can generate inflammation, accelerate aging, create serious autoimmune diseases such as Crohn's disease and ulcerative colitis,[39] and have dramatic damaging effects on brain function.

DEFICIENCIES OF EPA AND DHA ARE ASSOCIATED WITH

Lower intelligence

Poor school performance[40]

Aggression and hostility[41]

Depression and suicide[42]

Memory loss and cognitive decline[43]

Brain shrinkage and dementia[44]

Too many Americans damage their brains when they are young by eating Frankenfoods, and then as they get older they suffer from chronic diseases and premature aging and finally risk losing their minds almost completely through dementia. The constellation of factors present in and missing from the modern fast food diet, as well as deficiencies in omega-3 fatty acids, accelerates brain deterioration.

The number of new cases of Alzheimer's disease, which is directly linked to an unhealthy diet, is expected to triple between 2010 and 2050.[45] The number of people living with dementia worldwide is currently estimated at 47.5 million and is projected to increase to 75.6 million by 2030. In the United States, compared with their Caucasian counterparts, African Americans are about two times more likely and Hispanic Americans are about one and one-half times more likely to develop Alzheimer's and other forms of dementia. African Americans and Hispanics are at much higher risk, and diet is the only factor that can

Omega-3 and omega-6 are both fatty acids; they are very similar, but their effects on the brain are very different. The cell membranes in the brain are made out of DHA. When we don't have adequate reserves, the body will substitute an omega-6 molecule called docosapentaenoic acid (DPA), which is similar to DHA.[46] Even though DHA and DPA are interchangeable, they are not identical. DHA is more flexible than DPA. This property is called *membrane fluidity* and is very important for proper cell function. In the brain, these membranes surround the neuron and allow more neuro-chemical signals to get passed back and forth. DHA-impregnated membranes allow more nutrients to get into cells and more toxins to get out. High levels in the brain of n-6 DPA are associated with poorer cognitive function.[47]

Humans are extremely adaptable. Ideally, we should consume healthy amounts of both short-chain omega-3 ALA and the longer chain DHA, as well as EPA through our diet or high-quality sup-plements. But when this is not possible, our genes are intelligent enough to make use of omega-6 fatty acids. This comes at a price, however, because omega-6 triggers inflammation and alters the composition of our brains in unfavorable ways.

account for these differences; no known genetic factors can explain the greater prevalence of Alzheimer's and other forms of dementia in these two populations. Alzheimer's is a disease that is often diagnosed late in life. We now know that it is also a progressive ailment that is present and can be predicted from mild cognitive and emotional problems decades before diagnosis.

WHAT YOU EAT AFFECTS YOUR PERSONALITY, AND YOUR PERSONALITY AFFECTS WHAT YOU EAT

Studies confirm that children who consume a superior diet perform better academically compared with those who are nutrient deficient.[48]

Well-fed children are also less hyperactive, less moody, and better behaved.[49] Furthermore, recent research has documented that increasing consumption of vegetables and fruits can significantly elevate psychological well-being and people's "happiness levels."[50] This study is one of the first major scientific attempts to explore psychological well-being beyond the traditional findings that more fruits and vegetables can reduce the risks of cancer and heart attacks. Researchers followed more than twelve thousand randomly selected individuals for more than two years. Happiness benefits were detected for each extra portion of fruit and vegetables consumed, up to eight portions a day. They found that people who changed from consuming almost no fruits and vegetables to consuming eight portions a day experienced an increase in life satisfaction that was equivalent to moving from unemployment and poverty to employment and financial adequacy. This improvement in a sense of well-being occurred within twenty-four months.

This study ran in conjunction with the Australian Go for 2&5 campaign, which promoted the consumption of two portions of fruit and five portions of vegetables per day. Commenting on the findings, Dr. Redzo Mujcic, one of the researchers from the University of Queensland, said: "Perhaps our results will be more effective than traditional messages in convincing people to have a healthy diet. There is psychological payoff now from fruits and vegetables—not just a lower health risk decades later."[51]

WE AREN'T RATS, BUT WE BEHAVE LIKE THEM

Scientists at the Scripps Research Institute in Florida found that feeding rats junk food progressively degraded their brains' reward systems.[52] They tested two groups of rats: One was fed a diet of high-fat, high-calorie foods, and the other received a normal diet. The rats fed the unhealthy diet quickly became obese, less active, and developed a preference for unhealthy foods. But more significantly, the structure of their brains changed. The number of dopamine neuroreceptors in the brains of the junk food rats plummeted, and some areas of the brain shrank, decreasing learning capacity.[53] At mealtimes, mild electric shocks were administered to all rats. The rats fed the normal diet immediately stopped eating, but the rats eating junk food continued eating even while they were being shocked. They had become desensitized and compulsive. This relates to how fast food induces compulsive eating, and the diminished brain function, in turn, affects how poor eaters behave socially.

Like the rats fed fast food, too many Americans have diminished dopamine function as a result of overconsumption of junk food. They also experience diminished chemosensory perception, which means that they are less able to smell and taste. This is especially evident in the elderly, who have a reduced ability to enjoy the subtle flavors of real foods, so they become more reliant on using salt and sugar to boost flavors.[54] Alzheimer's patients show even greater olfactory deficits than other elderly, an effect related to the degree of dementia. Our inability to enjoy healthy foods is linked to alterations in the brain that ultimately become permanent as we progress toward dementia. It is a direct consequence of an impaired metabolism caused by an unhealthy diet. It is ironic that eating unhealthy foods damages us in a way that makes healthy eating unappealing. The good news is that we can recover, but that recovery requires conscious effort because of the way in which unhealthy diets alter our personalities and taste preferences.

After chronic overstimulation with concentrated and rapidly absorbed calories, we develop cravings. Eventually, after habitually eating fast food, the enjoyment that we once had from eating these foods weakens and instead we experience cravings—that intense desire that is so difficult to satisfy. Interestingly, this loss of self-control in eating and the loss of self-control that impulsively violent people experience have similar causes. Unhealthy diets simultaneously impair the function of dopamine, serotonin, and other neurotransmitters in the brain, and these changes correlate with anger and violence in both animal studies and human studies.[55] People who consume an unhealthy fast food diet have less self-control, have a reduced ability to control food intake, and also are more hostile and easily angered. Unnatural Frankenfoods destroy us from the inside out and affect how we treat each other. In contrast, a healthy diet with adequate phytochemicals, nutritional diversity, and omega-3 fatty acids elevates serotonin levels and normalizes receptor sensitivity, which can improve mood and eliminate the need to eat for emotional reasons.[56]

SCIENTIFIC STUDIES RELATE INTELLIGENCE TO NUTRITIONAL ADEQUACY

Human intelligence is higher, on average, in some places than in others around the world. Scientists analyzed IQ scores from 113 countries worldwide and found lower scores in countries with higher exposure to parasites and infectious disease, especially when such diseases impact nutrition during vulnerable periods of brain growth and development. Parasites often create micronutrient deficiencies in the host. The health and nutritional status of a region is the single largest determinant of the intelligence of its population; and aside from widespread infection and parasites, the single largest determinant of regional health is diet. Poor diet is a problem we can solve if we put our minds to it. Populations that have reduced infectious parasites and have instituted better sanitation and better nutrition have already seen higher scores on IQ tests in subsequent generations.[57]

The Avon Longitudinal Study of Parents and Children (ALSPAC), hosted by the University of Bristol, demonstrated that the micronutrient content of a diet plays a vital role in the development of childhood intelligence. The U.K. study started in the early 1990s, when more than fourteen thousand pregnant women were examined, followed by the long-term outcomes of their offspring. Researchers found that intelligence, measured by a Wechsler Intelligence Scale IQ test, was significantly affected by the quality of diet. Toddlers in this study who consumed a healthier diet had higher IQs by 8.5 years of age compared with those who consumed a low-nutrient diet.[58] Those who ate more junk food and fewer fresh fruits and vegetables also had more behavioral problems by age 7.[59] The fact that early childhood nutrition can have lifelong consequences indicates that nutrients affect the expression of genes that govern brain development.[60]

Other studies have corroborated such results. An eye-opening 2015 study demonstrated that improved diet and more physical activity during adolescence predicted better verbal intelligence in early adulthood.[61] This means that nutrition (and exercise) has positive effects on physical health, brain health, and intelligence in later life and it is not only the diet eaten during the first five years of life that determines ultimate intelligence.

Ninety percent of lunches packed at home contain desserts, chips, and sweetened beverages that would not pass muster to be served at schools under new nutritional guidelines. With $700 million a year spent on marketing fast food to kids, nearly one in three American children between the ages of 2 and 14 eats fast food daily. This is especially relevant in light of a recent study of twelve thousand students between fifth and eighth grades that showed those who ate processed and fast foods had the worst skills in math, reading, and science. The researchers concluded that "high levels of fast food consumption are predictive of slower growth in academic skills."[62]

Let's stop for a moment to reflect on this scientific data: *The junk food diets that our children eat directly affect their academic performance.* And yet, fast food is being served to kids at breakfast, lunch, and dinner all around the country. It is high time that this information becomes public knowledge so that we can change these accepted "normal" patterns.

Children who do not eat a wide variety of fruits and vegetables lack protection and are more vulnerable to many serious diseases. We know that diets rich in leafy green vegetables and fruits are anti-inflammatory because the wide array of protective antioxidants and phytochemicals work to counteract inflammation and prevent autoimmune disease, but this same biological effect also counters free radical activity in the brain benefiting brain function.[63] Infants who consume fruits, vegetables, and home-prepared meals have been shown to have higher verbal IQs and better memory performance by 4 years of age.[64]

Excellent nutrition has positive effects on intelligence, and fast foods and junk foods have powerful negative effects on intelligence. A 2012 study showed that fast foods and high-fat foods, such as hamburgers, onion rings, oily pizzas, and other regularly consumed fast foods, scar the brain and damage the hypothalamus in both rodents and humans.[65] In school-age children, low-nutrient diets that include fast food and fried foods are linked to the poorest academic performance.[66] Unfortunately, the fast food–inflamed brain results in detrimental effects continuing into adulthood.[67]

Many people know that these types of diets are the recipe for obesity, diabetes, and heart disease, but it is not as well-known that our fast food environment leads to a continuing cycle of destruction inside the brain. Subtle brain damage routinely occurs in childhood, leading to a poor-quality life. Then, if one lives long enough, dementia happens with aging. Thus, opportunity and happiness are ruined along the full spectrum of life.

PARENTS ARE THE MAJOR CULPRITS IN LOWERING THEIR CHILDREN'S INTELLECTUAL POTENTIAL

The amount of scientific evidence is irrefutable that junk food, candy, soft drinks, fast food, and commercial baked goods damage the brain. Unfortunately, well-meaning parents and grandparents are the biggest culprits, poisoning the health and future intellect of the nation's children. Children don't shop and buy their own food. Adults reward children with doughnuts and chips for playing well in sports; adults support their children's Halloween candy collections; adults make holiday cookies and cakes; adults take their children on fast food excursions— lots of traditional American practices and social norms damage the brains of our precious children. It is time to change this, especially because the right food choices lead to higher intelligence, emotional stability, and happiness.

It is not only the diet early in life that affects intelligence and mental health; fast food that mothers consume before giving birth affects the mental health of their offspring. Conduct problems and ADHD often exist together and are linked to both fast foods eaten early in life and the prenatal diet of mothers. Such problems include antisocial behavior, the inability to follow rules, bullying, fighting, cruelty to others or animals,

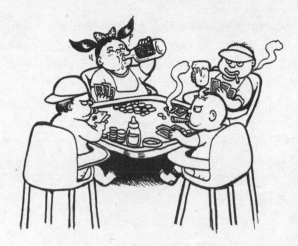

stealing, and poor performance in school. These problems are associated with diets high in oils and sugar during pregnancy.[68] Abnormal DNA methylation within the brain, leading to poor learning capacity and antisocial behavior, can accumulate both during pregnancy and in early childhood in response to fast food.

Autism spectrum disorder is a neurodevelopmental condition characterized by severe deficits in intellect, socialization, verbal and nonverbal communication, and behavior. Since the 1960s prevalence rates of this disorder have increased dramatically; this increase cannot be explained entirely by changes in diagnosis practices, with one in sixty-eight U.S. children now affected, according the U.S. Centers for Disease Control and Prevention (CDC).

Methylation defects refer to carbon-based molecules that attach to sites on our cells' DNA, altering the function of the DNA; as these defects accumulate, cells become more prone to abnormal function and eventually cancer. Even childhood leukemia and brain cancer in children has been linked to the unhealthful diet their mothers eat not only during pregnancy, but also before conception.[69] Someday in the near future, obstetricians won't advise against just drugs, cigarettes, and alcohol—fast food will be equally off-limits.

Fast food intake, obesity, and diabetes have also risen to epidemic levels in women of reproductive age over the same time period. Though the link between fast food and obesity and diabetes is well-established, it is not common knowledge that fast food exposure is linked to autism as well. Fast food, maternal obesity, and pregestational diabetes have all been shown to be associated with autism—each as an independent risk factor—but in combination the risk is more pronounced, increasing more than fourfold.[70] Our nation's eating habits are simply damaging the brains of the children of the next generation, even before they have their first fast food meal.

FAST FOOD PROMOTES THE USE OF ILLEGAL DRUGS AND CRIME

A randomized, placebo-controlled trial in a British prison tested the association between antisocial behavior and nutritional status. Compared with the test group, prisoners whose diets were supplemented with vitamins, minerals, and essential fatty acids had 26 percent fewer reports of antisocial behavioral incidents.[71] A research team in the Netherlands replicated the study and had similar results.[72] Findings were also similar at a high school for troubled youth. When candy and soda were removed from the school and better food was made available, negative behaviors such as vandalism, drug and weapons violations, dropout and expulsion rates, and suicide attempts became virtually nonexistent.[73] After decades of studies, it appears that the hypothesis that nutrition and violence are related is gaining momentum. A 2009 article in *Science* about diet and violence in prisons quotes behavioral psychologist Iver Mysterud saying, "The [nutrition-violence] effect is obviously real and it has been researched for 30 years; the policy implications are obvious: Get rid of sugar and highly processed foods, improve the diet." This joins the chorus of others recommending that prisoners with nutritional imbalances and deficiencies receive supplements of minerals, vitamins, and fatty acids.[74]

It's becoming more and more clear that the consumption of sweets and fast food in childhood is associated with violence and crime in adulthood. In 2009, a British study showed a powerful association between candy consumption in childhood and violence in adulthood. Researchers found that children who were fed more candy at age 10 were significantly more likely to be convicted of a violent crime by age 34; this relationship was found to be robust even when controlling for environmental and other individual factors. Not even economic hardship, parental attitudes, education, and personality traits in early life showed as strong a correlation with adult violent crime as did eating candy.[75] It's time for parents to rethink the practice of rewarding their children with junk food and candy. And don't forget Halloween—the ultimate junk food orgy. This is akin to recreational drug use for the young.

Illicit drug use, another major problem in some urban areas, is directly linked to nutrient-related dysfunction in the brain. Studies show that substance abusers are malnourished.[76] Former addicts who received drug counseling combined with nutrition education had significantly better outcomes than those given counseling alone.[77] The fact that drug users are malnourished doesn't prove that malnutrition led to their drug use; however, the fact that good nutrition enhances recovery suggests that the lack of nutrition contributes, and more evidence is accumulating every day. More and more scientists are coming to the conclusion that eating fast food can lead to changes in brain chemistry that can increase addiction and drug-seeking behavior later.[78] The issue here is high sugar consumption, and fast food functions as a "gateway drug" to harder, more powerful brain-altering chemicals. This is especially critical today when you consider that about half the people in federal prisons were incarcerated for nonviolent, drug-related offenses.[79]

Well-known musician Eric Clapton has said that his drug addiction started with sugar: "It [the pattern of addiction] started with sugar. When I was 5 or 6 years old I was cramming sugar down my throat as fast as I could get it down. Sweets, you know, sugar on bread and butter . . . I became addicted to sugar because it changed the way I felt."[80]

A brain under nutritional stress seeks ongoing stimulation, creating the increasing tendency for dependence on sugar, alcohol, and drugs. As the brain's health deteriorates, susceptibility to chemical stimulation

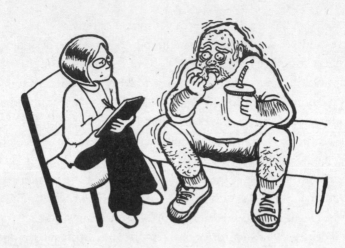

"Heroin was my gateway drug!"

with junk food, alcohol, and legal and illegal drugs as a means of coping with a difficult life increases. Fast food keeps our nation sick and it keeps our poor people poor; they become unable to escape the cycle of poverty and face reduced achievement in their lives. In order to solve this problem of disease, crime, and the disenfranchisement of a segment of our population, we must assure that everyone is aware of these issues, has access to healthy food, and understands the importance of eating healthfully. Equal opportunity can only begin with the gift of a healthy brain.

Diabetes, heart disease, and cancer are recognized diseases linked to diet. In sharp contrast, increased aggression, reduced learning capacity, and depression are not generally recognized as diet-related problems because the effects are subtle. Consequently, the only way to fully grasp the dangers of an unhealthy diet is to examine the extreme behavioral effects on large populations. Not everyone who eats unhealthy foods gets cancer; likewise, not everyone who is disruptive, less forgiving, and has a decreased ability to concentrate becomes a violent criminal. Fewer than five people out of one hundred thousand commit murder in any given year. To understand the effects of bad diet on criminal behavior, we have to look at large studies encompassing entire populations.

Of course, food is not the only factor implicated in violence and drug use, but it is the most overlooked, and possibly the most important, factor in this equation. High rates of violence and crime are not only problems in urban inner cities. A less publicized crime problem prevails in the American South to this day. According to FBI crime statistics, the Southern region of the United States experiences violence at rates nearly double that of the Northeast, which includes high-crime cities such as Camden, New Jersey; Philadelphia; Washington, D.C.; and New York City.[81] According to 1993 crime data, white males in the rural areas of the South were about four times more likely to commit homicide than white males living in the Mid-Atlantic region.[82] These days, increased violence in these rural areas continues, and they can be considered food deserts because the diet is so poor. There is a cluster of 644 counties in fifteen states, mainly in the Southeast, where diabetes is so prevalent that the area has been called the "diabetes belt."[83] It is precisely the same region that has the bulk of violent crimes. The numbers tell the story. In areas where diets are worse and diabetes rates are higher, so are rates of violent crime.

A 2015 study by the CDC found that vegetable and fruit consumption was consistently lower in Southeastern states compared with the rest of the country.[84] Overall, 13.1 percent of Americans ate the recommended amount of fruit; Tennesseans consumed the least, with only 7.5 percent meeting recommended levels compared with nearly 18 percent of Californians. Fewer than 9 percent of Americans met recommendations for vegetable intake; the state with the lowest number was Mississippi, with 5.5 percent compared with California, where 13 percent of the population ate vegetables. These statistics are even more shocking when one considers the fact that the government's recommendations for fruit and vegetable consumption are too low to guarantee superior health and hence optimal brain function.

THE HAVE-NOTS IN AMERICA LIVE ON FAST FOOD

International studies comparing health differences in the United States, the United Kingdom, Canada, and Australia found that disparities in birth weights existed between the highest- and lowest-income groups.[85] However, the disparities in the United States were the most pronounced of all the countries studied; low birth weights were consistently associated with low-income levels. The poor diet of the have-nots is more pronounced in our country, and this is not just observed in inner cities, but also among rural communities.[86]

Correlational data such as the established relationship discussed above between high oil intake, sugar, and crime do not signify cause and effect, and certainly there are other contributory factors to the development of chronic diseases, brain disease, and personality. More comprehensive studies performed with proper methodology are needed and will be invaluable. However, the lack of conclusive evidence should not permit the continuation of nutritional negligence keeping communities prisoned in a stressful and unhealthful life. The concept that behavior, mental health, intellectual potential, and aggression are separate from the parameters affecting bodily health is illogical, and even ridiculous.

Some of the most intractable problems we face in the United States are the result of subtle brain damage that goes largely unnoticed because we don't associate problems in the brain with unhealthy diets. The SAD is making too many of us prone to chronic depression, anger, impaired decision-making, and diminished learning capacity. These are, in fact, early signs of dementia, but they are also the symptoms of a society that has been fundamentally altered by its diet. Clearly, this area deserves substantial funding support for further scientific research, but this doesn't mean we shouldn't act now on the information we already have available. This crisis deserves urgent action because poor nutrition leaves a wide path of human suffering.

Imagine if we could significantly increase intelligence and reduce poverty and crime by simply changing how people eat. This is not such an unreasonable dream. Malnutrition not only prevents ex-offenders, drug addicts, and truants from turning their lives around, but it is probably the reason they went astray in the first place. Our failure as a society to consider the evidence and confront this fast food genocide makes us like proverbial lemmings that see the abyss but still march off the cliff.

CHAPTER THREE

LET FOOD BE THY MEDICINE

When the facts change, I change my mind. What do you do, sir?

—ATTRIBUTED TO JOHN MAYNARD KEYNES

What we eat matters. I hope I have made this very clear, having covered the ways in which fast food has created a sickly nation and perpetuated medical dependence. I have discussed the ways in which high-fat processed foods are dangerously addictive and negatively affect our poorest communities the most radically. And I also have delved deep into how nutrient-lacking food affects the brain and results in life-altering behavioral changes.

But there is good news. We can end this genocide. We can take back our lives from the tyranny of fast foods permeating the globe. But first let's take a moment to look at how nutrient-rich foods save lives.

The facts about nutrition have changed in recent years. Fortunately, we now have on hand hundreds of thousands of studies with clear evidence that nutritional excellence can effectively prevent disease and extend the human life span. Unfortunately, only a very small percentage of people take advantage of these life-giving findings.

Recent discoveries in nutritional science have revealed that it is not merely excess sugar, white flour, and oils that accelerate aging and premature death; too many animal products in the diet can also have detrimental effects. It has been well-established that as animal protein is consumed in higher amounts, particularly above 10 percent of total calories, insulin-like growth factor-1 (IGF-1) levels rise. IGF-1 is a growth-promoting hormone that, at higher levels, can promote aging, cell replication, cancer, and the spread of cancer.[1] With levels of animal products approaching 30 percent of calories, IGF-1 levels can run dangerously high, accelerating the development of both cancer and heart disease.

Many books and nutritional gurus promote a high-protein diet with lots of animal products. However, an increasing number of scientific studies have accumulated evidence that demonstrates the folly of this viewpoint and the dangerous outcomes that occur from following such ill-conceived advice. Higher intake of animal products in the diet is associated with twelve different types of cancer, as determined by data from the GLOBOCAN project of the International Agency for Research on Cancer. Researchers investigated populations in eighty-seven U.S. counties that had high-quality data available and demonstrated an association with cancer in the overwhelming majority of counties in which pasture-raised or naturally raised animal products were used, as opposed to feedlot-fed commercial meats, which are likely even more detrimental.[2]

More protein from animal products encourages the growth and spread of cancer. But when people modify their diets to include more natural, higher protein plant foods, such as beans, greens, seeds, and nuts, and fewer high-protein animal products, they achieve dramatic health and life span benefits, especially fewer deaths caused by heart attack.[3]

People in the nutritional arena make all types of claims, and they always have some studies to back up their views. Eggs are good; eggs are bad; fat is good; fat is bad—in each case, someone finds and quotes a different study to support a predetermined position. People can claim almost anything and always find some study somewhere that supports their viewpoint. The public is left with no choice but to believe whomever they want and just pick the diet they prefer to eat.

So why am I giving extra credence to the three studies I am highlighting as examples below? Why not accept other studies that show animal products are not so dangerous, and could even be helpful for some people? The main reason is the large number of participants in these studies and the significant number of years the study subjects were followed. Short-term studies can be manipulated to show benefits when a person loses weight, even if the diet is not ideal for cancer protection or longevity in the long run.

Blood test markers may improve, but these are *soft endpoints,* meaning they are suggestive of benefits but may or may not translate into fewer heart attacks, fewer strokes, less cancer, and a longer life down the road. *Hard endpoints,* such as a cardiac event, a cancer diagnosis, or a death, are more powerful indicators and need to be granted more weight and legitimacy. The data from many long-term studies with hard endpoints have accumulated recently, making the science definitive.

STUDY NUMBER ONE

Scientists followed more than 85,000 women and 44,000 men for twenty years or more (twenty-six years in women and twenty years in men), none of whom had prior diabetes, heart disease, or cancer. More than 12,500 deaths were recorded. This study demonstrated a 43 percent increased rate of death from all causes in those participants eating a "low-carbohydrate diet" that was high in animal products, compared with those eating a high-vegetable diet.[4]

This huge and convincing study, with more than twenty-five years of follow-up in women, clearly showed that a high-protein diet was much more dangerous than even the SAD; and of course the opposite approach, with fewer animal products and more plant vegetation in the diet, demonstrated a significant enhancement of life span. The study essentially puts an end to all debate about a high-protein diet. It simply is irresponsible to advise such a diet, because it kills people.

This massive study was published in 2010, meaning that we have known for years—without question—that these popular high-protein diets are deadly. It makes you wonder how authors can write books glorifying the benefits of high-protein, meat-based diets when such studies are available for everyone to review. Clearly, some authors pander to the masses' desire to eat meat despite the known dangers.

STUDY NUMBER TWO

A 2012 study looked at the relationship between a low-carbohydrate, high-protein diet and the incidence of cardiovascular diseases in Swedish women. More than forty-three thousand 30- to 49-year-old women were followed for more than fifteen years.[5] This study was notable both for the large number of participants and for the care taken to access the degree of dietary adherence to the high-protein, low-carbohydrate diet protocol. Participants with the highest proportion of animal protein in their diets were also found to be consuming more animal fats, compared with those who consumed fewer animal products.

The researchers gave the subjects a diet score from 1 to 20 based on how closely they adhered to a low-carb, high-animal-protein dietary pattern. Those who were following the old Atkins-type or Dukan/Paleo diet most closely, with lots of animal products and severe restriction of carbohydrates, were given a score of 20. Those who followed a diet restricting animal products significantly and liberally eating plant foods rich in carbohydrates were given a score of 1. The researchers gave every participant a score to indicate how much that participant's dietary pattern favored plants or animals.

Researchers tracked cardiovascular events (per ten thousand woman-years) and found a dose-dependent increase in risk: a 5 percent increase in risk of cardiovascular events (heart attack or cardiovascular-related death) per 2-point increase in the low-carb, high-protein diet score. Overall, a 60 percent increased risk of cardiovascular events and deaths occurred in those women adhering to a low-carb, high-protein diet with a diet score higher than 16.

The results showed a gradual and consistent increased risk of developing cardiovascular disease and experiencing a cardiovascular-related death when the consumption of animal products increased and consumption of plant-food carbohydrates decreased. The study's conclusion? *Low-carbohydrate, high-protein diets are associated with an increased risk of cardiovascular disease and cardiovascular-related death.* The researchers also compared their results with four other studies that looked at the same issue. They found that their results were consistent with earlier, smaller, long-term studies and that all these studies collectively showed that diets low in protective plant foods and high in animal products are exceedingly dangerous.

STUDY NUMBER THREE

In the third study, more than six thousand people eating high-protein diets that were low in sugar were studied and compared with people eating fewer animal products and more carbohydrates. They were followed for eighteen years and were in the 50–65 age range. Following deaths over those eighteen years, the researchers found a fourfold increase of risk of cancer death and a 75 percent increase in overall death in the group eating more animal products.[6]

It is interesting to note that the people in the high-animal-protein group were consuming the average level that most Americans consume— that is, about 18 percent of calories from animal protein, or about 27 percent of calories from animal products when you add in the fat calories. This means that high-protein diet gurus, who advocate much higher levels of animal protein than investigated in this study, may be dispensing more dangerous cancer-promoting advice compared with even the shocking higher death rate seen in this study. The lowest-protein study group consumed 5 percent of calories from animal protein, or less than about 8 percent in animal products, which is considerably less than what Americans currently consume.

It is also interesting to note that there was a seventy-three-fold increased risk of developing diabetes in the higher-protein group, and a twenty-three-fold increased risk in the moderate-protein group, compared with the lower-protein group. This increased risk of diabetes with higher animal protein intake was consistent at all ages.

It's important to note that the study included data on elderly people that showed that animal protein in the diet was beneficial with advancing age, likely because of decreased digestive capacity and increased frailty with aging. However, that aspect of the study did not examine participants eating high-protein seeds, nuts, beans, and greens, which can increase the protein concentration of the diet without the known drawbacks of increasing animal products. Regardless of the question surrounding the ideal diet for the elderly, we know that the goals to maintain body muscle and skeletal mass and to maintain immune function as we age can be best achieved with a diet mostly of natural, nutrient-rich plants. If animal products are needed, they should be used judiciously.

WE ALL MUST AGREE TO AGREE

Over the past decade, we have garnered an overwhelming amount of evidence regarding the dangers of the SAD and the protective effects of eating more natural plant foods. In fact, most nutritional scientists throughout the world agree on three basic tenets of healthy eating:

1. Foods that are highly refined and processed lose their natural structure, fiber, and micronutrients. They also are generally highly glycemic, resulting in increased insulin production. These foods promote disease and premature death.

2. Eating more colorful fruits, vegetables, beans, nuts, and seeds protects against disease and reduces all-cause mortality, extending human life span.

3. Eating excess animal products can shorten life span and promote chronic disease and premature death. Some animal products are safer than others, but even safer ones should be consumed in only limited amounts.

Hundreds of studies have looked at the relationship between eating whole plant foods and chronic diseases such as cardiovascular disease, diabetes, and cancer. For virtually every disease, studies have shown that people who eat the most vegetables, fruits, legumes, nuts, seeds, and whole grains always have the lowest risk, no matter what disease is being investigated.

Large-scale, population-based studies document these effects. The more vegetables people eat, the better their health. For example, researchers analyzed sixteen prospective studies from the United States, Europe, and Asia that reviewed the effects of fruit and vegetable consumption on death from all causes, cardiovascular disease, and cancer.[7] The studies involved a combined total of 833,234 subjects, with a follow-up period ranging from 4.6 to 26 years. This large-scale study showed that the risk of all-cause mortality decreased by every serving of produce eaten per day. The authors concluded: "The results support current recommendations to increase consumption [*of whole plant foods*] to promote health and overall longevity. The benefits of eating right are unparalleled by any medication on the market." Dr. Kim Williams, former president of the American College of Cardiology, has called heart disease "a 99 percent food-borne illness."

With the accumulated evidence available today, it is clear that heart disease, the leading cause of death in the United States, is the result of nutritional folly. This fact makes almost every cardiac-related hospitalization, every death, and every stroke victim's injuries the more tragic. We know this is all needless suffering and needless premature death, because these people could have learned to eat differently. We could revolutionize health care, add decades to life expectancy, and solve our health care problems—and much of the modern world's economic difficulties—if people just ate better and followed the lead of the nutritional science community.

AMERICA: LAND OF THE FREE AND HOME OF THE OBESE

The facts regarding human nutrition have evolved so that we know how to save millions of lives. Yet people choose to ignore, twist, and vilify the science that has conclusively demonstrated that for excellent health, we need to eat a diet that consists predominantly of natural plants. Most people have not changed their behaviors, and dangerous eating and drinking are the norm. People are entrenched in their various dietary camps and do not want facts to interfere with their acquired food preferences.

We have a serious health care crisis, and things are not getting better—they are getting worse. Throughout the United States, we have a growing population of people suffering from obesity and diabetes, and others who have serious dietary-induced diseases. Though health varies widely depending on where one lives and what one eats, most people in this country are overweight and sickly by the time they reach middle age. For example, the average adult woman in the United States is 5-feet-4-inches tall and weighs 166 pounds; a dangerous and foreboding statistic. And that means half of all women weight more. This ubiquitous ill health has devastating effects on the productivity of our workforce and the health of our economy, as well as contributing to poor living conditions in our cities. The explosion in the number of people suffering from diabetes, as well as the deterioration of mental and physical health, leads to despondency.

More than 40 percent of Americans between the ages of 40 and 59 are now obese. The number of overweight and obese people has never been so high in all of human history, and this explosion of waistlines

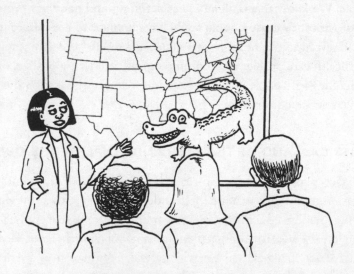

"We have finally determined, based on geographical correlation,
that the cause of obesity is alligators."

has occurred relatively recently, so the full damage is just beginning to unfold. The future looks bleak, with a predicted eruption of Alzheimer's disease as our current obese population becomes older. Furthermore, Alzheimer's is occurring at younger and younger ages.

A study looking at this issue concluded that for an obese person in his or her 40s, the likelihood of that person developing Alzheimer's disease is 74 percent higher than for someone of normal weight, and if that person is obese by his or her 30s, the risk is much higher.[8] Americans are eating themselves into brain atrophy and dementia, which will place an increasing stress on the younger generations who have to care for these individuals.

A serious problem in our country—and in the modern world generally—is the lack of acceptance that chronic, dietary-induced diseases such as diabetes, obesity, heart disease, stroke, and dementia are almost totally preventable through superior nutrition. Our economy is being weighed down by an expensive and largely ineffective medical system—a system that relies on expensive tests, treatments, and last-minute heroics to combat the effects of a nation poisoning itself with a rich, disease-causing diet.

Heart disease is the leading cause of death for both men and women, yet it can be almost entirely prevented. I say "almost," because some people's health conditions have deteriorated so much before they switch to a healthy diet that a heart disease–induced death cannot be prevented. Also, some people have rare congenital and valvular heart diseases caused by infections or other nonnutritional factors.

According to the World Health Association, "Americans have one of the worst life expectancy" scores of all modern countries.[9] But what is even worse is our very poor "healthy life expectancy score," which takes into account not merely how long we live but also that our quality of life is so poor if still alive, because people are sickly, with both physical and mental deterioration. If you eat like other Americans and live long enough, the result is often dementia and stroke, which cripple the elderly and force them into long-term-care facilities where their quality of life is limited.

YOUR HEALTH IS IN YOUR HANDS

A Nutritarian diet is the "gold standard" eating style to maximize health and longevity. It contains at least 90 percent natural plant foods, including fresh fruit, vegetables, beans, mushrooms, onions, sprouted grains, nuts, and seeds. If much of our nation ate this way, we would be able to invigorate our economy, improve emotional intelligence, and increase productivity. Chronic disease, such as heart disease, would rarely be found, and—after decades of change—we would halt the explosion in cancer rates that has occurred in the past century, and the number of new cancer diagnoses would fall precipitously. Such diseases would be as unusual as they were earlier in human history.

A Nutritarian diet is an eating style in which the vast majority of calories are obtained from eating natural, colorful, nutrient-rich plant foods. Refined, processed foods are avoided or reduced, and the use of animal products is kept to less than 10 percent of calories consumed. A Nutritarian diet style has a specific purpose: to maximize how long we live and to minimize the possibility of our suffering from heart disease, stroke, dementia, and cancer. It is not a fixed or rigid platform of rules, but a changing body of recommendations that moves with the preponderance of evidence to protect human lives from disease and to maximize health.

A Nutritarian diet is also effective, and sometimes modified specifically, for the treatment of diabetes, autoimmune disease, irritable bowel syndrome, gout, kidney stones, and migraines. It can be used therapeutically to enable recovery from most chronic diseases.[10]

The body is a miraculous, self-healing machine when fed properly. Through dietary excellence, high blood pressure, high cholesterol, and diabetes melt away, and even advanced cases of atherosclerosis (coronary artery disease) resolve, removing the need for expensive, invasive, and usually futile medical care. **Most diseases that plague modern America are the result of nutritional ignorance and are best remedied with superior nutrition, not drugs.**

I was the principal investigator on a 2015 study on a Nutritarian diet documenting the benefits for reducing weight, lowering cholesterol, and reducing blood pressure.[11] The results were remarkable. Out of 443 individuals, the average drop in systolic blood pressure was 26 mmHg—much more than drugs accomplish and more than any other diet ever tested. Patients routinely reversed their heart disease, even when the cases were very advanced. This eliminated their need for coronary artery bypass surgery and angioplasty.

As we have increased our waistlines in the United States, we are facing an exploding epidemic of type 2 diabetes. What once was a relatively rare disease now affects almost 10 percent of all Americans, and that percentage continues to increase. Yet a Nutritarian diet also reverses type 2 diabetes in approximately 90 percent of compliant individuals.[12]

It would be very difficult for a person to become overweight eating mostly fruits, vegetables, beans, nuts, and seeds. Being overweight is predominately the result of consuming disease-causing processed foods, especially flours, oils, cheeses, and sweeteners. Heart disease and diabetes simply do not exist in populations that eat mostly natural plant foods. The "Blue Zones" around the world—where people enjoy comparitively healthy and long lives—are a testament to this concept.[13]

There are also populations eating natural diets that have no recorded heart disease. For example, the Kitava study documents an island population with about 2500 inhabitants, with no recorded heart disease.[14] The people have plenty of food to eat, and they are well nourished; they are very lean (despite food abundance), have low blood pressure, and no cardiovascular disease. It was particularly fascinating that many of them smoked cigarettes but still did not develop heart disease. Fast foods, processed foods, sweeteners, dairy, oils, sugar, cereals, and alcohol are absent from their diet, and their salt intake is very low—hence, strokes and heart disease are not found in this population. We have no reason *not* to cut the junk out of our diets. The benefits are literally life-giving.

HEALING AND PROTECTIVE FOODS: G-BOMBS

When we eat foods containing all the nutrients humans require, as well as an adequate amount of phytochemicals and antioxidants, the self-repair mechanisms in our cells function normally to prevent disease, and our immune systems can more effectively protect us against dangerous infections and immune system disorders.

Some natural foods have more disease-protective nutrients than others. Though one could accurately state that all fruits, vegetables, beans, nuts, seeds, and whole grains are "good for us," it would be inaccurate to think they are all good for us to the same degree. By recognizing some "superstars" in this field of celebrities, we can have a more powerful impact on our health destiny. To win the war on cancer, we must design an anticancer diet that focuses on the foods with the most powerful anticancer effects and floods our bodies with the protective substances contained within them.

The acronym **G-BOMBS** is an effective tool to help people remember to eat these superstars regularly—even daily if possible. It stands for **G**reens, **B**eans, **O**nions, **M**ushrooms, **B**erries, and **S**eeds. Scientific evidence demonstrates that each one of these foods has significant cancer-protective effects, but the most powerful protection occurs when the portfolio of foods you regularly eat includes all of them.

G = GREENS

Green vegetables contain more micronutrients per calorie than any other food, and they also contain the most plant protein per calorie. About half of the calories in green vegetables, including leafy greens, comes from protein, and this plant protein is packed with thousands of beneficial phytochemicals, as well as folate, calcium, and small amounts of omega-3 fatty acids. The consumption of green vegetables is associated with protection against cancer and heart disease as well as life span enhancement. The green cruciferous vegetables, such as broccoli, kale, and cabbage, are also well-known for their isothiocyanates (ITCs), which have potent protective effects against cancer.[15] This family includes green vegetables like collard greens and bok choy plus some nongreen vegetables like cauliflower.

EAT CRUCIFEROUS VEGETABLES FOR HEALTH:

- Arugula
- Bok choy
- Broccoli
- Broccoli rabe
- Broccolini
- Brussels sprouts
- Cabbage

- Cauliflower
- Collards
- Horseradish
- Kale
- Kohlrabi
- Mustard greens

- Radishes
- Red cabbage
- Rutabaga
- Turnips
- Turnip greens
- Watercress

Cruciferous vegetables contain *glucosinolates,* and in a different area of the cell, an enzyme called *myrosinase.* When we blend, chop, or chew these vegetables, we break up the plant cells, allowing myrosinase to come into contact with glucosinolates, initiating a chemical reaction that produces these beneficial ITCs. These compounds have been shown to detoxify and remove carcinogens, kill cancer cells, and prevent tumors from growing.[16]

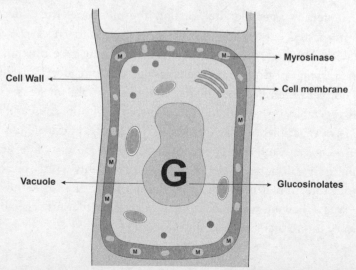

Glucosinolates + Myrosinase → Isothiocyanates (ITCs)

Cruciferous vegetables are especially helpful for preventing hormonal cancers like breast cancer because some ITCs, such as indole-3-carbinol (abundant in broccoli, Brussels sprouts, and cabbage), can even help the body excrete estrogen and other hormones. In fact, research has shown additional anti-estrogenic effects of hundreds of these green food compounds, which blunt the growth-promoting effects of estrogen on breast and cervical cancer cells.[17]

In a 2009 study, Chinese women who regularly ate one serving per day of cruciferous vegetables had a 50 percent reduced risk of breast cancer.[18] A 17 percent decrease in breast cancer risk was found in a European study of participants consuming cruciferous vegetables at least once a week.[19] Plus, breast cancer survivors who eat cruciferous vegetables regularly have a lower risk of cancer recurrence—the more cruciferous vegetables they eat, the lower their risk.[20] In men, twenty-eight servings of vegetables per week decreased prostate cancer risk by 35 percent, but just three servings of cruciferous vegetables per week decreased prostate cancer risk by 46 percent.[21] One or more servings of cabbage per week reduced the risk of pancreatic cancer by 38 percent.[22]

The active ingredient in broccoli, is broccoli.
—DAVID KATZ, M.D., PRESIDENT, AMERICAN COLLEGE OF LIFESTYLE MEDICINE

Cruciferous vegetables are not only the most powerful anticancer foods in existence; they are also the most micronutrient-dense of all vegetables. Although the National Cancer Institute recommends five to nine servings of fruits and vegetables per day for cancer prevention, it has not yet established specific recommendations for intake of cruciferous vegetables. I recommend three to six fresh fruits and eight total servings of vegetables per day, including two servings of cruciferous vegetables—one raw and one cooked. Consuming a variety of vegetables within an overall nutrient-dense diet can provide us with a profound level of protection against cancer. And don't forget: Eat some raw and chew well. Chewing well, blending, or juicing cruciferous vegetables is necessary to produce the most anticancer ITCs.

B = BEANS

Beans and other legumes are the most nutrient-dense carbohydrate source. Like green vegetables, beans are also high in protein, but unlike animal protein, they do not promote unfavorable cancer-promoting hormones. In fact, beans are a powerful anticancer food, because of their high phytochemical content and also because they are a very low-glycemic food. The starch they contain is mostly a mixture of slowly digestible starch and resistant starch, which means that their calories enter the bloodstream slowly over several hours, preventing an insulin surge. This has a stabilizing effect on blood sugar, which promotes satiety and helps to prevent food cravings.[23] The high amount of resistant starch (which is not broken down by digestive enzymes) reduces the total number of calories absorbed from beans and is also fermented by intestinal bacteria into fatty acids that help to prevent colon cancer.[24] Combined with the high amount of soluble fiber, beans also lower cholesterol.[25]

O = ONIONS

Onions, along with leeks, garlic, chives, shallots, and scallions, make up the *Allium* genus of vegetables, which play a powerful role in fighting cancer, are anti-diabetic, and have beneficial effects on the cardiovascular and immune systems. Allium vegetables are known for their characteristic organosulfur compounds, which are released when onions are chopped, crushed, or chewed. Studies have found that increased consumption of allium vegetables is associated with a lower risk of gastric and prostate cancers because they contain compounds that detoxify carcinogens, halt cancer cell growth, and block angiogenesis (the growth of new blood vessels).[26]

M = MUSHROOMS

Mushrooms may not be the most dense in vitamins and minerals, but they have unique compounds that influence human health and immune function. They are rich in angiogenesis inhibitors.[27] Cancer cells secrete angiogenesis promoters to secure a robust blood supply to fuel their growth and metastatic process. This process is prevented by the angiogenesis-inhibiting compounds found in mushrooms, which hinder cancer cell growth and promote cancer cell death. Angiogenesis promoters are also secreted by fat cells to enable fat growth on the body. Mushrooms inhibit the growth of fat on the body through this same mechanism.

White, cremini, Portobello, oyster, shiitake, maitake, and reishi mushrooms all have anticancer properties. Some are anti-inflammatory; others stimulate the immune system, prevent DNA damage, slow cancer cell growth, and cause programmed cancer cell death.[28]

Mushrooms also contain aromatase inhibitors, which can limit the production of estrogen and protect breast tissue from excess estrogen stimulation.[29] Other anticancer compounds in mushrooms collectively account for their powerful effects against breast cancer. One study found that Chinese women who regularly ate about 10 grams of mushrooms a day had a 64 percent lower risk of developing breast cancer.[30]

Note that you should always cook mushrooms before you eat them because they contain small amounts of a mild toxin called *agaritine,* which is greatly reduced in the cooking process.[31]

B = BERRIES

Blueberries, strawberries, raspberries, and blackberries are true superfoods. Berries are low in sugar and high in nutrients, and their vibrant colors mean that they are full of phytochemicals and antioxidants, including flavonoids. Flavonoids affect gene expression and detoxification, inhibit cancer cell growth and proliferation, and hinder inflammation and other processes related to cancer and heart disease.[32] Notably, berries have the highest nutrient-to-calorie ratio of all fruits.

Antioxidants provide cardioprotective and anticancer effects and stimulate the body's own antioxidant enzymes. Berry consumption has been linked to reduced risks of diabetes, cancers, and cognitive decline and has been shown to improve both motor coordination and memory.[33]

Several studies have shown that high flavonoid intake lowers the risk of heart disease by up to 45 percent.[34] Flavonoids and polyphenols in berries, cherries, and pomegranates act in several ways to maintain heart health, including by reducing inflammation; by improving blood lipid, blood pressure, and blood sugar levels; and by preventing plaque formation.[35]

The antioxidants in berries, cherries, and pomegranates help to protect against cancers. In the 1980s, ellagic acid, another type of antioxidant abundant in berries, was found to block the formation of tumors, providing the initial evidence that these fruits had strong anti-cancer benefits.[36] The anticancer effects of flavonoids include reducing inflammation, preventing damage to genetic material, preventing cancer cells from multiplying, slowing the growth of cancer cells, preventing tumors from acquiring a blood supply, and stimulating the body's antioxidant enzymes.[37]

Berries are excellent foods for the brain. Substances present in blueberries can both reduce oxidative stress and improve communication between brain cells. Blueberries, strawberries, raspberries, and blackberries have all been shown to slow or reverse age-related cognitive decline in animal studies, and blueberries have now been tested for their effects on human memory.[38] Older adults with mildly impaired memory were given wild blueberry juice as a supplement, and after as few as twelve weeks, measures of learning and memory had improved.[39]

In summary, berries, cherries, and pomegranates are important components of a natural, high-nutrient diet. I recommend eating them daily to provide the body with protection against free radicals, inflammation, heart disease, and cancers. Include them as part of your variety of fruits, in addition to a bounty of vegetables, beans, nuts, and seeds, which together can provide an abundant and varied mix of antioxidants, further protecting your health.

S = SEEDS AND NUTS

Seeds and nuts are rich in a spectrum of micronutrients including phytosterols, minerals, and antioxidants. The healthy fats in seeds and nuts also aid in the absorption of micronutrients when eaten with vegetables.[40] Countless studies have demonstrated the cardiovascular benefits of nuts, and in addition they aid in weight maintenance and diabetes prevention.[41] Seeds are similar to nuts when it comes to healthy fats, minerals, and antioxidants, but seeds are also abundant in trace minerals and are generally higher in protein than nuts. Sunflower seeds are about 20 percent protein. Flaxseeds and chia and hemp seeds are also good sources of omega-3 fats, and flaxseeds, chia seeds, and sesame seeds are rich in lignans, which have strong anticancer effects.[42]

Flaxseeds are the richest source of plant lignans, having about three times the lignan content of chia seeds and eight times that of sesame seeds (note that flaxseed oil does not contain lignans because lignans bind to the fiber in the seed). Kale and broccoli also contain lignans, but only about one-tenth the amount in sesame seeds per serving.[43] Plant lignans are classified as phytoestrogens, and there has been much interest in the potential contribution of lignan-rich foods to reducing the risk of hormone-related cancers, especially breast and prostate cancers.[44]

Lignans inhibit the production of aromatase (an enzyme that converts other hormones into estrogen) and estradiol, lowering serum estrogen levels.[45] Plant lignans also blunt the effects of estrogens.[46] These benefits were documented when forty-eight postmenopausal women consumed 7.5 grams per day of ground flaxseeds for six weeks, then 15 grams for six weeks, and significant decreases in estradiol, estrone, and testosterone were noted. When you are overweight, the fat cells produce more estrogen, increasing your risk of breast cancer, so the finding that the overweight women saw the greatest lowering of estrogen from the flaxseeds demonstrates how important these seeds are to limiting breast cancer in our population.[47]

This protection against breast cancer was demonstrated in a double-blind, randomized, controlled trial of dietary flaxseed. Women daily ate either a control muffin with no flaxseeds in it or a muffin containing 25 grams of flaxseeds starting at the time of breast cancer diagnosis for just thirty-two to thirty-nine days until surgery. Tumor tissue analyzed at diagnosis and surgery demonstrated surprising benefits even in this short time. There was significant tumor cell death (apoptosis) and reduced cell proliferation in the flaxseed group in just the one month.[48] Longer trials confirm such benefits. Women with breast cancer, eating more dietary lignans (flaxseeds have the most of all foods) and followed for an average of six years, were found to have a 42 percent reduced risk of death from postmenopausal breast cancer and a dramatic (40 percent) reduction in all causes of death.[49]

One study on flax that followed a group of women with breast cancer for ten years found a 71 percent reduced risk of breast cancer–related deaths in the group that consumed the most lignans.[50] **Flaxseeds are clearly superfoods; even with a mediocre diet they offer powerful protection against breast cancer.**

The bottom line: Don't forget to eat your seeds, especially some ground flaxseeds (or chia seeds) every day. I sometimes forget to do this, too, but reviewing the science encourages me to remember. When seeds and nuts are eaten in conjunction with greens, beans, onions, mushrooms, and berries, dramatic reductions in the risk of breast and prostate cancers are possible.

MEDITERRANEAN DIET NOT SO MUCH, BUT TOMATO SAUCE IS A KEEPER

The "Mediterranean" diet typically includes tomatoes and tomato sauce and is generally higher in fruits and vegetables compared with the SAD. But it should not be considered an optimal diet because it was not carefully designed to comprehensively include the most protective anticancer foods. It also often contains white flour, oil, and too many animal products. It is a step in the right direction compared with the SAD, but too many people are touting its benefits without a complete understanding of its negative features—especially white flour products. However, its inclusion of tomatoes and tomato sauce is one of its most powerful benefits.

Tomatoes are packed with *lycopene,* which is one of six hundred *carotenoids,* and the carotenoid level in your body is an important indicator of your overall health. Your carotenoid level generally parallels the levels of other plant-derived phytochemicals circulating in your body. In a study of more than thirteen thousand American adults, low levels of total carotenoids and lycopene in the blood were linked to increased risk of death from all causes.[51] And of all the carotenoids, lycopene at low levels in the blood was the strongest predictor of premature death.

Overall, people with very low levels of carotenoids are at risk of developing autoimmune disease, headache, fatigue, and cancer.[52] Lycopene is the signature carotenoid of the tomato, and it helps protect against prostate cancer, skin cancer (in the skin, lycopene helps prevent damage from the sun's ultraviolet rays), and heart disease.[53] Many observational studies have found a connection between higher blood lycopene levels and lower risk of heart attack. One study found that low serum lycopene was associated with increased plaque in the carotid artery and a triple risk of cardiovascular events compared with higher levels.[54]

In another study, women were split into four groups according to their blood lycopene levels. Women in the top three quartiles were 50 percent less likely to have cardiovascular disease compared with the lowest quartile.[55] A 2004 analysis of the Physicians' Health Study data found a 39 percent decrease in stroke risk in men with the highest blood levels of lycopene.[56]

Lycopene is more absorbable when tomatoes are cooked—a cup of tomato sauce contains about ten times the lycopene of a cup of raw, chopped tomatoes—so enjoy a variety of both raw and cooked tomatoes in your daily diet. Of course, lycopene is not the only important nutrient in tomatoes. They are also rich in vitamins C and E, beta-carotene, and flavonol antioxidants, in addition to many others nutrients.[57] Antioxidants usually exert their protective effects in concert with each other; they work synergistically.[58]

THE YOUNGER YOU EAT BETTER, THE BETTER

By 2030, the global cancer burden is expected to nearly double, with dramatic increases in countries having low rates in the past that have now adapted to fast foods and American eating habits.[59]

For many years, evidence based on hundreds of studies has shown that the SAD promotes cancer; this is because it is high in both highly refined foods and animal products and low in colorful produce. Study after study show that eating lots of fruits and vegetables protects against cancer. It should be clear to everybody that if we want to avoid getting cancer, we should change our diets.

But wait—when looking at modern studies based on dietary patterns in adult American women, one sees that these patterns have not been so clear. The women in these studies made significant dietary improvements by cutting fat and increasing produce, yet their rates of developing cancer are only slightly reduced. What's going on here?

The reason why scientists have failed to show a radical effect on reducing cancer from including more healthy plant foods in the diet is that some of the protective effect is blunted when you incorporate these dietary modifications too late in life. Cells are most sensitive to damage when they are young; so for dietary modification to offer the most powerful anticancer effects, to mimic the very low cancer rates we see in areas of the world where people eat more produce, *these changes must be started earlier in life.*

Today's science is fascinating. It shows that the major effect of diet as a cancer promoter occurs much earlier in life than anyone has thought before. The first seven years are critical to create or prevent cancer—and we are talking about the most common cancers that generally occur after one is 50 or 60 years old.

Several cancers, especially colon cancer, are associated with obesity, but this association is still not strong. The association becomes powerful when we look at the age when a person becomes overweight. Excess body mass in early childhood is most ominous.[60]

Recent studies have confirmed the idea that most adult cancers are strongly associated with overeating and increased calorie consumption in children, but especially consumption of empty calories. Although childhood growth and early maturity have been hailed as successes of the twentieth century, the scientific data question these common parental objectives. Childhood diets with lots of milk, cheese, and meat as well as bread, oil, and sweeteners may be effective in producing big adults, but they also are extremely effective in producing sick adults who are prone to cancer.

EARLY MATURATION AND BREAST CANCER

Experimental evidence suggests that the susceptibility of mammary tissue to cancer promoters is greatest in early teenage and early adult life. The time during breast growth and development is a particularly sensitive period in a young woman's life, affecting the development of breast cancer later in adulthood.

Of particular concern is a pattern linking breast cancer to the early age of puberty we are witnessing in modern times. In the nineteenth century, the average age of puberty, as marked by the onset of menstruation, was 17 years, whereas in the past fifty years in Western industrialized countries, such as the United States, the average age of puberty is 12 years.[61] Earlier age of puberty is considered a risk factor for developing breast cancer.[62]

Endocrinologists are seeing more and more girls with precocious sexual development, even before today's average age of 12, and medical studies confirm that the trend is real and getting worse. Estrogen unquestionably stimulates the development and growth of breast cancer cells; however, it is the timing of this exposure that is most crucial and highly complicated. But one thing we know for sure is that girls who experience puberty earlier have much higher estrogen levels and maintain these significantly higher levels for many years.[63]

The heightened levels of estrogen and IGF-1 initiated by poor food choices early in life remain heightened throughout the critical years when the breast tissue is developing and most sensitive to damage. Most dangerous is the diet pattern that combines sweets and meats—in other words, a diet that results in high levels of insulin, IGF-1, and estrogen. The levels of these three hormones, which are affected by diet and body fat correlate well with the geographic distribution of breast cancer worldwide.

It is particularly important to note the most significant age range at which diet most critically affects the age of puberty. A study published in 2000 followed children since birth and reported that the girls who consumed more animal products and fewer vegetables between ages 1 and 8 were prone to early maturation and puberty, but the best predictor was an animal protein–rich diet before age 5.[64]

Fat cells produce estrogen, so excess fat on the body during childhood results in more estrogen exposure. Higher intake of calories, milk, and total animal protein has been linked to earlier puberty.[65] In contrast, a high intake of fiber-rich fruits, beans, and vegetables lowers circulating estrogen levels. Diet can powerfully modulate estrogen levels in childhood. A 2003 study illustrated that 8- to 10-year-old girls closely followed with dietary intervention for seven years dramatically lowered their estrogen levels compared with a control group without dietary modification.[66] As we get older, the opportunity to lower this risk diminishes.

This pathological early maturation of today's children is threatening. Cancer occurrence has been shown to arise many years after precancerous changes occur in the breast. Ominously, these changes are visible more and more in teenagers before their 18th birthdays.[67] The evidence is clear that breast cancer is a disease caused disproportionally by childhood and teenage eating practices.

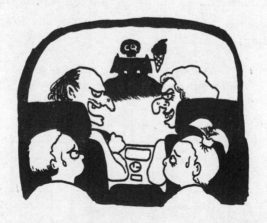

"Let's stop at "Cancer Queen" so the kids can
have one of their ice cream sundaes."

A 2013 study followed almost one hundred thousand women between the ages of 26 and 46 and found that the younger the women, the greater effect diet had on later breast cancer incidence. These researchers noted that the consumption of dairy foods and meat was best associated with the occurrence of breast cancer.[68] Prostate cancer shows the same causative relationship with early life events.[69]

This does not mean that once we have passed the age of 30 our goose is cooked. But it does mean that moderate improvements in dietary practices incorporated later in life are insufficient to drive cancer rates to very low levels. Nothing less than nutritional excellence is needed to repair the early-life DNA damage and methylation defects that accumulate throughout life from eating the SAD, resulting in higher risks of developing cancer.

The Nutritarian diet, the gold standard of dietary excellence, is specifically designed to dramatically lower cancer risk and extend life span, even in people who have not eaten very healthfully earlier in life. When consumed consistently for many years in adequate quantity and variety, phytochemicals work together to detoxify cancer-causing elements, deactivate free radicals, and enable DNA repair mechanisms.[70] Nevertheless, full protection against cancer and the full potential for human longevity can be realized only from a lifetime of healthy eating.

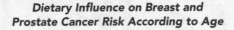

Dietary Influence on Breast and Prostate Cancer Risk According to Age

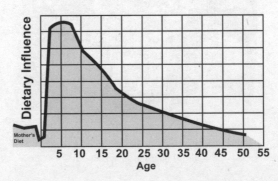

Today, new cancer diagnostic techniques are emerging, including blood tests that are able to diagnose breast cancer 10 years or more before mammograms can. Breast cells become abnormal many years—even decades—before mammograms can detect a collection of cells that are large enough to be seen by the human eye. Even at the very early stage with comparatively few abnormal cells, protein markers are shed into the blood. What these new tests are discovering is that about 40 percent of adults in the United States over the age of 40 already have cancer cells in their body.[71]

This is an important reason why the Nutritarian diet style has become so popular among Americans who are looking to repair such damage and prevent cancer. *Now* is the time to eat very healthfully—not after a cancer diagnosis. Nevertheless, the younger you begin eating well, and the earlier in the process of cancer development that you initiate an anticancer nutritional protocol, the greater the probability that a disease process or cancer can be reversed.

My philosophy of health and health care involves the underlying principle that genetics play a smaller role in the etiology of most chronic diseases than do environment and nutrition. A properly nourished body is highly resistant to infection, has natural defenses against cancer, and is naturally slim and muscular. It cannot be denied that heart disease, strokes, obesity, and even most common cancers can be avoided and prevented. However, it would most likely take embracing a healthful diet throughout life, not just after age 50, to really reduce cancer to a very rare occurrence.

I claim that nutritional excellence can:

- Prevent high blood pressure and even reverse it in the vast majority of cases

- Prevent type 2 diabetes and even reverse it in the vast majority of cases

- Prevent heart attacks and even reverse advanced heart disease in the vast majority of cases

- Prevent breast cancer, prostate cancer, and colon cancer, if adopted early enough in life, and even reverse these cancers in many cases of early cancer

- Prevent childhood cancer and autism if dietary excellence is adopted early enough before conception

- Improve the overall health, intelligence, and emotional stability and happiness of our population

The fact that these claims seem so radical speaks to how uninformed and misled our nation's people are—because these claims are not radical, nor are they outrageous. As far as the idea that these claims are too extreme—well, that just speaks to the extreme (unhealthy) nature of the SAD and the extent of people's ignorance about the critical importance of proper nutrition. When a person develops brain cancer or multiple sclerosis in his or her 30s, or a parent dies in his or her 40s of a heart attack, leaving children with only one parent or no parent at all, eating healthy to prevent such tragedies doesn't seem so extreme. It only seems extreme because the medical community thrives in a drug culture in which we are taught that drugs are our tickets to health and that the SAD is not the cause of our diseases.

The incidence of obesity and diabetes is still climbing, and it is worse among those of lower economic means and education. The number of kids diagnosed with autism is exploding. More people are developing diabetes at younger ages, and we are seeing more heart attacks and strokes in young people. This represents unacceptable human tragedy and foreshadows higher rates of cancer and dementia, as well as an even greater strain on our costly, ineffective, and inefficient health care system—including our overburdened nursing homes and hospitals. This is the genocide I am talking about. What are we waiting for?—things to get even worse?

CHILDHOOD OBESITY

Time trends since the 1980s

	PERCENT PREVALENCE		PERCENT PREVALENCE
1976–1980	5.7	2005–2006	15.4
1988–1994	10	2007–2008	16.8
1999–2000	13.9	2009–2010	16.9
2001–2002	15.4	2011–2012	16.9
2003–2004	17.1	2013–2014	17.2

Sources: Ogden CL, Carroll MD, Lawman HG, et al. Trends in obesity prevalence among children and adolescents in the United States, 1988–1994 through 2013–2014. *JAMA.* 2016;315:2292–99; *Childhood Obesity in the United States, 1976–2008: Trends and Current Racial/Ethnic, Socioeconomic, and Geographic Disparities.* Health Resources and Services Administration, Maternal and Child Health Bureau. Rockville, MD: U.S. Department of Health and Human Services, 2010.

TRUE HEALTH CARE IS SELF-CARE

Social norms, economic incentives, and the development of our pharmaceutical-centered approach to chronic disease have encouraged the masses to transfer responsibility for their health to doctors, and to equate health care with medical care. When we absolve ourselves of personal responsibility for our health, and accept the myth that diet doesn't matter and genes dictate our health future, we lay the groundwork for health tragedies.

The historical rise of a pharmaceutical-based system of health care, instead of one that is based on lifestyle medicine, has been a foundational deficit in our health care system that can never be improved by politicians or governmental regulations. Our present drug-centered health care system has contributed to the large segments of our population who are committing slow suicide with fast foods.

Things might begin to change if hospitals become protective enclaves where not merely smoking is prohibited, but also eating junk food and all foods that include white flour, salt, and oil. This would be a huge change from the current climate, in which hospitals install fast food restaurants on their premises, have fast food kiosks in their lobbies, and serve the likes of pancakes with syrup and white bread to their patients. If all physicians, health care workers, and health authorities in the United States were lean, were very healthy eaters, and advocated healthy living and eating, a trickle-down effect would reinforce the message of the dangers of commercially baked goods, fast foods, fried foods, processed meats, and commercially raised animal products.

There is movement in this direction. The American College of Lifestyle Medicine is a physician-specialty organization, with a rapidly growing membership, that puts lifestyle and nutritional medicine first. Its members generally talk the talk, and walk the walk. Defined: "Lifestyle Medicine involves the therapeutic use of lifestyle, such as a predominately whole food, plant-based diet, exercise, stress management, tobacco and alcohol cessation, and other non-drug modalities, to prevent, treat,

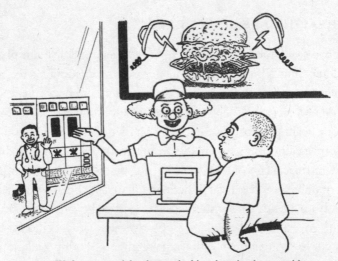

"We have a special today on the big whopping burger with bacon-macaroni and cheese. It comes with a free ride to the hospital!"

and, more importantly, reverse the lifestyle-related, chronic disease that's all too prevalent."[72]

This sensible approach, with doctor as teacher and motivator for healthier habits rather than merely prescriber of medication and doer of procedures, is not "alternative medicine" or "holistic medicine"; rather, it is *progressive medicine*. It is where medicine should have gone—and would have gone—if the financial incentives and political and economic power of the pharmaceutical industry were not so massive and influential. All physicians should receive extensive training in lifestyle medicine and nutritional science, and nutritional healing should be heavily embraced in medical schools and residency programs. This is a critical skill set that is missing in the training of health care professionals. The medical profession should have incorporated it years ago, and should embrace it today.

Doctors should not smoke. They should not drink alcohol; they should not drink soda; they should not eat fast food or junk food. They should be pillars of health in our communities, and they should fight for healthy habits among their patients and in their communities.

You do not have to follow my nutritional advice—that is up to you. My mission is not dependent on what you do, but I am committed to making sure that you, and others, know that you don't have to be sick: You can live a better, happier life without the fear of heart attacks, strokes, dementia, and even cancer. I hope that becomes your future.

CHAPTER FOUR

THE LESSONS OF HISTORY

Not ignorance, but ignorance of ignorance, is the death of knowledge.

—ALFRED NORTH WHITEHEAD

Our society is a reflection of the foods we eat. This isn't a new concept. In fact, history has shown us this truth with frightening accuracy. That's why the pages that follow are as much a history lesson as they are a discussion of nutrition and health. I've included the examples you're about to read because they reveal the ways in which our society has suffered from nutritional deficiency in the past, and why it is so crucial that we change this for the future. I hope that the information in this chapter will lead you to greater understanding of and compassion for those people who are most affected by poor nutritional options, and will serve as a rallying cry for positive change. We cannot let the discoveries of nutritional science and what they reveal about the causes of death and disease remain a conversation "for another time." The time is now. As you'll see, the mistakes of history have carried over into our current reality.

THE TRAGEDY OF PELLAGRA

More than one hundred years ago, extreme violence plagued the South, especially against former slaves from the end of the Civil War. For example, the Freedmen's Bureau has a register of more than a thousand murders from 1865 to 1866 in Texas, mostly against former slaves.[1] After the war, racist groups emerged, such as the Ku Klux Klan, the White League, and the Knights of the White Camelia, which aimed to assassinate or intimidate African Americans and the white officials who tried to help them assimilate after they were freed from slavery. Such groups also used violence to prevent black people from voting. Violence was the way some tried to restore a system of white supremacy that was disrupted by the end of slavery.

Coinciding with this increased violence was an increase in cases of a nutrition-based disease called *pellagra*. And while it may seem peculiar in this context to mention pellagra, this now rare illness played a significant role in the postemancipation era. Pellagra is caused by niacin deficiency and was epidemic in the South. It could cause a form of dementia that made some people chronically depressed and angry and others impulsively violent.

Science ultimately traced the cause of pellagra to the Southern diet at that time. But because of sheer indifference and ignorance, local doctors chose to overlook the obvious connection between unhealthy diet, pellagra, impaired brain function, and violent behavior. Of course, this nutritional deficiency was certainly not the sole cause of violence and hate crimes, but there is no question now that there is a link between the foods people ate and the behaviors that ensued. And the severe and dangerous problems exacerbated by poor nutrition continued needlessly for decades. All the while, a vital lesson about the importance of nutrition was ignored.

Despite being a disease most Americans have never heard of, pellagra created a famous American stereotype. It had four distinct symptoms known as the four Ds: dermatitis, diarrhea, dementia, and death.[2] The dermatitis caused areas of the skin exposed to the sun to turn a bright red; one of the etymologies of the term "redneck" is that it referred to poor white people with this condition. Europeans called the rash a Casal necklace, after Gaspar Casal, who first described the disease in 1762. "Pellagra" comes from the Italian phrase *pelle agra,* meaning sour skin.

The Southern diet, which was rich in corn, flour, and sweeteners, traces its origins to slavery. Volumes have been written on this subject, but none has recognized the fascinating role these calorie-dense, low-nutrient foods played in shaping mind sets—and our nation's history. A diet lacking in fresh produce, specifically dark leafy greens rich in vitamins and nutrients, has the power to alter our physical state and mental faculties in such a way as to change the way we behave. We now know that poor nutrition can create violence, magnify racism and bigotry, and increase tensions between various populations of the world. It did in the past, and it continues to do so today.

A NUTRITIONAL DIFFERENCE

In the nineteenth century, African Americans, on average, died at a younger age compared with poor whites. However, this was not true of all blacks everywhere. Despite high infant mortality rates, a significant percentage of blacks outlived their poor white neighbors. Some enjoyed advantages that translated into superior physical health and optimal brain function.

Todd Savitt, a medical historian, examined Virginia mortality records in four counties and found that more blacks than whites died of old age between 1853 and 1860 and according to an 1850 census, there were more centenarians among blacks.[3] The same trend, according to Savitt, existed throughout the South.

Many historians have suggested that slaves received superior medical care because they were considered to be financial investments. However, this implies healing powers beyond those of nineteenth-century doctors, as medicine in those days was primitive and could not account for the kinds of differences observed in the mortality records. Even today, doctors cannot replicate those outcomes through medical means. A better explanation for this enormous health discrepancy and the longer life spans of slaves is not the deliberate effort by slaveowners or the skill of Southern doctors, but is the nutritional advantage of many slaves' diet compared with the diet of poor whites.

Southern agriculture focused on producing cotton and tobacco; feeding people was an afterthought. Most Southerners ate lots of corn products, because it was cheap and easily grown. It took hundreds of years, and the suffering of many, before modern science discovered that corn is deficient in niacin. Most poor Southern whites ate primarily corn, cornbread, pork fatbacks (like bacon), and molasses-flavored sweets. This resulted in insufficiencies in multiple vitamins and minerals, much like the fast food diet people eat today. But we no longer see cases of pellagra because we now have niacin-enriched junk food.

The diet of slaves living on plantations was different from that of poor whites, in many cases because they were permitted to grow their own food. By the mid-seventeenth century in Virginia, for instance, many slaves were growing kale, cabbages, mustard leaves, black-eyed peas (cowpeas), gourds, okra, spinach, squash, watercress, watermelon, yams, corn, pumpkins, and peanuts.[4] These foods fed slaves and plantation families and were not made available to those who didn't live on the plantation. The resulting health and life span of slaves who ate a healthier diet is a great example of a truth scientists have known for decades: Health and life span can be extended by packing in more micronutrients and more micronutrient diversity. During the late nineteenth and early twentieth centuries, there were no refined fast foods with concentrated calories to induce overeating and obesity. However, all the healthy vegetables and beans were not valued throughout the South.

In the 1930s, during the Great Depression, the Works Progress Administration employed writers through the Federal Writers' Project to produce a written history of the lives of slaves before the opportunity was lost. They fanned out across seventeen states, mostly in the South, to interview twenty-two hundred former slaves. Firsthand testimony revealed that slave diets varied from plantation to plantation. One former slave from South Carolina said that slaves ate potatoes, rice, corn pone, hominy, fried meat, molasses, a whole-wheat by-product called "shorts," turnips, collards, and string beans. The white plantation owners ate the white flour, leaving the bran, germ, and whole wheat for the slaves. A former Mississippi slave added: "We always had plenty of something to eat. Meat, cornbread, milk and vegetables of all kinds. The garden was made for the colored, and the whites together, so each person didn't have to worry with making one for hisself."[5]

In the years following the Civil War during Reconstruction, the federal government established the Bureau of Refugees, Freedmen, and Abandoned Lands, known as the Freedman's Bureau, to assist newly emancipated slaves in their transition to freedom. Over the five-year period from 1865 to 1870, the bureau established more than four thousand schools for blacks, employing nine thousand teachers and giving instruction to about a quarter of a million pupils of all ages. The thirst for knowledge of the newly freed community and their children was unquenchable. African Americans went on to sustain more than thirteen hundred schools; they built five hundred school buildings and made donations out of their own earnings to do so and pay teachers and further the cause of their children's education.[6] Unfortunately, an inaccurate vision of newly freed slaves as uneducated and helpless sharecroppers was perpetuated for many decades. On the contrary, many former slaves and their offspring, empowered by a nutritional advantage, embraced education and actively pursued the American dream.

Schools sprang up throughout the South, and literacy rates among African Americans soared, from an estimated 5 percent to 10 percent under slavery to 70 percent in 1910.[7] Among black people born after 1860, literacy rates were substantially higher. A significant number of freed slaves obtained college degrees, and a black middle class emerged.

The rise of the black middle class after slavery was a cause for great concern to many who felt threatened by this emergence. Ray Stannard Baker, an American journalist and historian born in 1870, was considered a muckraker because he exposed political corruption. He observed firsthand the surprising ascent of African Americans:

The eagerness of the coloured people for a chance to send their children to school is something astonishing and pathetic. They will submit to all sorts of inconveniences in order that their children may get an education. One day I visited the mill neighborhood of Atlanta to see how the poorer classes of white people lived. I found one very comfortable home occupied by a family of mill employees. They hired a Negro woman to cook for them, and while they sent their children to the mill to work, the cook sent her children to school![8]

Baker further reported that a Senator Thomas of the Alabama legislature stated that "he would oppose any bills that would compel Negroes to educate their children, for it had come to his knowledge that Negroes would give the clothing off their backs to send their children to school, while too often the white man, secure in his supremacy, would be indifferent to his duty."[9]

Not only did African Americans embrace education, they also embraced capitalism and employed the skills they learned as slaves—only now, they could profit from those skills. As Booker T. Washington described it: "If a Southern white man wanted a house built, he consulted a Negro mechanic about the plan and about the actual building of the structure. If he wanted a suit of clothes made he went to a Negro tailor, and for shoes he went to a shoemaker of the same race."[10] On plantations young black men and women were constantly being trained not only as farmers, but as carpenters, blacksmiths, wheelwrights, brick masons, engineers, cooks, laundresses, sewing women, and housekeepers.[11]

A VIOLENT BACKLASH

The efforts of African Americans to educate themselves was a direct threat to white supremacy. According to historian Leon Litwack, the response to black ambition was swift. Some whites employed terror, intimidation, and violence in response to black success because such success was unacceptable to a people who deemed themselves racially superior.[12] As W. E. B. Du Bois put it, "There was one thing that the white South feared more than Negro dishonesty, ignorance and incompetency, and that was Negro honesty, knowledge, and efficiency."[13]

For many poor Southern whites, the rise of an African American middle class was too much to bear. James Kimble Vardaman (1861–1930), a Mississippi governor and U.S. senator, famously stated, "If it is necessary every Negro in the state will be lynched; it will be done to maintain white supremacy."[14] He was not referring to criminals.

This emerging black middle class in the midst of a racially segregated and profoundly bigoted society speaks to an African American population of smart, industrious, and fearless individuals who were embracing their newfound freedoms in profound ways that were shifting the culture. And one rarely discussed aspect of this great charge forward was that African Americans were living with a nutritional advantage. As mentioned, African Americans were in general eating a more varied diet with vegetables, resulting in lower chance of pellagra and giving them adequate nutrition to aid these necessary and great steps forward.

And without question and as expected, this rapid development threatened the social status of whites, many of whom suffered nutrient deficiencies in their basic diets. Rather than working to elevate everyone, Southern authorities enacted Jim Crow laws, which suppressed African American advancement and segregated their housing, schooling, and access to public places. It institutionalized the basis for white supremacy. Jim Crow laws were America's version of South African apartheid, keeping blacks separated from whites and prescribing how they were to behave.

White supremacy and Jim Crow laws were established to diminish the status of African Americans, even if it meant resorting to violence and suppressing educational opportunity for all. In 1896, the U.S. Supreme Court decision in *Plessy v. Ferguson* introduced the doctrine of "separate but equal" and made Jim Crow practices the law of the land. The effect of the *Plessy* ruling was immediate. There were already significant differences in funding for the segregated school system, which continued into the twentieth century; states consistently underfunded black schools, providing them with substandard buildings, textbooks, and supplies. States that had successfully integrated elements of their society abruptly adopted oppressive legislation that erased Reconstruction-era efforts at reform. Jim Crow practices were encouraged and spread to the North in response to a second wave of African American migration from the South to Northern and Midwestern cities that started around 1941.

Jim Crow laws and white supremacy were motivated by racist ideologies and by competition over jobs and economic opportunities. In a 1965 speech following the Selma to Montgomery March, Dr. Martin Luther King Jr. explained how Jim Crow manipulated blacks and poor whites alike:

You see, it was a simple thing to keep the poor white masses working for near-starvation wages in the years that followed the Civil War. Why, if the poor white plantation or mill worker became dissatisfied with his low wages, the plantation or mill owner would merely threaten to fire him and hire former Negro slaves and pay him even less. Thus, the southern wage level was kept almost unbearably low.

. . . the southern aristocracy began immediately to engineer this development of a segregated society. . . . If it may be said of the slavery era that the white man took the world and gave the Negro Jesus, then it may be said of the Reconstruction era that the southern aristocracy took the world and gave the poor white man Jim Crow. He gave him Jim Crow. And when his wrinkled stomach cried out for the food that his empty pockets could not provide, he ate Jim Crow, a psychological bird that told him that no matter how bad off he was, at least he was a white man, better than the black man. And he ate Jim Crow. And when his undernourished children cried out for the necessities that his low wages could not provide, he showed them the Jim Crow signs on the buses and in the stores, on the streets and in the public buildings. And his children, too, learned to feed upon Jim Crow, their last outpost of psychological oblivion.[15]

By the turn of the twentieth century socially promoted white violence against blacks had become common throughout the South, and it coincided with a rampant epidemic of pellagra, which we have seen can make people more aggressive, confused, and eventually demented. Southern authorities turned a blind eye toward or tolerated the violence, and Southern doctors rejected the possibility that the violence might be intensified by a disease.

In 1902, a Georgia farmer became the first American diagnosed with pellagra, which by 1912 was epidemic in the South. He had suffered for fifteen years before his diagnosis. Each spring when the weather warmed, blisters erupted on his arms and legs, and he became severely depressed and suicidal. By 1912, in South Carolina alone, thirty thousand cases were recorded, with twelve thousand deaths. Three million

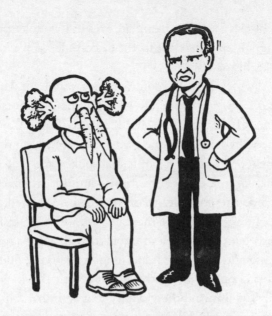

"In my professional opinion, you are not eating correctly."

cases were recorded in the early twentieth century in the South, but this greatly underestimates the problem, because it is thought that only one in six people suffering from the disease sought out a physician.[16] It was not a new disease; by the time medical authorities detected it in the United States, it had been a recognized epidemic in Eastern and Southern Europe for nearly two hundred years.

Pellagra, which is mostly caused by a lack of niacin in the diet, was a result of what is called the "3M diet," meaning meal (that is, cornmeal mush), meat (mostly pork fat), and molasses. White flour was not "enriched" with B vitamins and niacin until the 1940s. In the Southern United States many poor whites relied on this diet. Angry white supremacists were not all poor or hungry; they were also wealthy landowners and community leaders. But pellagra-affected males were already primed by the rampant racism and heightened tensions in the South. It is no wonder that the increased aggression the disease can cause led them to join angry and violence-prone social groups and networks directing their anger against blacks. Far from being an excuse for violent crimes and murders, pellagra is an important factor to consider as we look back at this time in U.S. history.

Most U.S. doctors refused to consider the psychological implications of pellagra and viewed it as merely a skin ailment. A notable exception, James Woods Babcock (1856–1922), a native South Carolinian and Harvard-trained physician, was one of the only American doctors who appreciated the scope of this epidemic. Babcock noted that "apparently healthy persons commit crimes of various kinds for which they cannot be rightly regarded responsible, according to the accepted views as to culpability because they are not mentally sound."[17] He examined old medical records back to 1828 and concluded that pellagra had been continuously present, undetected, and ubiquitous in the South.[18]

While most people will rightly disagree with Babcock's assertion about culpability, racism and the violence that went hand in hand with it should never be excused. Racist crimes shattered lives and tore the fabric of this country. But we should not dismiss or ignore the ways in which nutritional deficiency has real and lasting effects on individuals and society. To ignore nutrition is to ignore a critical aspect of how we function in the world. We must not make this same mistake again.

A nineteenth-century French psychiatrist, Henri Legrand du Saulle, was one of the first doctors to draw attention to pellagra's criminal implications. He described how the disease could result in acts of violence, including homicide and suicide. He noted how people afflicted with this disease "commit the most reprehensible acts, and this is the most convincing proof of [their] insanity."[19] Many other European physicians echoed Legrand du Saulle's findings. Unfortunately, according to Henry Fauntleroy Harris, a physician from Georgia, U.S. doctors mostly ignored the connection between pellagra and violence and generally ignored the European reports. Harris noted that throughout the South, people "plagued with a multitude of both physical and mental ailments, were often driven to acts of violence and even homicide."[20]

As one early-twentieth-century writer noted, "Pellagra is a universal scourge which attacks all races and has millions of victims; which provokes crimes, insanity, and suicide; and fills our prisons and asylums."[21] Pellagra affected the character of the South. Research has demonstrated that areas with higher levels of the disease also had higher rates of violence and social dysfunction.[22]

There is no way to prove that specific acts of violence that happened more than one hundred years ago were the result of pellagra or nutritional deficiencies. The important issue here is that a time of extreme violence coincided with the presence of a disease that made people more violent and when deficiencies of niacin and other nutrients were rampant.

A nutrient-deficient, corn-based diet creates a constellation of problems. It impairs serotonin function, a neurotransmitter needed for emotional stability.[23] Corn is deficient in omega-3 fatty acids and niacin. Omega-3 DHA and vitamin D also control the synthesis of serotonin. Researchers who discovered this relationship explain that "serotonin plays an important role in inhibiting impulsive aggression toward self, including suicide, and aggression toward others." These researchers also noted that "experimentally lowering brain serotonin levels in normal people has a wide range of behavioral consequences: impulsive behavior, impaired learning and memory, poor long-term planning, inability to resist short-term gratification, and social behavioral deficits characterized by impulse aggression or lack of altruism."[24] Studies also show that low serotonin combined with high testosterone leads to increased aggressiveness.[25]

The ideology of white supremacy created a catastrophe. It empowered people with low status and nutrient-deficient dysfunctional brains to be violent toward African Americans. A constellation of mild nutritional deficiencies, even without full-blown pellagra, still affects emotional stability. Subclinical pellagra can also create mental symptoms and induce anger, even without a skin rash. Despite our increased understanding of the relationships between diet and brain chemistry, and brain chemistry and behavior, we still fail to acknowledge how inferior diets can help to create dysfunctional communities today.

I'd like to take a step back here and talk about how this example from history relates to the experiences we have with nutrition in our world today. It's hard to believe that diet can play a role in how we treat one another, that it can escalate our prejudices and amplify our belief systems, that it can even lead to murder and violence. The prevalence of pellagra in the American South is a devastating example of a moment in time when the accepted diet in the area made matters much worse. While good, nutritious food isn't a cure for racism, bigotry, misogyny, or any other prejudice, and while nutrient-deficient food isn't an excuse for prejudice, it is a powerful driver that affects how we interact with one another. You'll learn more about this in the next chapter, but it's important that I make this clear now: Pellagra may not be around today, but we have new nutritional disasters amplifying tragic issues in our lives.

PERVASIVE INDIFFERENCE AND DENIAL

Because of Southern indifference, outsiders from the North eventually set up research facilities to find a cure for pellagra. In 1912, the New York Post-Graduate Medical School and Hospital established the Thompson-McFadden Pellagra Commission based in the South. The school chose Joseph F. Siler, a physician with the Army Medical Corps, and Philip E. Garrison, a Navy surgeon, to head the commission. The following year, Dr. Charles Davenport (1866–1944), a Harvard-trained biologist from the Eugenics Record Office in Cold Spring Harbor, New York, joined the commission to study pellagra from the viewpoint of heredity.

Eugenics has been called a form of scientific racism because eugenicists encouraged selective breeding to improve the human race. Davenport was a eugenicist who opposed the idea that poor nutrition or disease could affect brain function. He did not join the commission out of a concern for the poor. Instead, the existence of a disease like pellagra threatened the very foundations of eugenics; that is, the idea that violence could be caused by a bad diet would reduce the idea of being superior to simply being better fed.

The Pellagra Commission surveyed more than five thousand people and found no relationship between diet and the occurrence of the disease.[26] In 1914, the U.S. Public Health Service Hygienic Laboratory, which would become the NIH, started a competing commission on pellagra to find a cure. The U.S. surgeon general appointed Dr. C. H. Lavinder to lead the government commission.

By 1914, the Thompson-McFadden Commission concluded that pellagra was likely an infectious, insect-borne illness. In the same year, Lavinder was replaced by Joseph Goldberger, a trained researcher and medical pioneer from New York City.

Goldberger advocated for the poor and tested solutions. He visited places where the disease was most prevalent: orphanages, asylums, and prisons. In these institutional settings, only the orphans, patients, or inmates got sick with pellagra; workers were rarely affected. The disease was not contagious; he noted that the only difference between the two groups was what the workers ate—their diet was not as restricted as that of the orphans and inmates. Goldberger suspected that some essential missing factor in corn caused the disease. In the fall of 1914, Goldberger supplemented the diets at three institutions: two Mississippi orphanages and a Georgia state sanitarium.

By the following spring, of the 172 cases in the orphanages, only one recurred; no new cases developed. In the sanitarium, all 72 cases in the test group were cured. Pellagra recurred in half of the control group. This was proof enough for Goldberger, who concluded that a balanced diet cured pellagra. In his 1915 annual report, Goldberger wrote that a change in diet cured all of the children and made them healthier than ever before: "There can be no doubt that the cause of pellagra is dietary."[27] After Goldberger published his results, Siler and Garrison both resigned from the Pellagra Commission, leaving Davenport in charge.

For the next six years, Goldberger continued to conduct experiments and tried to persuade the authorities to take action. In 1921, he wrote the U.S. surgeon general describing how poverty and a poor diet led to pellagra. President Warren G. Harding responded by urging the Red Cross to provide aid and suggested that Congress make a special appropriation to address the problem. But this offended politicians throughout the South.[28] One remarked that news reports of "famine and plague" were "utter absurdity."[29] Southern leaders were not interested in curing pellagra.

The United Daughters of the Confederacy, who voted at first to thank the president, ended up sending him a letter of protest a month later. Southern leaders not only rejected the president's offer, but also rejected the idea that people in the South were suffering from the effects of poverty or malnutrition. For his part, James Babcock, the one doctor who had described the connection between pellagra and crime, was fired in 1914 by the South Carolina legislature for, among other things, having "caused injury to the reputation and progress of South Carolina by calling attention to the prevalence of pellagra in that state."[30]

Most people today have no knowledge of pellagra or Goldberger's efforts to combat this disease. The entire episode was swept under the rug. Goldberger spent the rest of his life trying in vain to persuade the medical community of his findings. He died unheralded in 1929. Eight years later, in 1937, Conrad Elvehjem discovered nicotinic acid, or niacin, a B vitamin—the missing factor in corn. By then, the pellagra epidemic had largely subsided because of the Depression and public feeding programs.

THE BIRTH OF A LIE: EUGENICS

The indifference of Southern politicians to this horrible ailment was in part due to the efforts of Charles Davenport, who rejected the idea that human differences were linked to nutritional differences. He advocated an alternative ideology that continues to dominate our thinking to this day. Davenport was one of the leaders of eugenics in the United States. This ideology was first conceived in 1863 by British mathematician Sir Francis Galton, the half-cousin of Charles Darwin. Galton assumed that observed differences in humans were the result of heredity. He believed that healthy offspring could be produced only if healthy and talented people married other healthy and talented people. Eugenics, from the Greek meaning "well-born," was based on the premise that humanity could be perfected through better breeding; it was part religion and part science. Nutrition did not enter into the eugenics equation.

Violence in the South did not go unnoticed; it in fact inspired the American eugenics movement. The deteriorated physical and mental condition of nutrient-deficient Southerners was well-known. Many nineteenth-century travelers and writers observed the high prevalence of nutritional illness in the South, describing white skin, rashes, a sunken chest, and a sinister countenance; many people lived in squalor, with a high incidence of insanity, epilepsy, and tuberculosis as well as pellagra.[31]

In 1916, one year after Goldberger reported that pellagra was a nutritional disease, Davenport perpetrated his greatest crime: He published an article in the *Archives of Internal Medicine* on the hereditary causes of pellagra.[32] Davenport presented detailed tables and pedigree trees to establish his view that pellagra was a hereditary disease.

Davenport's paper was readily embraced because of its length, scientific complexity, and "authoritative" tone. But the different standards of medical education in those days did not require that physicians question the report's veracity. Davenport persuaded the medical community that pellagra and all of the social problems it caused were not the result of bad diet, but of bad genes. It confirmed that people who didn't have this disease were superior. It was precisely the lie that most people wanted to hear.

Not everyone was swayed by Davenport. Some of his methods were so flawed that even his fellow eugenicists criticized him. His methods had been questioned before: In 1913 and 1914, members of the Galton Eugenics Laboratory in England, including Karl Pearson and David Heron, published a response to an earlier paper critical of Davenport's methods and of his organization, the Eugenics Record Office.[33] Heron noted that Davenport had essentially falsified data in order to support his claims. Pearson believed that Davenport's deception would cause eugenics to be discredited. But it had precisely the opposite effect, at least in the short term.

Pellagra was an unpopular disease shunned by doctors, politicians, and eugenicists. Eugenics shifted scientific focus away from the study of nutrition, instead advocating remedies of violence, sterilization, and segregation. Even the idea of extermination was floated as an acceptable means of "keeping up the standard of the race."[34] Eugenics, which was the alternative hypothesis for diseases like pellagra, took the place of nutritional wisdom.

A NEAT, PLAUSIBLE, AND WRONG SOLUTION

H. L. Mencken said "There is always a well-known solution to every human problem—neat, plausible, and wrong." The assumption that all human problems resulted from heredity led to the belief that all human problems could be solved by eliminating the people with the problems. This is flawed logic of the so-called eugenics solution. The popularity of eugenics in the early twentieth century was a direct consequence of a failure to learn from the medical examples of pellagra, hookworm, and iodine deficiencies. In a real sense, we are all victims of Charles Davenport's deception, which would have global consequences. By promising racial superiority, eugenics lured many prominent Americans, such as Madison Grant, a lawyer, conservationist, and religious postmillennialist. Grant helped preserve the California redwoods and the American bison; he founded the Bronx Zoo, fought for strict gun control, built the Bronx River Parkway, helped to create Glacier and Denali National Parks, and worked tirelessly to protect whales, bald eagles, and pronghorn antelopes—all while advocating for the sterilization of humans.

In 1916, Grant published *The Passing of the Great Race,* an international best seller that influenced a generation of scientists, academicians, and businesspeople. In it, Grant presents the eugenic solution to all the world's problems:

Those who read these pages will feel that there is little hope for humanity, but the remedy has been found, and can be quickly and mercifully applied. A rigid system of selection through the elimination of those who are weak and unfit—in other words, social failures—would solve the whole question in a century, as well as enable us to get rid of the undesirables who crowd our jails, hospitals, and insane asylums. The individual himself can be nourished, educated and protected by the community during his lifetime, but the state through sterilization must see to it that his line stops with him or else future generations will be cursed with an ever-increasing load of victims of misguided sentimentalism.

This is a practical, merciful and inevitable solution of the whole problem and can be applied to an ever-widening circle of social discards, beginning always with the criminal, the diseased and the insane and extending gradually to types which may be called weaklings rather than defectives and perhaps ultimately to worthless race types.[35]

Grant was referring to poor whites from the American South and Eastern Europe who filled U.S. prisons and insane asylums—80 percent of whom were later found to have pellagra. Around this same time, Davenport's assistant at the Eugenics Record Office, Harry H. Laughlin, began lobbying for eugenics laws. He developed model legislation for compulsory sterilization and immigration restrictions based on eugenics "science." A group of Virginians devised a plan to enact Laughlin's law, launching a preemptive "friendly suit" that would ultimately end up in the U.S. Supreme Court. This lawsuit sought to preempt future challenges by deliberately compromising the rights of Carrie Buck, a young mother who gave birth to a daughter after being raped by a relative of her foster family. To avoid prosecution, the family placed her in the Virginia Colony for Epileptics and the Feebleminded, whose superintendent, Albert Priddy, advocated for the sterilization of the "feebleminded." Priddy previously had been sued for forcibly sterilizing patients against their will.

Priddy eventually persuaded the Virginia legislature to pass the 1924 Sterilization Act, which empowered the state to legally sterilize its citizens on the basis of a finding of feeblemindedness. A confederate of Priddy immediately filed suit on Buck's behalf contesting the state's right to perform involuntary sterilizations. In the course of the litigation, Priddy died. His successor, John Hendren Bell, was named in the suit. Buck's lawyer, who was also her guardian, was in cahoots with the state. He deliberately lost and appealed the case in order to get a higher court to affirm the lower court ruling. His goal was to preempt someone else from effectively challenging the law. The case finally reached the U.S. Supreme Court in 1927.

Laughlin wrote a scientific analysis of Carrie Buck for the court, concluding that Buck and her mother "belong to the shiftless, ignorant and worthless class of anti-social whites of the South.... The evidence points strongly toward the feeblemindedness and moral delinquency of Carrie Buck being due, primarily, to inheritance and not to environment."[36] Justice Oliver Wendell Holmes Jr., in writing for the court, opined that "it is better for all the world, if instead of waiting to execute degenerate offspring for crime, or to let them starve for their imbecility, society can prevent those who are manifestly unfit from continuing their kind."[37]

The 1927 Supreme Court decision in *Buck v. Bell* made eugenics the law of the land. Thirty-three states ultimately adopted eugenics laws. California applied the law most vigorously, conducting the most prodigious number of involuntary sterilizations. Sixty thousand Americans would be forcibly sterilized; the vast majority were white. About one-third of the sterilizations were carried out in California. It was the beginning of what would soon become a global catastrophe.

Three years earlier, in 1924, a young Adolf Hitler was inspired by the German translation of Madison Grant's manifesto—a book he would later call his "Bible." Hitler's Nazi Party seized power in 1933 and modeled its Nuremberg Laws after California's eugenics code. The California sterilization efforts further inspired the Nazis and their Final Solution. In 1934 E. S. Gosney, founder of the Human Betterment Foundation to support compulsory sterilization, received a letter from C. M. Goethe, a prominent California eugenicist visiting Germany, that said:

You will be interested to know that your work has played a powerful part in shaping the opinions of the intellectuals behind Hitler in this epoch-making program. Everywhere I sensed that their opinions have been tremendously stimulated by American thought, and particularly by the work of the Human Betterment Foundation. I want you, my dear friend, to carry this thought with you for the rest of your life that you have really jolted into action a great government of 60 million people.[38]

The Nazis sterilized an estimated four hundred thousand people. A Virginian eugenicist complained that "they are beating us at our own game."[39] Nazis would ultimately exterminate five and a half million people under the guise of eugenic science and launch a world war whose impact continues to haunt us to this day.

At the military tribunals at Nuremberg after the war, Major General Karl Brandt, who was Hitler's personal physician, was charged with heinous crimes relating to the slaughter of the Jews during the Holocaust. In his defense, Brandt's lawyers introduced into evidence a copy of Madison Grant's book. During the trial, Nazis also quoted Oliver Wendell Holmes's opinion in *Buck v. Bell* in which he had stated, "Three generations of imbeciles are enough."

The scope of Hitler's crimes cannot be overstated. Yet the Nazi Party also seemed to be aware of things that were actively hidden from the American public. They understood that nutrition matters. The Nazis didn't just profess to be the master race; they sought to actively achieve it by implementing the most progressive public feeding programs the world has ever seen. The Nazis collaborated closely with U.S. scientists, including Davenport, who held editorial positions at two influential German journals. They banned everything that was unhealthy, including carcinogens such as asbestos and food dyes. They established policies that promoted healthful food while opposing excessive fat, sugar, and alcohol in the diet and a sedentary lifestyle. Otto Flössner, a nutritional physiologist at the Reich Health Office, believed that a whole food diet complemented racial hygiene.[40]

Nazi researchers suggested that improper dietary habits led to an increased risk of cancer decades before scientists in the United States reached the same conclusion. They encouraged consumption of fresh fruit, vegetables, and whole grain bread as well as the avoidance of meat-derived fat.[41] A 1930s Hitler Youth manual titled *Health Through Proper Eating* discussed the dangers of empty calories and championed legumes such as soybeans as a healthier alternative to meat. In 1939, Hitler invaded Poland, launched the Holocaust, and started a world war.

This is a surprising and mostly untold story of the role of nutrition in the lead-up to this tragic historical moment. It is also a warning about allowing "facts" to remain unquestioned. The contradictory arguments made by the Nazis were not the first or the last time that science and fake science have been used to promote evil.

As we move closer to the present day, we will see the ways in which technology seemed to displace some of the gains made in nutritional science. The war came home to U.S. soil in many ways.

THE MILITARY LAUNCH THE FAST FOOD INDUSTRY

A generation after World War II, in the 1960s, crime rates exploded in the United States. Nowhere was this catastrophe felt more than in African American communities. The war had transformed the country economically, socially, and physically. It created the longest economic boom in U.S. history, which turned the country into a global superpower. The G.I. Bill enabled millions of vets to get a college education; in 1947 G.I.s made up 47 percent of college enrollments. G.I. benefits also helped returning vets to buy new homes, farms, and businesses. The war elevated the entire nation. In 1949, the desegregation of the military had launched the civil rights movement. However, what was perhaps the most significant change was also the least recognized: World War II fundamentally altered how Americans ate.

While the Nazis were advancing nutritional science, American scientists were operating under the faulty premise that nutritional adequacy could be achieved by chemical means. Medical experts at the turn of the twentieth century had failed to learn from the pellagra outbreak. The general presumption that all calories are created equal perpetuated the flawed conclusion that people are not created equal. By simply recognizing how poor nutrition leads to chronic illness and impairs human brain function, we could have avoided many tragic and lasting consequences.

Two years after Hitler invaded Poland, Japan launched an attack on Pearl Harbor on December 7, 1941, and pulled the United States into the global conflict. In response, the country transformed its industry into the greatest war machine this planet has ever seen. The military needed weapons and a way to feed troops in far-flung parts of the globe. Feeding an army on foreign soil is an age-old challenge. A frustrated Napoleon Bonaparte once said, "An army marches on its stomach." In 1795, the French Army offered 12,000 francs to the first person who could invent a new way to preserve food. Fifteen years later Nicolas Appert presented his idea for canning food, using the same basic process in practice today.

The Hormel Company introduced canned Spam (short for shoulder of pork and ham) in 1937. It seemed like the perfect military food solution. By the end of the war, the U.S. military had purchased more than 150 million pounds of Spam, and it had quickly become a staple in cuisines around the world, especially in the Pacific region. In addition, products such as M&Ms, Tootsie Rolls, and instant coffee, designed to feed U.S. soldiers, became staples of the American diet. The military required nonperishable foods that soldiers could carry onto the battlefield. Veterans who ate these foods during the war desired more after the war. Candy bars, commercial baked sweets, such as Twinkies and Devil Dogs, and fast food chains such as McDonald's sprang up and profited from this demand.

At the same time, American diets improved briefly during the Depression and World War II because of farm-to-table programs and meat rationing, which led to an increased consumption of vegetables. However, by failing to learn from the mistakes of the past, Americans created the modern U.S. diet and became victims of their own success and ingenuity. Like a diet predominant in corn, bacon, and molasses leading to subclinical pellagra, a diet dominated by processed and fast foods increases physical, psychological, and intellectual problems and creates the illusion of genetic inferiority. Presently, impoverished communities, both urban and rural, have less access to fresh foods and are more acutely affected by these nutrition-related issues.

The year 1945 brought an end to the war and a big stockpile of ammonium nitrate, which had been used to make explosives during the war. But ammonium nitrate doesn't just make bombs explode; it also makes certain crops grow faster. The government wanted to turn the war machine into an instrument of peace, so U.S. Department of Agriculture officials had a good idea: Turn the main ingredient of explosives into a fertilizer. Furthermore, nerve gases, which worked as well on insects as on people, became pesticides. The remnants of war were modified and dispersed into the U.S. agricultural system. As the Indian environmental activist Vandana Shiva points out, "We're still eating the leftovers of World War II."[42]

Ammonium nitrate as a fertilizer works best on corn. This ingredient of explosive bombs during the war led to an explosion of corn production after the war. Enterprising people found creative ways to make use of the surplus corn, and ranchers began feeding it as a primary food to livestock. These days, corn-fed livestock is deceptively referred to as "conventionally fed." Such conventionally fed cattle grow significantly faster compared with grass-fed cattle, but they are also profoundly unhealthy. A corn-fed cow loses its natural immune function, so to reduce its risk of developing bacterial infections, ranchers mix high doses of antibiotics into its food.

Corn-fed beef is chemically different from grass-fed beef; for instance, it has significantly lower levels of omega-3 DHA. Raising cattle on corn dramatically lowered the cost of beef; more cattle can be raised on less land and in less time. Government farm subsidies for growing corn further aided the development of cheap meat, leading directly to the explosion of fast food restaurants and a dramatic rise in the consumption of DHA-deficient meat. And as we have seen, people who consume processed foods, fast foods, and excessive amounts of conventional meat will tend to have very low levels of DHA. A global survey revealed that Americans have extremely low levels of omega-3 DHA and EPA in their bloodstreams,[43] and this directly affects serotonin function and resulting crime rates.

US Meat Consumption Per Person 1900–2012[44]

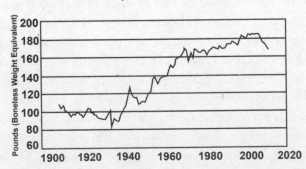

Another new use for corn came out of the postwar Japanese Agency of Industrial Science and Technology (AIST), which was founded in 1952 to redirect Japan's military scientists toward civilian research. In 1971, an AIST scientist, Yoshiyuki Takasaki, patented high-fructose corn syrup (HFCS), which ended up being a bomb that landed on the American public. HFCS is produced by using an enzyme from bacteria to break down cornstarch. After World War II, corn became the most abundant food on the planet; most of it is now consumed by Americans, who are also the largest consumers of HFCS. Today, the average American consumes 60 pounds of corn syrup every year, and the percentage of Americans with diabetes has grown with this increased consumption.[45] Policymakers focus almost exclusively on the short-term consequences of unhealthy diets, while generally ignoring the long-term effects, such as diabetes.

SHELF-STABLE, CONCENTRATED, PORTABLE, AND ADDICTIVE

Industrializing the food industry and feeding the Allied troops were massive undertakings during World War II. After the war, the military established a policy of military preparedness that promoted food technology. The U.S. military actively shaped the SAD to ensure a population that could be ready at a moment's notice to produce army rations or to create consumer products that met military standards. Modern commercial foods were created by the military so we could effectively wage war. The technology to make these foods was then handed over to the food industry, and the basic ingredients were made cheaply so these foods became widely available and consumed in large quantities. The primary purpose of fast food was first developed to energize military personnel on the battlefield, not to maximize long-term health.

Energy bars, canned goods, deli meats, and even goldfish crackers all have military origins. In her 2015 book *Combat-Ready Kitchen: How the U.S. Military Shapes the Way You Eat,* Anastacia Marx de Salcedo describes how many of the packaged, processed foods we find in today's supermarkets started out as science experiments in an army laboratory. Many modern processed foods can be traced back to the Natick Soldier

Systems Center, a U.S. Army research complex in Natick, Massachusetts. This federal laboratory investigates how to improve the taste and shelf life of soldiers' rations. The processed cheese now found in the likes of goldfish crackers and Cheetos is just one of the ingredients that was developed at Natick. The center is also behind longer-lasting loaves of bread and the energy bar, which are designed to be sources of quick energy. It is the policy of the military to get the science that it uses for rations into the public food supply. It is part of a broader policy to ensure a powerful industrial base as the foundation of national defense preparedness.

World War II changed how Americans ate. People became accustomed to highly flavored, processed foods with long shelf lives. In 1943, the War Food Administration enacted Order Number 1, which mandated the enrichment of all bread. The order would be repealed in 1946 after the war, but the enrichment of bread continued. Vitamin enrichment masks long-term problems, as it replaces a select amount of lost nutrients, ignoring hundreds more. Modern nutritional science has

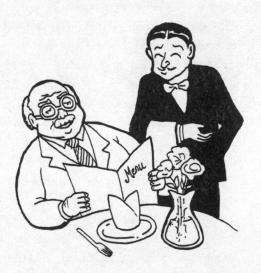

"I'd like the large high fructose corn syrup liquid with added phosphoric acid, caffeine, salt, and artificial caramel coloring and a side of deep fried potato batter with corn syrup emulsifiers, MSG and yellow dye #4."

uncovered hundreds of complex compounds (called *phytochemicals* or *phytonutrients*) in natural plants that humans need which are not vitamins and minerals, and not all of them have yet been identified.

The government is subsidizing the very foods that are destroying us because of our failure to learn from the nutritional mistakes of the past. The simple truth is that people require a broad assortment of colorful plants in conjunction with exposure to DHA-containing (wild) animal products, to maximize overall health and brain health. And for those few nutrients not sufficiently available in plants, specifically vitamin B12 and DHA, supplements are available today.

The food industry creates an astonishing array of foods from a tiny group of plant species. Today, only four crops—corn, soybeans, wheat, and rice——account for two-thirds of all calories humans eat. Add those calories to the heightened consumption of commercially produced animal products in the United States and it is clear we have crowded out fruits, vegetables, nuts, and seeds from our nation's plates. Since World War II, meat, dairy, and processed food products have become increasingly available, and the nutrient diversity of our diet has shrunk.

We now have more food than ever and yet nutritionally, the SAD is astonishingly reminiscent of the Southern 3M diet of molasses, meat, and (corn)meal, which led to the pellagra epidemic. Food fortification efforts have eliminated such acute nutritional deficiencies and their associated diseases (for instance pellagra, rickets, and beriberi), but those efforts have also led to life-shortening, chronic health problems such as obesity, diabetes, and mental illness. The incidence of psychotic dementia has been overshadowed by ADHD, other learning difficulties, subclinical aggressiveness, and reduced impulse control.

Despite the growth of nutritional science, the physical and emotional health of Americans suffers greatly. The low cost, appeal, and profitability of packaged and fast foods have led to the expansion of the consumption of those foods. Many contributory influences confound this problem, including, as we have seen, the addictive nature of processed foods and the appeal of using drugs for medical problems instead of changing the dietary habits that cause chronic disease.

CHANGE CAN HAPPEN

Leaded gasoline caused a catastrophe in recent history that is similar to the one being caused by fast food today. In the 1920s, petroleum companies added tetraethyl lead, a known toxin, to gasoline to increase the octane level, enabling cars to run more efficiently. The economic boom following the war dramatically increased the number of cars on the road, and all of those cars were fueled by leaded gasoline. But studies show that the use of leaded gasoline caused brain damage that affected behavior and learning capacity.[46] People in densely populated urban areas were subjected to concentrated dosages because of traffic congestion and the canyons created by high-rise buildings. This disproportionately affected poor people with already poor nutritional status. People who are deficient in iron will also metabolize more lead.

The rise of lead in the atmosphere is associated with an increase in violent crime rates, just as the drop in atmospheric lead was followed by

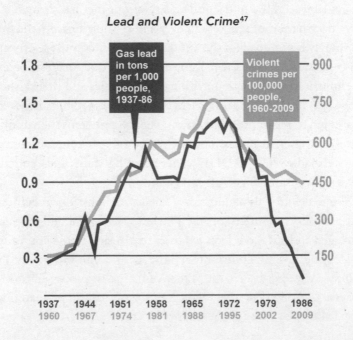

Lead and Violent Crime[47]

a similar drop in the violent crime rate. The removal of lead from gasoline and paint was one of the most successful public health initiatives of the twentieth century. Antioxidants from fresh fruits and vegetables also reduce the toxic effects of lead.

The government was slow to act on evidence suggesting that lead contamination was a significant problem because it thought the solution was impractical. But this was not the case. According to studies cited in a 1989 paper published in the *World Health Statistics Quarterly*, the benefits of eliminating leaded gasoline outweighed the costs 10 to 1. The authors concluded with the following bit of wisdom: "The environmental health calamity caused by lead in petrol could have been avoided if the initial warnings had been heeded and better preliminary research of the health issues had been carried out. Nevertheless, incontrovertible proof of causality should not be required before regulations are made to protect public health."[48]

Research evidence, although not conclusive, suggested that lead pollution caused violence. Lead was removed from gasoline, and violent crime rates dropped. However, crime rates did not drop to pre-1960 levels because the lead problem coincided with a dietary problem. A similar problem has occurred from the use of soft drinks, fast food, and junk food. This has been made worse by the rapid increase of not just HFCS-sweetened soft drinks, but also the tremendous increase in oil consumption. Oil is an empty-calorie junk food; in other words, it supplies a huge load of concentrated calories but no micronutrients or fiber. The excess of omega-6 fats in oils also increases omega-3 insufficiency.

There is no easy fix to the health problems created by the SAD. Policymakers consistently make decisions that favor the commercial food industry over public health, and the food and drug industry have tremendous influence in Washington, D.C., that slows and inhibits change for the better. Nutritional mistakes made by health authorities have also taken their toll. For instance, in 1961, the American Heart Association advised Americans to reduce their intake of saturated fats by replacing animal fats, such as butter, with vegetable oils, shortening, and margarine.[49] People replaced one dangerous food with another. Soybean oil

Consumption of Soybean Oil[50]

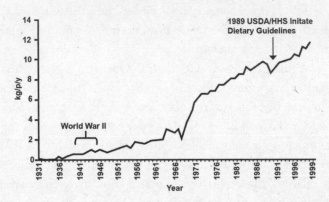

became the primary source of fat for most Americans. Government subsidies made it a cost-effective ingredient for cost-conscious makers of processed foods. Vegetable and seed oils, such as soybean oil, are generally very high in omega-6 linoleic acid and low in omega-3 ALA.

The rise in crime also directly corresponded to the rise in the consumption of linoleic acid, and this has had an effect that we have yet to address. The sharp rise in linoleic acid consumption from increased use of food oils also directly correlates with the rise in murder rates that began in the 1960s.[51] This problem has been studied and systematically ignored, reminiscent of the problem that occurred with lead. The CARDIA (Coronary Artery Risk Development in Young Adults) epidemiological study of four thousand subjects found that people with lower tissue levels of omega-3 fatty acids were more hostile.[52] Oily, processed, and fast foods are rich in omega-6 linoleic acid and low in omega-3 fats. And the more omega-6 fat consumed, the more omega-3 fats are needed and the more the formation of the brain-protective omega-3 fats is inhibited. Another study found that greater intakes of seafood rich in EPA and DHA were correlated with lower rates of homicide mortality across thirty-six countries.[53] Young developing brains across the United States are suffering multiple nutritional stresses simultaneously.

LEARNING FROM THE PAST

The status quo resists change. Remember, there was huge opposition to the claims that smoking cigarettes was harmful. Some people will never consider evidence to be conclusive. It can't be denied that nutrient deficiencies create immediate effects that can destroy human potential. Low-nutrient diets stress the brain and influence decision-making by impairing brain metabolism. In the past, and today more than ever, society's greatest problems of poverty, violence, criminal behavior, drug abuse, and devastating health tragedies have their roots in the diet style of the population under duress.

Unhealthy eating feeds inequality, bigotry, racism, and intolerance. Today, we know that modern dietary practices cause much human tragedy and affect society on every level—from autism, to childhood cancer, to learning difficulties, to medical dependence and premature death, and yes, to drug addiction and crime. It is time to end this tragedy.

CHAPTER FIVE

DNA, SOCIAL ENERGY, AND FAST FOOD

In a real sense all life is interrelated. All men are caught in an inescapable network of mutuality, tied in a single garment of destiny. Whatever affects one directly, affects all indirectly. I can never be what I ought to be until you are what you ought to be, and you can never be what you ought to be until I am what I ought to be. . . . This is the inter-related structure of reality.

—MARTIN LUTHER KING JR.

Transforming the health of the nation will require a multifaceted effort. Our genes are programmed to protect us and allow us to flourish. These protections are hard-wired and yet unfortunately can be completely undermined by our unnatural, processed food diet. And this is exactly what is happening. In addition, humans are social creatures, and we are learning more and more about how our interactions affect our decisions and behaviors. In the following pages, we explore the vicious cycle that shows how the wrong food choices undermine our genetic tendencies and behaviors and in turn make it that much more difficult for us to break away from bad dietary and social choices. Understanding the complexities of these issues is the first step in creating the necessary change.

Be forewarned, the consequences of fast food consumption may be more ominous on our children and grandchildren. Evidence is accumulating that an unhealthful diet, excess body weight, and especially overeating protein create adverse consequences that are imprinted on genes and passed on to future generations.[1] For instance, researchers examined the grandchildren of people born in Överkalix parish in northernmost Sweden where few plant crops grow. They also examined historical records of harvests, food prices, and other data to determine food availability. The main crops grown in this subarctic region are barley and oats, which were used primarily as animal feed. In 1905, residents ate lots of meat because they did not have access to imported fruits and vegetables. After years of good harvests, when food was abundant, they ate more meat; after periods when food was scarce, meat consumption declined.

Amazingly, the diet had health effects on three generations. Researchers compared people who had lived through periods when there was an overabundance of meat with those who lived through periods when food was scarce. They found that people who ate lots of meat in their childhoods produced children and grandchildren who were significantly more likely to develop cardiovascular disease as adults. Likewise, meat-deprived grandparents had grandchildren who lived considerably longer. Those people who ate the most meat produced children and grandchildren whose life spans were cut decades short.

The lives of these people were not shortened by junk food, but by genes that were altered by the excessive consumption of animal proteins. They passed those genetic alterations (called *epigenetic modification*) on to their offspring and their offspring's offspring. At first glance, it doesn't make sense that children whose grandparents had better access to food would have their lives cut short, while those whose grandparents struggled to get enough would live longer. It doesn't make sense until you view it from the perspective of systems, which enables us to see how the parts of a system fit together to form a whole.

Predators and their prey coexist in a circle of interdependence; what happens to one, affects the other. Nature allots a certain amount of each prey to each predator because if predators ate too many of their prey, they would exhaust their food supply and could eat themselves and their prey into extinction. The size of predator populations are closely linked to the population size of their prey. For instance, the number of Canadian lynxes in a given area is directly related to the number of hares. Canadian lynxes exist in a subarctic environment where there are few other prey species. They eat snowshoe hare and little else. Snowshoe hare cope with the seasonal absence of vegetation by eating bark, which enables them to survive harsh northern winters. Every ten years, the population of snowshoe hare explodes, which always follows a period of decline of the lynx.[2] This decline of the lynx always occurs after a period of plenty caused by increased populations of the hare.

By examining a large number of these relationships, researchers found that if a predator eats more than its allotment, its life is shortened from excess consumption.[3] When too many hares are consumed, too few will remain to replenish their numbers; that is, there are fewer prey animals (hares) to produce offspring when too many are eaten. Nature protects against extinction. Too much protein changes the DNA of the predators, and their lives and the lives of their young are shortened, which in turn curtails the eating of more hares in the future, assuring that enough hares survive into the future.

The lynx population doesn't immediately recover; the reduced life span remains lower for two generations, which gives the hare population a chance to replenish itself. If the lynxes recovered too quickly, they would prevent the hares from replenishing their numbers. They could eat themselves into extinction. The altered expression of lynx genes caused by the excessive consumption of snowshoe hare is passed on to the lynx's offspring and their offspring's young, resulting in the shortened life spans. This example shows that nature maintains ecological equilibrium by diet-induced DNA changes that alter the expression of predator DNA in response to how much food the predator eats. This evidence for the evolutionarily conserved nature of protein-mediated longevity is extremely strong, ranging from invertebrates to humans.[4]

Natural law is enforced within the DNA of the predator. It penalizes the individual and its offspring so that it may ensure the survival of the collective. This same law applies to other mammals, including humans. When too much is available to eat, many people will simply eat too much. We don't normally see ourselves as predators because we buy our meat neatly packaged from the grocery store. However, if we eat meat, we are predators; our genes don't care where the meat comes from. Excessive meat consumption shortens human life span, too. And that shortened life span may be passed on to future generations.

Proponents of the Paleo diet are seemingly unaware of the complexity and depth of the supportive evidence. They mistakenly believe that humans will be healthier if they eat more meat because they believe that's what Paleolithic humans ate and Paleolithic humans were healthier than people are today. However, analysis of Paleolithic skeletons has shown that few people at that time survived beyond middle age.[5] In certain regions and periods when Paleolithic humans did become apex predators, eating hunted animals for most of their calories, evidence suggests that they usually died young. Of course, early humans ate what was available to eat in their local habitats and did not have one type of diet, but certainly their diet was not scientifically formulated to maximize longevity, and they ate merely to survive and reproduce.

Today's science has uncovered more about the fascinating relationship between overconsumption of meat and shorter life span. We now know that IGF-1 production increases as we consume more animal protein and this, in turn, also shortens life spans in humans.[6] Plant-eaters produce far less IGF-1 and are not subject to this life-shortening form of predatory control. We know from credible studies that as we eat more plants and fewer animal products, lifespan increases in length.[7]

These studies become more trustworthy and important because they include thousands of individuals followed for multiple decades, and they use the hard endpoint of death. And, as shown in the scientific studies cited in Chapter 3, plant phytochemicals do the opposite: They slow aging, strengthen immune function, and protect against cancer. Methylation damage to our DNA, which can promote aging and cancer, is cumulative and exacerbated by eating too many animal products and too much fast food.[8] Further, this meat-heavy dietary approach inhibits the consumption of natural, colorful plants rich in phytochemicals necessary for optimal health.

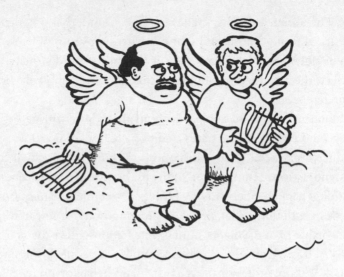

"I said to Dr. Fuhrman, I'd rather be dead than eat vegetables,
but that was before I found out there was no food at all up here."

We are a long way from fully understanding how DNA works. Nevertheless, it is becoming increasingly obvious that DNA not only makes life possible for individuals but also preserves and safeguards life for future generations in order to protect the species. People who seek to maintain good health later in life, while consuming large amounts of meat, are waging an unwinnable battle. Those who shift from a junk food diet rich in sweets and processed carbohydrates to a meat-based diet in midlife may see some health improvements—not because meat is inherently healthy, but because junk food is fundamentally worse. The benefits of such diets are short-lived, and ultimately life span is unfavorably affected.

OUR GENETIC MATERIAL IS DYNAMICALLY MODIFIED BY ENVIRONMENT AND SOCIAL INTERACTIONS

Positive social energy promotes good health. **Social energy** is a form of power derived from interaction with others. It is an invisible force that grows from encouraging social interactions that connect us to one another.[9] Even though we can't measure it directly, we can measure its effects. The absence of this vital energy is an underlying contributor to obesity, chronic disease, and many hard-to-explain problems. Social energy is not some New Age concept but rather an identifiable force that affects the activity of genes responsible for governing behavior and food preference.

The term *social status* applied to humans conjures images of social privilege and elitism. Social status traditionally implies position, wealth, and education. Social energy, in contrast, is built by goodwill toward others and action. Humans get status by harnessing social energy to make things happen. Social energy enables us to build organizations, start businesses, and build social circles. A growing body of research reveals how favorable or unfavorable human interactions affect the activity of our DNA. It is why more socially accomplished people live longer.

Mark Wilson, professor of psychiatry and behavioral science at the Emory University School of Medicine, has studied the connection between social interactions, behavior, and gene activity, which are all surprisingly linked to nutrition. The way we eat determines how we interact with each other and vice versa. Wilson not only revealed how this process works, but he also showed how the presence of unnatural foods corrupts the natural order and leads to behavioral mayhem.

Social hierarchy in the animal world is purposeful. It performs an essential function that ensures the survival of entire species by systematically allocating limited resources to those responsible for producing offspring. Consequently, high-status animals pursue healthy resources, while low-status animals are biologically programmed to stay out of their way, even if it means going hungry. We live in a world where resources are sometimes limited. In the absence of an efficient means of allocating resources, life, as we know it, would have vanished long ago. If all animals competed for food equally when food was scarce, there would not be enough for any single mating pair to produce healthy offspring.

Wilson and his colleagues taught a group of monkeys how to eat junk food.[10] They then housed the monkeys together in a shared environment until a social hierarchy formed. The researchers provided unlimited access to healthy monkey chow and also to high-calorie junk food. Two types of monkeys emerged out of this study: One type spent significant amounts of time socializing with and grooming other monkeys, and the second type continued to be isolated even though they were surrounded by others. Not only did each type exhibit different social behaviors; each behaved differently with food. The high-status monkeys, which exerted more social energy, only occasionally dabbled in the unhealthy fare. They consumed a predominantly high-nutrient diet and instinctively regulated their caloric intake, even in the presence of unhealthy options. In sharp contrast, the subordinated, low-status monkeys ceased to consume healthy foods and dined exclusively on junk. They lost their ability to regulate their caloric intake and became compulsive binge eaters. However, they didn't do so openly; they waited until late at night to eat after the other monkeys went to sleep. High-status monkeys managed their stress by engaging in social interactions. The low-status monkeys under the added stress of hierarchical subordination managed theirs by self-medicating with low-nutrient, high-calorie foods. They ultimately became obese.

In a second study conducted on well-fed monkeys, Wilson and his team found they were able to manipulate status by moving monkeys from one group to another and train them to improve their behavior and social status. These researchers were able to show that manipulating social hierarchy could actually alter the expression of genes that regulated social interactions and food preferences.[11] The activated genes resulted in better immune function and better health, and those primates that obtained better social positions were simply less likely to become addicted to junk food.

OUR PRIMATE-WIRED BRAINS

Humans also have genetically driven behaviors that can be modulated by our environment. Social energy is determined by how others treat us. Like monkeys, we are more likely to behave impulsively and prefer junk food when socially deprived. Furthermore, socially accepted people with a close circle of friends live longer than those who are lonely.[12]

The longest-lived, healthiest people in the world share some common traits; among them is having good relationships with other people. The Australian Longitudinal Study of Aging showed that people with good social relationships were 22 percent less likely to die during the following decade.[13] Close contact with just children and relatives had little effect on survival; those people with the strongest network of friends and acquaintances were the most likely to live the longest.

The portfolio of studies examining this question corroborate the data: Positive social interactions with other people in our communities improves health and lengthens life span.[14] Likewise, people who think of themselves as victims or feel routinely rejected have a significantly increased risk of chronic disease and are more likely to become depressed and obese.[15] Social rejection causes depression to set in faster than other forms of adversity. Depressed people then instinctively seek out unhealthy foods and are more likely to gain weight as a result.[16]

Scientists studying primates find the same outcome. As we have seen, monkeys with higher social status receive more attention, are more social, and therefore eat a superior diet, resulting in superior immune function. Furthermore, the aforementioned experiments have demonstrated that low-status animals and animals under the stress of dominance by higher-status animals may become biologically wired to eat alone. When exposed to unnatural, unhealthy, artificially flavored Frankenfoods, they become addicted easily, avoid nutritious foods, and remain socially isolated.

Low status in the animal kingdom is not a mark of physical inferiority, nor is it a permanent condition. Primate research has demonstrated that low-status monkeys that do not socialize do not require as much nutrition as their sexually active peers. In the wild, low-status monkeys would be calorie-restricted and thin. Caloric restriction is well-established and shown to slow the aging process and extend longevity.[17] Wild primates eating less food do not have worse health or survival compared with their better-fed peers, though they may be less able to produce offspring. However, this situational behavioral pattern can spontaneously change. Low-status animals are like reservists in the military who can be called into active duty when needed. A sudden increase in the availability of nutritional resources, or the death of a high-status peer, represents an opportunity to ascend. As Wilson's research team observed, a change in status led to a change in the expression of genes that altered behavior, diet, and immune function.

In the animal kingdom, low-status animals ascend when the opportunity presents itself. Nature guards the health of both high-status and low-status individuals by providing various and overlapping ways of maintaining health and life span. Eating a nutritious diet extends life, as long as too much animal protein is not eaten; however, not only does eating fewer calories and less animal protein extend life, so does eating less frequently (intermittent fasting), thus preserving the health and life span of the lower-status animals.[18]

Unlike wild animals that use social function as a means of survival, humans exploit social hierarchies for personal gain. Our species has unwittingly created large numbers of disenfranchised individuals who have been thrust into a dangerous food environment, and the unintended consequence is fast food genocide.

BRAIN FUNCTION AND IMMUNE FUNCTION ARE INTERTWINED

Status differences can become biological differences. The emerging field of human social genomics studies this phenomenon. Researchers Gene Slavich and Steven Cole of UCLA point out that our genome appears to encode a wide variety of "potential biological selves," and which "biological self" gets realized depends on the social conditions we experience over the course of our lives.[19] Cole identified socially activated genes in humans that regulate immune function. People with high social energy have strong anti-inflammatory immune responses that are absent in those with low status.

The immune system benefits greatly from plant phytochemicals and intermittent fasting. Low-status animals in the wild normally consume micronutrient-dense, calorie-restricted diets, so they do not suffer from chronic inflammation, as do low-status humans. In sharp contrast, lonely people or people with primarily negative social interactions in Western countries consume too many low-nutrient calories (fast food), which transforms a mildly compromised immune response into chronic inflammation and very serious illnesses. Being low status or not having positive social connections does not make wild animals innately more susceptible to pathogens. We humans do that to ourselves by eating unhealthy foods.

Negative social energy diminishes brain function in both monkeys and people. Social energy empowers us to rise above our circumstances by enabling us to increase our status and purpose. We create this energy by being altruistic and compassionate, conversing with others, and helping others. People with this type of social energy are more likely to be healthy, accomplish things, and be financially secure because they are not satisfied with just getting by or maintaining the status quo. A favorable social environment and adequate nutritional intake are the primary determinants of higher socioeconomic potential in life.

Taste preferences and eating behavior can be manipulated and are excellent barometers of self-esteem and connectivity to others. A study has shown that socially isolated people with poor self-esteem and people exposed to toxic social environments are more likely to prefer high-fat, sugary, and salty foods that are low in fiber. People who were the least educated were found to have the strongest dislike for fruits and vegetables.[20] Young children exposed to adverse social circumstances develop unhealthy food preferences long before they are old enough to use money or have gotten an education. Exposure to fast food determined these preferences and did so at an age that can destroy their educational opportunity.

We can surround our children with positive social energy; we can teach the importance of eating nutritionally superior foods. Undoubtedly, favorable social energy and the importance of eating nutrient-rich foods can be taught, and children given the opportunity to learn communication skills and good nutrition have greater opportunity for happiness and success in life.[21]

In modern human populations, low social status predisposes a person to seek out unhealthy processed foods, which fundamentally can alter that person's character as well as lead to diabetes, obesity, chronic depression, and anger. The pervasive availability of these foods tips the balance and transforms low social status into a disease that affects entire communities. In our modern fast food world, children raised in socially oppressed homes, who may not have role models for correct expression of social energy, are further damaged by their disease-promoting food environment; this affects their genes and their brains, and as they age, they lose the will to climb out of the oppression they have experienced.

SOCIAL ABILITY AFFECTS GENE ACTIVITY IN HUMANS

For years, scientists operated under the erroneous assumption that the "law of the jungle" prescribed survival of the fittest and that genes determined traits independent of other factors. This idea originated from the Darwinian premise that some genes were better than others. Such concepts created an unprincipled view of the world that treated excessiveness, brutality, and selfishness as natural consequences of being superior. The idea that gene expression can be altered challenges many deeply held beliefs. Scientists dating back to Charles Davenport have viewed genes simplistically as unchanging containers of heredity that define individual traits independent of all other influences. However, scientists now know that genes operate in ways that are far more complex. Areas of human DNA that were previously thought of as "junk DNA" are now known to be important software that can direct cell function. These small areas of our DNA can be turned on or off and dramatically affect the expression and function of genes and in turn other biological functions.

Social environments influence the biological expression of genes throughout the body and in specific regions of the brain.[22] Compassion and acceptance create positive social energy that has favorable biological effects. Favorable human interaction alters chemicals at the cellular level, resulting in beneficial effects on behavior, food choices, and health outcomes. Humans increase their likelihood of survival by cooperating and collaborating with other humans. Our adaptable DNA "software" also enables our cells to adjust to environmental changes, but this can be positive or negative depending on both social environment and nutritional exposure.

The discovery that core traits are determined by socially regulated genes challenges some of our most basic assumptions about people. Food choices, food quality, food diversity, and food availability all interact with social forces and human-to-human interactions to affect our behavior and health. These discoveries should have fundamentally altered how we think about problems of crime, poverty, and chronic disease, but because of our ignorance, we search for solutions in all the wrong places. Author Thomas Kuhn explains why important discoveries such as this often go unnoticed. He notes that scientific advances occur in a "series of peaceful interludes punctuated by intellectually violent revolutions"; in each revolution, "one conceptual world view is replaced by another."[23] Breakthrough discoveries in science are rare because even the brightest minds are often reticent to embrace new ideas that violate accepted worldviews. Max Planck, who won the Nobel Prize for Physics in 1918, once said, "A new scientific truth does not triumph by convincing its opponents and making them see the light, but rather because its opponents eventually die, and a new generation grows up that is familiar with it."[24] Though it's not easy, we must be willing to change our beliefs in light of new information.

Our DNA responds to changes in the environment and to the food we consume; however, it doesn't do so randomly. Chronic disease and poverty do not generally result from inferior genes or DNA malfunction. Rather, these are predictable responses to negative social and dietary influences that can spread like an infectious epidemic throughout a community. When humans individually or collectively experience increased psychological stresses, their genes are affected and their stress-eating behaviors and addictive tendencies are enhanced.

As discussed, species' genetic makeup can react to stabilize the survival of interrelated species when food is plentiful and when it is scarce. However, DNA was not designed to operate in the presence of fast food or junk food in the midst of a toxic social environment. Obesity does not occur in the wild. Like any device, our DNA will not operate as intended when its environment is abused.

Hundreds of years ago, the leading causes of death were infectious diseases and malnutrition. Today, in developed countries, most people die from conditions that arise because of overeating a low-nutrient diet. The ubiquitous presence of unhealthy foods transforms entire populations, creating negative physical and social symptoms with global consequences.

Teaching and practicing empathy, compassion, and goodwill toward all, especially those who are different from our social "gang," is an important goal of health education and is also important for a shrinking earth with a growing population that is straining our limited resources. Compassion benefits us personally and collectively. We know from a growing number of studies that people who are more hostile and uncompassionate often have a reduced ability to control food intake.[25] They are also more likely to indulge in snacks, fast food, and alcohol consumption.

In clinical studies, people with eating disorders are routinely shown to be anxiety-prone, pessimistic, immature, irresponsible, hostile, and vengeful.[26] The connection between diet and personality is not a random convergence. Specific eating patterns and social situations have very specific effects on behavior and perceptions. These effects from eating nutritionally compromised fast food are linked to specific compounds and structures in the brain that make people more apathetic, lonely, compulsive, and aggressive. Fast food exposure can unravel the very social fabric that holds us all together.

It doesn't matter which comes first—social oppression, social isolation, or dangerous eating. This human-created vicious cycle of fast food and social stress creates a downward spiral of increasingly injured individuals and populations.

We must strive to understand the interaction between the social environment, our genes, and fast food. Fast food is not just altering our future health, but weakening us genetically and magnifying this damage in a frightening way in future generations. This means more unintended consequences for our children and grandchildren. This issue demands serious attention by our nation's population, including the media, health professionals, nonprofit organizations, and politicians.

CONUNDRUMS OF HUMAN ACHIEVEMENT

Diet and social status have been intertwined in ways that are not immediately obvious. As we saw in Chapter 4, in the years following the Civil War, nutritional deficiencies from a corn-based diet made Southerners more violent. However, this by itself did not explain the systematic violence directed at the upwardly mobile, black middle class that followed—a tragedy that historians have struggled to explain. According to scholars, deliberate acts of mass violence always involve conducive environments, destructive leaders, and susceptible followers.[27] Unmet needs and a negative social environment make people susceptible to committing such acts.

At the close of the Civil War, poor white people in the South did not have good food, educational opportunities, or hope for a better future. Southern leaders responded by doubling down on the idea of white supremacy. This in turn gave the illusion of status to otherwise low-status people. In the animal kingdom, socially disconnected individuals stay to themselves. In sharp contrast, in human social circles socially disconnected people can sometimes rise to authoritative positions while displaying and utilizing contempt, bullying, and arrogance.

Antisocial behavior starts in childhood; school-aged bullies oppress nearly six million school children every year.[28] Bullies seek status and empower themselves at the expense of others, whereas the most popular kids acquire status by engaging in more favorable cross-gender interactions.[29] Research indicates that children who engage in friendships with a mixture of males and females in their peer groups lack the desire to bully others. Research confirms that these bully-resistant kids are more empathetic and more socially perceptive.[30] They can effectively interact with children outside of their immediate social circles; this is the essence of social energy. But what is more fascinating is that this enhanced social energy leads to healthier eating habits, while bullying is strongly associated with unhealthy diets.[31] It works both ways: Good nutrition leads to a healthy brain, which results in proper social functioning; but poor social functioning can make people susceptible to the attraction of addictive eating and poor nutrition.

Without positive social energy, effective dietary change becomes very difficult. Most Americans have a choice about what they eat, but in many impoverished communities around the country people simply don't have a choice because healthy food options are not available.

Regional opportunity and outcomes vary not just in the United States, but worldwide. The Global School-Based Student Health Survey (GSHS) carried out among middle school students in nineteen low- or middle-income countries showed that the prevalence of bullying ranged from 7.8 percent in Tajikistan to 60.9 percent in Zambia.[32] These rates mirrored the broader levels of violence in each of these cultures, which suggests one or more common causes. According to the United Nations Office on Drugs and Crime, the intentional homicide rate in Tajikistan in 2011 was 1.6 per 100,000; in Zambia in 2012 it was 10.7, or nearly seven times higher.[33] The diets of people in Zambia and Tajikistan are very different. The Tajikistan diet consists of a variety of foods, including carrots, turnips, apricots, melons, and dried fruit.[34] According to the United Nations Food and Agriculture Organization, Zambians subsist predominantly on maize, a kind of corn.[35]

Unhealthy diets adversely affect all of our social relationships, including those between parents and children, and poor social relationships affect the quality of our diets. Parents are supposed to lead their children gently into adulthood by teaching them how to relate to, appreciate, and care for other people. However, social divisiveness and poor nutrition have weakened the potential of human culture for peace and happiness.

Researchers compared the interactions of middle-class parents and their children with those of lower-class families.[36] Their interaction styles differed dramatically. In comparison to lower-class mothers, middle-class mothers were less controlling, less disapproving, and more informative. Middle-class mothers told their children what they were doing right, while lower-class mothers told their children what they were doing wrong. Researchers found that the better the diet and the more the family ate healthfully, the better the children were raised. Studies also reveal that low-income families are less likely to eat together,[37] which is relevant when you consider that researchers have found that eating together as a family makes children more resilient.[38] Once again, we see how the cycle of social energy and diet can work to either improve quality of life or lead to increased suffering. Unfortunately, if nothing is done to change things, poverty will continue to perpetuate poverty.

We have seen how World War II altered how people around the globe ate. Besides leading to the rise of fast food restaurants, the war also contributed to an increase in the number of women working outside of the home and this trend continued in the 1960s and 1970s. The family meal became another casualty that researchers say led to a number of problems, including the deterioration of diet quality, especially among the young, an increase in eating disorders, and a decline in family relationships.[39] The family meal is an opportunity for positive social contact. Fewer family meals translates into increased antisocial behavior outside the home. For example, problematic school behaviors, early sexual activity, risk of suicide, and increased alcohol and drug consumption have been associated with kids eating alone.[40] Other research reveals that families of gang members are less likely to eat together and are less likely to express positive feelings toward one another.[41]

A twenty-year study using data collected from the European Prospective Investigation into Cancer and Nutrition (EPIC) found that social isolation radically affected food choices and health outcomes of adults too.[42] People who ate alone ate fewer fruits and vegetables and were more likely to be lonely. Loneliness shortens life span, promotes obesity and diabetes, and impairs neurogenesis, the ability of the brain to grow and repair itself.[43] It reduces a person's desire to eat healthy foods or to connect socially. Such people then become drawn to unhealthy foods and negative influences, which further alters brain structures, making people compulsive, insensitive, and aggressive.

Americans are more alone than ever.[44] One-third have no contact with those living near them. Today, poor people of all races are increasingly concentrated in high poverty areas with less access to social resources, which is creating an environment for catastrophe.

THE POWER TO CHANGE

Fast food genocide is happening now and creating many of our nation's problems, and the potential is there for further deterioration of subsequent generations. Only multifaceted solutions can stop it:

- Increasing positive social interactions

- Expanding educational and motivational efforts in communities

- Encouraging all ages to say "No" to fast food

- Demanding availability of and access to not just produce, but quick and easy healthy food options for everyone

All of these are necessary parts of an effective overall solution. A healthy diet will not only prevent and reverse serious chronic disease, but also enable millions to rise above adverse circumstances. There is evidence that tremendous benefits can come to those in most need.

Such evidence comes from prisons. Few places demean and debilitate people more than prisons. But multiple studies on prison populations show benefits when inmates' nutrition, self-worth, and social interactions are constructively addressed. For example, there are efforts across the nation today to have prisoners raise organic fruits and vegetables. In California, Washington state, and the city of Philadelphia, some prisons have state-of-the-art composting systems, farms, and organic agriculture vocational programs. On both coasts, rehabilitation is literally taking root as prison yards are transforming into thriving patches of strawberries, squash, cabbage, lettuce, eggplant, and peppers. Some of the produce feeds the inmates, and the rest goes to feed the poor. Early studies of gardening programs in California prisons found that fewer than 10 percent of participants returned to prison—a dramatic improvement from the U.S. rate of more than 60 percent.[45] The curriculum includes not just gardening and farming instruction, but classroom lessons on ecology, emotional intelligence, and leadership.

Even nutritional supplements have been shown to make a difference. A randomized, placebo-controlled trial in a British prison tested the association between antisocial behavior and nutritional status. Compared with the test group, prisoners given micronutrient supplements had 26 percent fewer violent incidents.[46] The supplements included vitamins, minerals, and the critical omega-3 fatty acid DHA. A research team in the Netherlands replicated the study with similar results.[47] These short-term studies reveal that missing micronutrients are a significant factor affecting behavior. In the long term, nutrients are best obtained from a healthy diet. But we know that without positive social interaction, people will likely have trouble adhering to a healthy lifestyle.

Another prison program produced even more dramatic results. In 1997, Terry Mooreland, the CEO of Maranatha Private Corrections, took over a five-hundred-inmate private prison in California's San Bernardino County, where prisons had become a revolving door for career criminals.[48] Inmates were given the option to enter a program called New Start where they agreed to adopt a healthy vegan diet, study religion, receive occupational training, and learn how to manage their anger. The San Bernardino recidivism rate had languished at 95 percent before Mooreland took over. During the seven years the New Start program was active, the recidivism rate fell below 2 percent. Inmates who opted for the traditional California Department of Corrections (CDC) routine continued to be fed the standard prison rations, did not participate in rehabilitative programs, and were housed in a separate unit in the prison. An astounding 85 percent of inmates agreed to room on the "vegan" side of the complex. The impact was amazing; fighting and racial strife ceased on the New Start side. On the CDC side, racial tension and gang violence, like the food, remained unchanged. The difference on the New Start side didn't end with the food; prisoners were also taught social skills while their counterparts in the other wing were left to their own devices. Social energy in the new wing increased as inmates became more friendly. More importantly, the odds of inmates from the New Start side returning to prison were significantly reduced.

Inmates experience a lack of positive social interaction long before they enter prison. According to the Justice Policy Institute, most inmates get caught up in what's called the school-to-prison pipeline.[49] In some schools, kids are treated more punitively and suspended and expelled at rates that far exceed the national average. This type of treatment leads to further isolation and decreased social health. Many of these kids come from homes where families don't eat together. Many end up on the streets and one step closer to prison.

One school decided it would no longer be a part of the pipeline. Appleton Central Alternative Charter High School (ACA) opened its doors in 1996 as a refuge for students who were severely at risk. Despite the fact that students who were struggling in conventional school settings got individualized attention, misbehavior, truancy, and failing grades were common. A local business began supplying ACA with free lunches in 1997. It brought in round tables, set up a lunchroom, and teachers ate with students. The following year, the business expanded the program to include breakfast. This wellness program provided healthy food to the school for five years.[50]

Before the implementation of this nutrition and wellness program, ACA had no kitchen or lunchroom with tables and chairs where students could sit and eat together. The only food and beverages available in the student lounge came from vending machines that sold sodas, candy bars, and chips. Students purchased this junk food from the vending machines throughout the day while sitting on couches or the floor, or they ate at computer stations.

ACA staff reported that students' disruptive behavior and health complaints diminished substantially after the wellness program was established. Students also seemed better able to concentrate. One social worker noted that the "reduced amount of sugar and processed food in the students' diets allowed them to be more stable and that this makes mental health and anger issues easier to manage." One teacher said she saw a decrease in impulsive behaviors, fidgeting, and foul language. Fewer students were referred to the office for discipline, and fewer students complained about headaches, stomachaches, and fatigue. In the classroom, teachers were able to cover a greater amount of material at a more challenging level. The principal recorded that negative behaviors, including vandalism, drug use, dropping out, expulsions, and suicide attempts, ceased. State reports filed on student behavior pointed to improved rates of attendance and lower rates of suspension and truancy.[51]

ACA stumbled upon a basic principle. The presence of unhealthy foods makes socially impaired students difficult to teach. Similar to merely making healthy foods more available to urban inner cities, the problem with fast food diets is not solved by simply making healthy foods more available. In most cases, obesity levels and other social problems remain unaffected.[52] ACA was different because it changed more than the menu: It simultaneously increased the school's positive social energy. Round tables where students and teachers could interact and eat together replaced vending machines. Though the ACA diet was less than ideal, it was a vast improvement over the way students had been eating before. They consumed more vegetables and fewer high omega-6 oils. The improved diet and increased social energy led to a change of behavior inside and outside of school. Many ACA graduates went on to college, including some who might have otherwise ended up in prison.

PUT ON YOUR OXYGEN MASK FIRST

The United States is a great nation because our citizens frequently enjoy a high standard of living, but we are collectively suffering from poor health. Our country has the highest rates of obesity in the world and the highest rates of almost every chronic disease, yet other nations are catching up as we export our fast food culture to them. What if we could create a nutritional advantage for every single American? By harnessing the power of social energy and making high-nutrient foods universally available, we can give every person a nutritional advantage. This in turn would enable everyone to rise above his or her circumstances and overcome life's adversities. This potential requires altruism, compassion, empathy, and knowledge.

We also have an obligation to take care of our own health. We need to be effective role models in order to maximize our favorable impact on others. We have to take care of our bodies and minds as we age to avoid becoming dependent on our children, so they don't have to give up their own lives and care for us when we become sick, demented, and debilitated from eating improperly. When we don't take care of our health, we don't just hurt ourselves; we place undue stress on those we care about the most.

Changing one's eating habits is not simple, and many people struggle with it. In my multiple decades of research and clinical practice, I have learned that the principal reason people struggle to adopt a healthy diet is because they have internal conflicts. One part of them wants to be healthy, while the other part wants to do something that results in the opposite of health. An unhealthy behavioral pattern, like eating a pint of ice cream, provides pleasure in the moment. In that moment when you hold the ice cream carton and spoon in your hands, you want to eat the ice cream; however, in the larger perspective, you want to be healthy and lead a long, productive life.

Adopting a healthy lifestyle generally requires change on many levels. Each level is controlled by a different region of the brain, and each level is like a different radio frequency or channel. To achieve permanent success in the health arena, we have to consider the complexity of human nature. We are physical, emotional, and social beings, and we must consider all of these factors when we seek to improve our health. If we don't, many people will reject incorporating or even learning more about a health-supporting lifestyle. Initial interest will dissipate. This is a physical manifestation of a subconscious process. Our brains are designed to dim awareness to information that causes us anxiety. For most people, the idea of overhauling the way they think about food and the way they eat is a source of anxiety. Plus, unhealthy foods are a slow-working poison. Many ailments related to the foods people eat take years to develop, and the only visible issue for most people is their excess weight. Studies have shown that most overweight people routinely underestimate the extent of their obesity and do not see themselves as significantly overweight. Consequently, it is not too difficult to imagine how so many people can ignore the evidence. They often don't see that it has anything to do with them.

The objections of those unwilling to change their diets can sometimes have very little to do with food. It is often the direct result of low self-esteem, which makes them vulnerable to negative peer pressure, addictions, and emotional overeating. Some may fear appearing different from other people, and they think changing the way they eat will result in a loss or weakening of their social relationships. This is a subconscious perception, but some people are unknowingly governed by it. Others overeat to a stupor, raising hormones in the brain so that they can dull the frustration and pain of their lives.

Our brains release certain hormones when we have positive social interactions. If these interactions are eliminated, the brain will seek out other ways to produce the hormones and pleasurable stimulation. This is why people with strong social ties are far less likely to be drawn into compulsive overeating and other addictive behaviors. For people who lack the emotional fulfillment that social relationships can provide, consumption of high-calorie foods gives the brain the surge it is looking for. Therefore, they are more compelled to engage in addictive eating behavior. It is important to work on all aspects of one's life simultaneously to successfully change eating behaviors.

Bad dietary habits can't solve anyone's social problems. Unhealthful behaviors lead to poor health, lower emotional well-being, and then advance this negative cycle. You have to address your beliefs, your thinking, your actions, and your diet because they work hand in hand. When you have a legitimate reason to believe in yourself, you will care for yourself better and be more inclined to eat right.

Feeling that you belong within a group of friends who help you to be a better person and with whom you have something in common raises your emotional health and self-confidence. It is far easier to change and transition into a healthy lifestyle when you have the support of others doing the same. The more your group embraces and supports you in your efforts to eat healthier and live a health-supporting lifestyle, the easier this becomes.

Our nation as a whole is eating itself to death. It is essential that we find smaller groups of support when attempting to move away from the deadly dietary norm. If you have a real and tangible positive social group, you are much less likely to be affected by the artificial ones created by advertisers, marketers, and technology.

If you want to get healthy, encourage others to join you and hang around other healthy people and those striving to be healthy.

Some people will try to make you feel uncomfortable because you are eating healthfully. Your change in behavior may make them uncomfortable because you are forcing them to examine their own unhealthy practices. If you look for approval from someone who is struggling on that issue, you will generally not get a positive response. Regardless of the illogical motives of the unconscious mind to "save face," you actually lower your social energy by letting these forces govern your life's choices.

Emotional health depends on feeling good about yourself. You need a legitimate reason to feel good about yourself and be enthusiastic about life. This can evolve from your efforts to make a difference and to value goodness around you—not trying to impress, not trying to make yourself look good, but rather trying to appreciate how much others have value and beauty in them. Feeling isolated and unconnected is worse than actually being isolated and unconnected. Fortunately nowadays, there are lots of ways to connect socially with others, particularly online. Online forums and various social media provide ways of communication and places where you can give and receive support. Obtaining peers who are also interested in healthy living is a great idea. Forming a support group or even joining a support group on the Internet can help you achieve personal success.

The good news is that you are not at the mercy of your genes or your subconscious mind, and you can control your health and weight. Heart disease, stroke, cancer, dementia, diabetes, allergies, arthritis, and other common illnesses are not predominantly genetic. They are the result of incorrect dietary choices. With knowledge, you can be empowered to make new choices by changing the way that you think.

It is important for all of us to understand the critical necessity to put in our mouths high-quality, nourishing food. Eat very little salt and fewer animal products. Eat mostly vegetables, beans, fruits, onions, mushrooms, nuts, and seeds. To paraphrase President John F. Kennedy, "It is not what your diet can do for you, it is what your diet can do for your country" (or something like that). By working together, we can become a healthier, more productive population. The burden of our health need not fall on our children, and the high cost of medical care should not be a fear that lives with us daily.

We are paying for this fast food genocide with our shared tax dollars. When people eat themselves into coronary bypass surgery or wind up in a nursing home, we all pay for it with our taxes and national debt. Our sickly population weakens our economy, and our businesses and industries can't compete within a world market given our exorbitant medical expenses. The cost of treating just heart disease and stroke is expected to triple over the next twenty years to $818 billion. Eating right will protect you and also help our neighbors, our country, and our planet. It is the right thing to do.

CHAPTER SIX

MAKING DESERTS GREEN AGAIN

We consider it normal to lose youthful vigor in our 30s, carry 30 to 40 extra pounds, live with chronic illness in our late 40s and 50s, and live our last decades completely dependent on others. But this should not be considered normal. This is the result of a lifelong pattern of unhealthful living and misguided information. We should look forward to enjoying an active life into our 90s. This seems like an outrageous expectation because most people spend a lifetime consuming an inadequate diet. They have yet to make the connection that we are what we eat and that ill health in the later years of our lives is the result of our earlier poor choices.

On the banks of the Delaware River, across from Philadelphia—the city of brotherly love—lies Camden, New Jersey, a city with a population of about seventy-seven thousand. It is one of the most violent cities in the country. It suffers from extreme poverty, high rates of obesity and diabetes, and low high school graduation rates. The problems plaguing Camden, and other urban areas like it, have baffled experts for years because it is a problem that hides in plain sight on almost every corner: Most residents of Camden do not live near a grocery store. Instead, they are surrounded by small neighborhood stores stocked with cigarettes, lottery tickets, highly processed snack foods, and few, if any, fresh fruits and vegetables. Camden is recognized by the U.S. Department of Agriculture (USDA) as a *food desert*.

The USDA defines a food desert as "a low-income census tract where either a substantial number or share of residents has low access to a supermarket or large grocery store."[1] When grocery stores, farmers' markets, and other healthy food providers aren't available, the corner store or fast food restaurant becomes the primary source of nutrition, particularly for people who don't own a car.

The rate of diabetes in a neighborhood is a barometer of its neighborhood-level deprivation of fresh produce.[2] Residents in urban areas like Camden suffer from diabetes at rates twice the national average.

Obesity and Diabetes by Zip Code

A report commissioned by LaSalle Bank in Chicago and undertaken by Mari Gallagher Research and Consulting Group with the help of the University of Michigan School of Public Health is titled "Examining the Impact of Food Deserts on Public Health in Chicago."[3]

Researchers gave each urban community a score called a Food Balance Score. They measured the distance from every block and community to the nearest grocery store and divided that number by the distance to the nearest fast food restaurant. The higher the number, the more out of balance healthy food access was.

They reviewed the death rates and age of death in those areas and were able to calculate the **Years of Potential Life Lost (YPLL),** which estimated the average years a person would have lived if he or she had not died prematurely. YPLL is a measure of premature mortality. As an alternative to death rate, this method gives more weight to deaths that occur among younger people. Death rate records deaths per 1,000 population at all ages.[4]

The results were shocking: The people who lived in areas with the worst food balance score were the most obese and had more than double the death rate from diabetes and cardiovascular disease compared with people who lived in areas with a better food balance score. The YPLL for diabetics in these locales showed that these people were losing more than *forty-five years* of life.

The amount of vegetables consumed in Camden is one of the lowest in the country, and this low consumption of vegetables is especially noted during the teenage years, the time when the influence of nutrition on behavior is profound.[5]

Food deserts are predominately located in low-income areas where people typically don't have easy access to transportation. People who can't afford to drive the mile or more to a grocery store are forced to rely on corner stores, bodegas, and fast food joints that sell commercial foods that create health problems. Imagine going into your local corner

DIABETES IN CHICAGO COMMUNITIES BY FOOD BALANCE SCORE

Food Balance Grouping	YPLL	Death Rate (per 1,000 population)
Worst	45.48	1.27
Middle	33.48	1.11
Best	25.36	0.56

CARDIOVASCULAR DEATH IN CHICAGO COMMUNITIES BY FOOD BALANCE SCORE

Food Balance Grouping	Death Rate	Food Balance Score
Worst	11.07	2.04
Middle	7.41	1.25
Best	5.72	0.87

store and finding that every item on the shelf is unsafe for prolonged human consumption. This is the stark reality for more than 29 million Americans and 8 million children.[6]

People with limited access to produce and healthy food are not starving for calories; in fact, most of them consume too many. Urban food deserts have plenty of fast food restaurants and convenience stores, and the population is generally overweight from the addictive nature of the available Frankenfoods. The problem is the absence or shortage of the delicate health-protective antioxidants and phytochemicals found in a variety of natural produce.

We routinely overlook the problem because we do not fully comprehend the role of nutrition in shaping what happens from the neck up. Nutritional opportunity determines behavior and intellect. A visit to local corner stores in Camden or Chicago reveals shelves of processed, nutrient-void foods that impair the normal functioning of the human body and brain. Numerous studies have found that the price of food goes down as the added sugar and oil content goes up. Consequently, inner cities in the United States have the lowest cost, lowest nutrient, most dangerous food supply in the world.[7]

Commercial foods that line shelves in corner stores are designed to have a long shelf life, look good, and taste good, but they are not compatible with human genetics. This deception is completed by the addition of synthetic nutrients, which prevent short-term vitamin deficiency disease, while the body and mind are slowly destroyed.

The SAD now derives more than half its calories from chemicalized processed foods, but in urban food deserts, the amount of fresh produce eaten by the local population is less than 5 percent of calories.

AMERICA'S WORST URBAN FOOD DESERTS

It is hard to generalize about the country's worst urban food deserts, as all these areas of concern are not effected equally; there are worse sections and better sections within the cities listed here. All have areas of poor access to fresh produce, with a heavy penetration of fast food restaurants and stores.

ATLANTA, GEORGIA

Few supermarkets are to be found in the poorest areas of Atlanta.

CAMDEN, NEW JERSEY

Only one supermarket serves an unhealthy populace in a city with one of the highest crime rates in the country.

CHICAGO, ILLINOIS

In certain areas of Chicago with little access to large grocery stores, largely African American neighborhoods have twice the death rate from diabetes and heart disease compared with neighborhoods that have adequate access to large grocery stores.

DETROIT, MICHIGAN

Detroit is the world's largest consumer of potato chips,[8] and more than half the city is considered a food desert.

MEMPHIS, TENNESSEE

A 2010 Gallup poll revealed a startling 26 percent of people in the Memphis Metropolitan Statistical Area who could not afford to buy adequate food for their families.

MINNEAPOLIS, MINNESOTA

Food deserts cover about half of Minneapolis and nearly one-third of St. Paul.

NEW ORLEANS, LOUISIANA

Since Hurricane Katrina in 2005, the lack of healthy food options in the poorest areas of the city have become critical, though it has been slowly improving.

WEST OAKLAND, CALIFORNIA

With healthy produce growers and farmers' markets only a few miles away, West Oakland has fifty liquor stores and hundreds of fast food restaurants and convenience stores selling junk food, with only a few supermarkets.

CONSIDERING THE FUTURE CHILDREN OF OUR COMMUNITIES

It is well-known that the incidence of obesity and diabetes are common in people who live in food deserts. But rarely do we consider the impact of fast food–infiltrated regions on the unborn. Full-term babies born with low birth weights are the result of *intrauterine growth restriction,* a term that refers to the poor growth of a baby in the mother's womb. Researchers have found that the farther an expectant mother has to travel to buy produce, the more likely she is to give birth to a full-term baby with low birth weight.[9] Low-nutrient diets create a wide range of physical and mental problems that start early in life. Low birth weights have been directly correlated with future learning problems, heart disease, high blood pressure, and type 2 diabetes later in life.[10]

Low-birth-weight babies are also more susceptible to developing future behavioral problems. One study found that 9-year-olds who experienced intrauterine growth restriction had more cognitive impairments, including difficulties with language, creativity, and executive functioning. They also had lower academic achievement and a diminished ability to "self-regulate," meaning difficulty in regulating attention, which leads to inappropriate behavior and academic problems, and difficulty in regulating negative emotions, which leads to irritability and aggressiveness.[11]

Typically during famines women become thin and stop menstruating. They do not become pregnant because of the lack of calories. Those unfortunate to be pregnant when famine strikes produce offspring with long-term health issues, but the damage in these cases is limited, as fewer women become pregnant when food is not available. But Frankenfoods have changed all of that, tricking the body into thinking that it is living in a time of abundance. Junk foods increase birth rates while simultaneously depriving offspring of required nutrients for full brain development.

The diets of mothers powerfully affect their unborn children. The brain is built in a micronutrient-intensive process that requires iron, iodine, zinc, magnesium, DHA, and a variety of vitamins and other micronutrients that are in low supply in many regions. Researchers in rural India evaluated the maternal nutrition of 792 low-birth-weight babies and found no association between size at birth and maternal calorie and protein intake. Instead, intake of micronutrient-dense foods and greens was strongly correlated with fetal growth and normal birth weight. Green leafy vegetables, fruits, and even milk were directly associated with healthy offspring, even after adjusting for potentially confounding variables such as socioeconomic status.[12] In other words, the nutritional quality of the mother's diet is critical.

Iron deficiency, the most common nutrient disorder in the world, also impairs growing brains. The effects of iron deficiency during infancy last a long time. In one study, children who had been treated for severe chronic iron deficiency in infancy still tested lower in arithmetic and writing achievement and motor function after treatment compared with children who had good iron status in infancy. The ratio of children who had repeated a grade or were referred for special education or tutoring was two to three times higher. The parents and teachers of formerly iron-deficient children rated their behavior as more problematic, with increased anxiety, depression, social problems, and attention deficits.[13]

Iodine deficiency is another major global problem. According to the World Health Organization, even mild iodine deficiency causes subtle mental impairment that leads to poor school performance, along with reduced intellectual and work capacity.[14] Iodine deficiency results in a global loss of 10 to 15 IQ points at a population level and constitutes the world's greatest single cause of preventable brain damage and mental retardation.[15] In extreme cases, iodine deficiency stunts physical and mental growth in developing fetuses. This condition, called cretinism, is rare in the United States, even though milder iodine deficiencies are not. In fact, they are on the rise; consumption of this vital mineral in the United States has declined by 50 percent since the 1970s. Fast food is low in iodine.[16]

Fast food and micronutrient deficiencies don't just promote infants with low birth weights and suboptimal brain function. The same foods are a major problem affecting all children throughout their developing years. Researchers tested two cohorts of children in Australia and Indonesia. The Australian cohort was well-nourished according to daily recommended allowances, while the Indonesian group was marginally nourished. Each child received either a placebo or multivitamin supplement that included iron, zinc, folic acid and vitamins A, B6, B12, and C, with DHA and EPA. Researchers found that supplements led to significant improvements in both the well-nourished and marginally nourished groups. In both cases, verbal learning and memory were increased in the test group compared with the control group.[17]

Though supplements have only a fraction of the micronutrient and phytochemical diversity of real food, this study was a testament to the essential role of nutrients in enabling our children to achieve

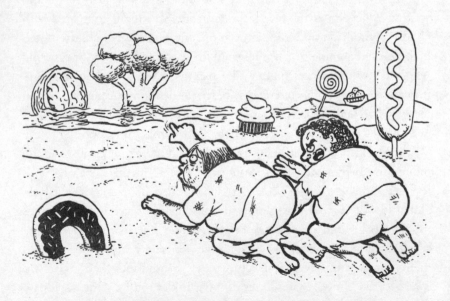

"You see healthy food ahead? No way! It must be a mirage!"

their maximum potentials. A gradual but full spectrum of intellectual damage from mild to severe is occurring, and this damage inhibits fast food–eating populations from reaching their potential and achieving the American dream of prosperity and happiness.

Commercial food makers do not and cannot replicate the wide variety of beneficial ingredients contained in whole foods, with their complex assortment of micronutrients and phytochemicals. The average American consumes a diet that is only marginally better than the diet of residents in Camden. Consequently, the problems in Camden are a bellwether of problems that threaten the health, welfare, and security of all Americans. This abysmal diet affects all areas of the country, but in the inner cities and the Southern states, things are worse.

NOURISHING BRAINS IN OUR CITIES

Revitalizing our cities and protecting the health of people in need not only involves building adequate housing, creating jobs, establishing adequate public transportation, and providing affordable access to medical care; it also must involve providing access to healthy food. A healthy population improves the economy, reduces demand for public welfare services, supports the tax base, and reduces crime; it elevates and supports all other initiatives to improve public good. This means that food policy and distribution must change significantly. People in impoverished communities and especially inner cities need produce, and they need public health authorities to encourage the consumption of produce through public health initiatives and messaging.

New York City is an example where significant improvements in food awareness, accessibility, and eating style have been made, resulting in improved health of the population in a relatively short time. Today, salad bars, chopped salads, vegetable bars, vegetable juice bars, and fruit and vegetable produce vendors can be found on the sidewalks throughout the city. More food markets are selling produce in lower income areas. The political discussions about reducing sugar and soft drink consumption and lowering salt intake initiated by former mayor Michael

Bloomberg had a positive effect on the social climate and health of New York. It is encouraging and even amazing that Bloomberg had such a powerful influence on saving lives in New York City, even when many of his initiatives were unpopular and rejected by the legislature.

The dialogue that Mayor Bloomberg opened among New Yorkers with his message about food on radio, on TV, and in print positively affected the way New Yorkers eat today. Since he first took office in 2002, Bloomberg unleashed a tsunami of public health initiatives: He attempted to cut sodium in prepared meals; he ordered that menus in chain restaurants include calorie counts; he posted restaurants' health department grades; and he worked to limit the use of tobacco products throughout the city. His first acts included a ban on smoking in restaurants and workplaces. In 2011, the restriction was extended to public parks and beaches.

Bloomberg's proposed restrictions spurred a backlash of criticism. Among other things, he was called Nanny-in-Chief and Big-Brother-in-Charge. Many people thought he went too far and that trying to legislate better health choices infringed on people's rights. Several of his efforts did not succeed legislatively. For instance, he tried to restrict the serving size of soda and failed. He also failed in his bid to get a soda tax adopted and to ban the use of U.S. government food stamps to buy soda. In their efforts to beat these proposals, soda companies staged rallies and gave millions of dollars to politicians and made other donations to hospitals to enhance their public image. However, the attention brought to these issues could not be silenced, and although the soda-tax efforts were defeated in both New York and Philadelphia, soda consumption still went down in these two cities by about 25 percent and has remained down in subsequent years.[18]

There is no question that the discussion raised about soda, sugar, and health in the media and government's role in encouraging better food choices had a positive result and are two of the primary reasons that New Yorkers started eating healthier. From the time that Bloomberg took office in January 2002, the city's smoking rate has dropped from 22 percent to just above 14 percent—one of the fastest declines in the country. Today, New York is most likely the healthiest city in the United States and certainly the healthiest large city because of what Bloomberg did and others have done since. A ten-year study by the New York City Health Department showed that New York's death rate fell 11.1 percent and life spans lengthened by more than 2.5 years, to 81.1 years, during the study period, 2004–2013, which ended with Bloomberg's third term in office. Premature deaths plummeted by 16 percent during the decade, and the racial gaps in death rates narrowed, according to the study.[19]

Mayor Bloomberg also started a program called FRESH (Food Retail Expansion to Support Health). Its mission is to help alleviate the lack of nutritious, affordable, fresh food in low-income New York City neighborhoods. This program offers tax incentives, density bonuses, grants, and loans to fresh produce retailers who open or expand in underserved parts of the city. Since launching in 2009, twenty-four FRESH projects have been approved. Thirteen new stores have completed their construction and are open to the public. These supermarkets are expected to provide more than sixteen hundred new jobs and represent a citywide investment of approximately $100 million.[20]

Certainly other factors played a role that developed increasing public demand, but in the past five years hundreds of healthy salad- and vegetable-friendly fast food places have opened in New York City. It is common to see a healthy salad takeout restaurant that offers assorted healthy toppings, including beans, seeds, and nuts, throughout the city. For example, in 2017 Just Salad has twenty-one locations in New York, Chop'T has six locations, fresh&co has fourteen locations, and sweetgreen has fifteen. Fast food establishments serving healthy options in New York City have exploded. And there are now many more small grocery stores that feature salad bars and offer a large selection of fresh produce.

New York City uses multiple strategies to improve the food environment, including enhancing access to and education on healthy eating. Green Carts is an important New York City innovation that helps vendors with mobile food carts offer fresh produce in neighborhoods that have limited access to supermarkets. The street vendor carts sell only fresh produce, including local vegetable favorites and tropical fruits. The program was launched in 2008 and since then, nearly five hundred vendors have opened Green Carts. Many of them have electronic benefits transfer (EBT) terminals (distributed for free to these vendors) to accept supplemental nutrition assistance program (SNAP) benefits. These efforts in New York have made a big difference.

It is interesting to note that Bloomberg's attempt to limit soda consumption was not welcome in some parts of the country. Mississippi—whose 34.9 percent obesity rate is our nation's highest, according to the CDC—passed an "anti-Bloomberg" law. Mississippi Governor Phil Bryant wrote, "It simply is not the role of the government to micro-regulate citizens' dietary decisions." But Bloomberg lashed back. "'Saturday Night Live' couldn't write this stuff," he said about Mississippi's move. "How can somebody try to pass a law that deliberately says we can't improve the lives of our citizens?" he asked. "It's just farce."[21]

As we improve the nutritional intake of our nation's inner cities, we will also have long-term positive effects on reducing chronic disease, poverty, violence, and crime.

WE ALL NEED TO WORK TOGETHER

One of the goals of the "Let's Move!" campaign led by former First Lady Michelle Obama was to eradicate food deserts by providing financial incentives to encourage supermarkets to open in these neighborhoods. Objectives of the program are to eradicate food deserts, fight childhood obesity, and encourage the consumption of fresh fruits and vegetables. Of course, what the national government can do is limited because of competing food interest groups and lobbyists (including the processed food industry), which derail the opportunity for dramatic changes and the ability to heavily influence food policies.

For example, on the Let's Move! website you can get information about MyPlate, a USDA program whose sample menus include dangerous fast foods, such as puddings, pretzels, tub margarine, and pork tenderloin with egg noodles. You won't see any raw nuts and seeds, no large salads with healthy dressings (made with real seeds and nuts), no bean chili or vegetable bean stew with greens, onions, cabbages, and mushrooms. It's just more semi-dangerous SAD recommendations that are a bit better than the typical fast food diets many inner-city children now eat. What a disappointment.

To significantly improve the nation's health, we must expose the truth about dangerous, low-nutrient foods such as white bread, pasta, and flour. Most importantly, we must share the latest nutritional science to showcase the necessity of eating greens, beans, nuts, and seeds. Government nutritional programs (if they continue to get funded at all) can be hindered by influential lobbyists. The government won't take a stand on strong initiatives such as reducing meat consumption, or cutting out added sugars, or eliminating sweetened milk from school lunches. It can't even support the basics, such as eating more fruit, veggies, and beans. It always purposefully confuses the message so as not to offend the food industry, especially the sugar, egg, meat, and dairy industries.

Though our national government is unlikely to advocate clear guidelines for excellent nutrition, these three are clear and well-supported by a consensus of nutritional scientists the world over. These three points need to be recognized everywhere, without confusion:

1. Eat more fruits and vegetables, especially vegetables of differing colors, beans, mushrooms, onions, seeds, and nuts.

2. Reduce or eliminate the consumption of fried foods, white flour, and sweeteners, including sugar, fructose, honey, and maple syrup.

3. Reduce all animal products to fewer than 10 percent of total calories, especially processed meats, barbecued chicken, and red meat.

Not thousands, but millions of people are dying needlessly every year in their 30s, 40s, 50s, and 60s, rather than living with good health into their 80s and 90s, according to the World Health Organization (WHO).[22] WHO is a global organization that includes more than seven thousand doctors and scientists from more than 150 countries. Its primary goal is to "build a better, healthier future for people all over the world." The findings and recommendations from this organization should be wake-up calls for the world.

Diseases linked to lifestyle choices, including diabetes and cancers, kill 16 million people prematurely (younger than the age of 70) each year according to a 2015 WHO report. This "lifestyle disease" epidemic "causes a much greater public health threat than any other epidemic known to man," said Shanthi Mendis, the lead author of WHO's Chronic Disease Prevention and Management report.[23]

WHO supports banning the advertising of tobacco and alcohol and taxing junk food and high-salt fast food. In Hungary, a heavy tax on unhealthy components of various foods and drinks led to a 27 percent drop in junk food sales.[24] Heeding the call of WHO, the United Kingdom announced the introduction of a 20 percent tax on sugar-sweetened beverages in 2017. The U.S. food industry argues that members of the public should be able to take "personal responsibility" for choosing what foods to eat, deflecting the blame to the consumer; but the truth is that the public lacks knowledge and choice.

This is a critical point. Is it really a choice if the information, let alone the healthy food itself, is not readily available? And while the general population may understand the basic distinction between healthy and unhealthy, I argue that most people don't truly understand the radical, detrimental life-altering and life-shortening effects of the highly processed, sugar-enhanced foods that they choose daily. This must change.

The costs of treating people who are sickly for years and then die in the prime of their lives are devastating. WHO has reported that $7 trillion will be sucked out of the global economy over the next decade by such premature deaths.

The current tactics of the sugar industry mimic how "big tobacco" was able to define its practices and promote tobacco use for years and years. Key in its strategy was paying scientists to plant doubt in the minds of the public, thereby confusing them, and financially supporting political allies.

WE CAN INITIATE CHANGE THAT SAVES LIVES

New innovations and initiatives for supporting better food availability are happening across the country. In New York state, a program called the Healthy Food & Healthy Communities Fund has provided $30 million in financing for produce markets since 2011. This program, along with some in New Jersey and Colorado, was modeled after the Pennsylvania Fresh Food Financing Initiative led by the Food Trust, the Reinvestment Fund, and the Urban Affairs Coalition. The goal of all these programs is to make it easier to develop full-service food retailers. This can happen through better loan terms, subsidies, tax incentives, and a host of other financial packages. In Pennsylvania, the financing program approved funding for eighty-eight new and expanded markets in the six years of the program.

In New Orleans, a city program called the Fresh Food Retailer Initiative was part of the financing that helped open several stores in target areas during 2013–2015. These included the reopening of Circle Food Store, a local landmark in the Seventh Ward that was devastated by Hurricane Katrina. It was and is again a needed mainstay of fresh food. A Tulane University study in 2014 showed that the number of supermarkets in New Orleans in that year had returned to more than thirty, after having been less than half that number in 2007.

Emerging research suggests that introducing supermarkets into low-income urban communities can improve dietary behaviors. An important 2002 study that followed ten thousand residents in Maryland, North Carolina, Mississippi, and Minnesota found that local food environments affected dietary intake. Researchers reported that African American residents increased their fruit and vegetable intake by 32 percent for each supermarket in their census area.[25] A similar study in the United Kingdom measured fruit and vegetable consumption as a marker of healthier eating behavior and found that 75 percent of the population increased their produce consumption after a supermarket was introduced into an area of need, doubling their average intake of fruits and vegetables.[26] The evidence shows that if quality food is available at reasonable prices, positive health effects occur for people at high nutritional risk.

But opening more food stores is not enough. People have to buy and eat those healthy foods. We need a grassroots-initiated food revolution. Old habits, ingrained food preferences, and food addictions are hard to break. Supermarkets on their own will not be successful in changing the eating habits of people who live in food deserts, so what else can we do? Well, we need to *educate* individuals about healthy choices and *provide creative incentives* for them to buy healthy foods. And education needs to target both children and adults.

For example, in New York City, the Department of Health and Mental Hygiene distributes "Health Bucks" that people can use to buy produce at all farmers' markets in the city that accept food stamps. Participants receive one Health Buck coupon for every $5 they spend at farmers' markets using food stamps. In other words, they get more food dollars if they spend what they have more wisely.

Clearly, we need to couple educational programs with financial incentives that encourage people to spend their food dollars wisely rather than buy fast food and junk food. This has begun to occur in some areas of the country. For example, seniors in New York City with yearly incomes of less than $30,000 can get vouchers that they can redeem at farm stands. Many farmers' markets will help collect produce and take it to food banks and pantries at the end of the market day. Tax deductions also can play an important role to encourage donations of produce to feed the hungry. The Good Samaritan Hunger Relief Tax Incentive Program allows farmers and small business owners to receive a tax deduction for donating food to banks, pantries, and homeless shelters. Look at Seattle: in 2008, seven neighborhood farmers' markets donated 40,343 pounds of produce to local food banks.

WORDS OF WISDOM FROM AKUA WOOLBRIGHT, PHD.:

We need an army of voices working with and within these communities to improve their health. Efforts have begun and it is starting to pay off, but it is a slow process that needs further innovation and support.

I have known nutritionist and educator Akua Woolbright for years, since she worked for Whole Foods Market on its healthy eating programs. We worked together to improve the health of Whole Foods Market team members and to set up educational initiatives for Whole Foods customers. Woolbright has a doctorate in nutritional sciences from Howard University. Today, she serves as the nutrition program director for the Let's Talk Food initiative in Detroit, a program sponsored by the Whole Cities Foundation.

When Dr. Woolbright went to Detroit in 2012 to work in this low-income community, she hit the pavement running. That first year she spent most of her time taking our nutritional message to the community. She went to health care centers, church basement meetings, hair salons, senior citizen centers, mosques, high schools—any place that would allow her to introduce herself and speak on their turf. She went to two to three different church services on Sundays to meet people and speak to pastors, asking whether she could lecture on healthy eating and present healthy cooking classes. Her work has won a steady and growing following of enthusiastic people, and her experiences teaching people who live in low-income areas in Detroit offer keen insight into changing the health of our country. Her insights below, which she shared to be included here, are invaluable.

The biggest surprise to me that I learned in the years I have been working in Detroit is the incorrect perception coming from public-health and medical authorities and the universities, stating that this message of plant-based, superior nutrition cannot work in a place like Detroit and that black people in large urban communities will not be receptive to healthy eating. I was told, "You won't make a difference, it is not worth the effort, and it is best just to prescribe medicine," because "these people just won't do it." We should not be making these false assumptions of what people can and cannot do.

It is not my decision to decide what people can and cannot do; my job is to bring people the right information so they can decide what they want to do for themselves. And the response has been overwhelming, and people have been transforming their health.

It is my responsibility to present sound nutrition information. Period. As an African American nutritionist, I feel an even more pronounced responsibility to make sure this life-saving information reaches my community.

The second most important thing I have learned is that the language we use is often inadequate. Whether it's New Orleans, Detroit, or Oakland, the people in these communities do NOT necessarily consider themselves under-served or disadvantaged and they may not like the term "food deserts." It is important that community health professionals reach a deeper understanding of the communities they serve so that the messages and approaches they apply will be more appropriate and effective. I have seen that people across all demographics are willing to apply the nutrition information they receive to make bold lifestyle changes.

People living in neighborhoods across Detroit are working every day to make our neighborhoods better, and I am happy that I've had the opportunity to make contributions toward the health and wellness of the people who reside in this city.

A different vocabulary is needed to speak about these communities in a way that is uplifting and respectful, to acknowledge the good that is here, and to add to the good that is already happening. This helps the community see you as an equal partner, not as someone looking down from an ivory tower of superiority, but as someone who is willing to meet them where they are and walk the journey with them.

Every day I talk to members of the black community with different socio-economic backgrounds, many of whom are living with some of the most serious health challenges and obstacles, and I work to help them get their lives back on track. Despite what some of my colleagues seem to think, this healthy eating message even works better in a community like this because folks have experienced and seen the negative effects of serious health conditions—the human tragedy that they are seeing with their own eyes every single day, so they are more ripe for a major nutritional overhaul. You don't have to show them the statistics of ill health in this community; they see it every day with their own family, friends, and neighbors.

The people that come to my classes come back and share— "my night sweats are gone," "I am sleeping through the night," "my fatigue, joint pain, or my *headaches are resolved." This is only the first tier of results that people experience early. And they never thought their suffering with these symptoms was linked to food and diet. Of course their sinuses clear up, and chronic sore throats and indigestion go away. But then the second tier of results starts to come into play and their chronic diseases gradually resolve. They are able to first reduce and in most cases eliminate the need for medication for blood pressure, diabetes, and high cholesterol. At one meeting, a person stood up who lost 100 pounds; a couple chimed in that had lost 40 together—so many losing and really keeping it off, because they are maintaining the lifestyle they were taught. They learned to make a permanent change in the way they eat.*

The beauty here is that this work is translatable to all these groups and populations; it crosses economic boundaries; it crosses race, cultural, and ethnic barriers. I am surprised that so much of what I learned in the university was wrong, and I found that cultural, ethnic, and racial differences were NOT an impediment to change—especially when [one is] given the opportunity to really spend time with and educate people properly. When [people were] given practical information and the lifesaving scientific information that supports it, so many were willing and able to change and not be helpless and frozen in their fast food habits.

I am talking to SNAP recipients; we have war veterans, single mothers, grandmothers, college students, government workers, auto industry professionals, office workers, and health educators who all attend my classes together, and that is the beauty of this movement—seeing the powerful interest that emanates across the entire spectrum. That has been the most important affirmation. If I had listened to the professionals in this field, I would have given up the first week. People everywhere and especially here want better for their families, and they want to enjoy the best quality health and happiness they can earn.

I have found that health practitioners must push the envelope and request more significant changes from their clients and patients. We have to go beyond portion control and moderation, which is not working. We have to get bolder in our approaches and expect more from people; if we don't believe it is possible, we are already lost. It starts with us, but it ends with people making positive changes in their lives.

Akua Woolbright's wisdom and work are critical for the future health of this country. The evidence is clear that good information and healthy food availability make a real difference in the lives of people in impoverished communities.

VOICES FOR HEALTHY KIDS

Voices for Healthy Kids is a joint initiative of the American Heart Association and the Robert Wood Johnson Foundation working to engage, organize, and mobilize people to improve the health of their communities and to help all children grow up at a healthy weight. Voices for Healthy Kids is dedicated to improving access to affordable healthy foods for children and families. They work to increase the number of healthy food outlets, grocery stores, supermarkets, and farmers' markets in underserved communities by increasing governmental support for financing initiatives.[27]

They are working on behalf of more than 1 million people in Alabama—including a half-million children—that live in areas without

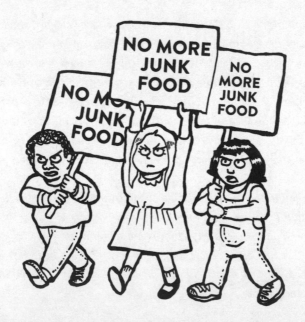

easy access to fresh and healthy food. That places Alabama among the top ten states in the nation in terms of a lack of access to healthy foods. But a group of health advocates under the leadership of Voices for Alabama's Children is working to change those statistics by creating a healthy foods access fund. The state-based program would establish a revolving-loan program that would provide financial incentives to grocers and other food retailers to locate their businesses in communities that have low or no access to healthy foods. Voices for Healthy Kids has also launched healthy food access initiatives in Texas, North Carolina, Oklahoma, Louisiana, and Ohio.[28]

The food and beverages and chain restaurant industries target children with intensive marketing.

In 2010, the food and beverages industry spent $40 billion lobbying Congress against regulations that would decrease the marketing of unhealthy food to kids and promote soda taxes. The fast food industry spends more than $5 million a day advertising sugary cereals, junk food, and fast food to children; and it's working.[29] It has been demonstrated that exposure to these advertisements induces children to eat higher amounts of sugar, fried food, and sweetened beverages. Advertising brain-damaging foods to children is no better than advertising cigarettes, alcohol, and addictive drugs to them. It's hard enough for parents to get their children to eat vegetables, but once they are hooked on commercial baked goods and sweets, it is, as we have seen, even more difficult.

Animals of all species will choose highly flavored, processed foods over real food and become highly addicted, obese, and sick when exposed to these food choices. In fact, animals will stop eating the produce they are habituated to eating in their natural environments and only consume calorically concentrated, highly flavored junk food when given the opportunity. Their palates and their brains can be captured to prefer high-tech, designer foods. Human children are no different. They don't like fruits and vegetables because their taste has been deadened and hijacked by highly palatable processed foods.

Of course, parents are ultimately responsible for what their children eat, but until communities and school systems prohibit these dangerous foods in public places, even well-intentioned parents become conflicted with societal pressures to conform to the dangerous eating practices placed on their children. Schools have to make clear that bringing cupcakes, doughnuts, cookies, and other junk food into school for parties, birthdays, and even for regular cafeteria consumption is not permitted. It's time to stand up to the big food companies and protect the health of our children. Advertising sweetened, processed foods to children is just not acceptable.

THE PROBLEM OF FOOD SUBSIDIES AND COSTS

Policy changes are needed; agricultural subsidies foster poor health. For more than eighty years, U.S. farmers have been the beneficiaries of a medley of subsidies and price-support programs to elevate and stabilize crop prices and keep fields productive. Critics and scientists say these policies have led to more obesity and disease by favoring the production of only corn, wheat, and soybeans. These crops are for feeding livestock rather than people and for use as sweeteners and additives in processed foods. These policies are now entrenched in America's heartland. They keep the foods fed to cows and pigs cheap and reduce the consumer costs of dairy and meat, thus keeping sugary, corn syrup–flavored fast foods cheap too, as well as corn oil, HFCS, soybean oil, and white flour. These policies primarily benefit huge agricultural corporations, fast food giants, and processed food manufacturers, not the family farm trying to grow fresh fruits and vegetables. While the overall price of fruits and vegetables in the United States increased by nearly 75 percent between 1989 and 2005, the price of junk food dropped by more than 26 percent during the same period.[30]

Food subsidies are one reason that the cheapest, unhealthiest, and most fattening fast foods are the most available foods in poor neighborhoods. Inexpensive, dangerous, and addictive foods have become the staple of an overweight and sickly population that faces an explosion of medical difficulties and medical costs. And these cheap foods do not come cheap—they burden a stressed population with tragic medical difficulties and unaffordable medical expenses.

If the United States is going to subsidize agriculture, it should at least subsidize healthy foods, not unhealthy ones. Rather than subsidize sugar, corn syrup, and beef, we should subsidize mushrooms, walnuts, almonds, broccoli, and bok choy. Subsidizing fruit and vegetable growers instead of commercial corn, dairy, and beef concerns would do a lot toward making our population healthier. It may not make a huge difference in the price of corn syrup liquid drinks at fast food outlets, but it would encourage large growers to think more about farming diversity and growing options. And, it would be a factor in educating our population about the value of fresh produce.

The fact that fresh fruits and vegetables are more expensive than processed snacks is perceived to be a major impediment to eating healthy food for many, particularly lower income, families. This is an issue that the USDA has studied. Hayden Stewart, an agricultural economist with the USDA's Economic Research Service, says that the USDA wanted to answer the question of how much it costs someone to meet fruit and vegetable recommendations. Her group found that an adult on a 2,000-calorie-per-day diet could satisfy recommendations for vegetable and fruit consumption in the 2010 *Dietary Guidelines for Americans* at an average cost of $2.00 to $2.50 per day, or approximately 50 cents per edible cup equivalent.[31] Stewart and colleagues also looked at costs associated with swapping out snack foods for fruits and vegetables and found that swapping is, at least, cost neutral.

Certainly, if a family cuts out fast food and processed food from their diet and spends those dollars sensibly on produce, they can eat healthfully with little extra cost, but those are acquired skills that Americans need to learn. And don't forget to factor in the costs of illness, chronic disease, excessive medical expenditures, and reduced work capacity that result from poor eating habits. The American College of Cardiology estimates that $22 billion in needless and excessive medical costs and $9 billion in lost productivity are related to improper eating in this country.[32]

We can see that efforts are under way to improve the way Americans eat, and this is happening near to me in Camden. The New Jersey Partnership for Healthy Kids launched a Get Healthy Camden initiative, and a Camden Food Innovation Grant Fund was started. But we need to do much more because we have passed the tipping point of danger. We need better nutritional guidance, and we need millions of new adult role models of healthy eating. Adults have to model healthy eating behaviors and get rid of fast food in their diets before they can expect kids to do the same. The efforts to promote the consumption of vegetables, beans, fruits, nuts, and seeds need to involve citywide agencies, joined by all areas of political and social influence, with heathy eating promoted in hospitals, medical clinics, and all public places. We need an integrated effort that involves celebrities and influential athletes promoting the consumption of fresh fruits, vegetables, beans, seeds, and nuts. Health professionals have to walk the walk and talk the talk. For instance, we can't continue to allow fast food restaurants in hospitals. Hospitals and public health facilities must remove white flour, pancakes, waffles, and other junk food from their menus. Every pebble of influence needs to come together to start and maintain an avalanche of good.

Imagine if we transformed America's inner cities into zones of excellent nutrition that grow healthy bodies and healthy minds. Instead of food deserts, they could be hotbeds of creativity and business opportunity; they could be transformed into Blue Zones of slim, healthy people living well and long, and being proud of their accomplishments. Improvements have already begun to happen in some areas of the country. With many people working purposefully together, we can stop fast food genocide.

CHAPTER SEVEN

FOOD FOR THE HEART AND SOUL

So far, this book has explored how a fast food genocide is destroying lives. We have examined food addiction, our brains on fast food, the historical legacy of ignoring poor nutrition, toxic hunger, food deserts, and several impressive organizations that are trying to help stop the vicious cycle of food inequality. The question now becomes: How do we start making the necessary dietary changes in our own lives? We cannot sit back and let disastrous dietary choices destroy our families, friends, and communities. In this chapter, I lay out the foundational components of a Nutritarian diet. This information will arm you for moving forward with a life-changing new perspective on how to eat. Millions of individuals have discovered these principals and regained their health and vitality. The movement, however, is just beginning. We can win the battle against processed foods once and for all, but it has to start with you!

We have seen how processed foods have become increasingly prevalent in the SAD. During the twentieth century, the consumption of fresh produce and whole grains plummeted, while the consumption of animal products increased. As a result, Americans now consume far more white flour, sugar, oil, salt, animal protein, and animal fats, and lots more calories, and far less fiber and plant-derived phytochemicals. The incidences of obesity, diabetes, autoimmune diseases, heart disease, and cancer have skyrocketed. With the advent and growth of the processed food industry and the fortification of foods with synthetic vitamins, a shocking thing happened: Cancer rates increased for seventy years, from 1935 to 2005.[1] Cancer rates and obesity-related mortality are continuing to climb worldwide as countries adopt the American-led consumption of fast food.

CHANGE IN PER PERSON FOOD CONSUMPTION	1900	2000
Sugar (lbs/year)	5	170
Soft drinks (gal/year)	0	53
Oils (lbs/year)	4	74
Cheese (lbs/year)	2	30
Meat (lbs/year)	140	200
Homegrown produce (lbs/year)	131	11
Calories	2,100	2,757

Fortified processed foods do not contain the comprehensive array of delicate nutrients that protect the brain. Calculating all the calories in the SAD coming from health-promoting foods such as fresh fruits, vegetables, beans, nuts and seeds, and whole grains, adds up to less than 10 percent of the calories Americans consume nationwide, though the numbers for inner cities and the southeast United States are much worse. This dangerously low intake of fresh produce guarantees a weakened immunity to infectious disease, leading to frequent illness and a shorter, more difficult life. The current medical system approaches this myriad of acute and chronic symptoms from the perspective of "pill for an ill" or "surgery for a fix." We are simply ignoring the primary cause of these symptoms and pushing temporary solutions that often intensify risk.

And, as we've seen, our fast food diets are even damaging our genetic code, which is passed on to future generations.

Many people cannot understand why, in all areas across the United States and among all economic groups, the consumption of calories has increased so much over the past seventy years and continues to do so. People don't want to be overweight, but they can't seem to help themselves. Have you ever been on a diet and find yourself losing and gaining the same 10, 20, or 30 pounds? Have you experienced how difficult it is to regain a favorable, healthy weight, once you've put on an extra 30 pounds? My findings over the past twenty-five years with more than fifteen thousand patients, along with thousands of supportive research studies, show that a poorly nourished body demands more calories, and those demands can be too powerful to ignore.

Most people eat too many calories because they don't eat enough nutrients. Nutritional inadequacy magnifies food addiction and the desire to overeat. It makes the craving to eat too frequently and too much feel overwhelming.

Eating more of the right foods to supply the nutrients the body needs can decrease overeating behavior and the desire for excessive calories. The information presented here will reduce your need for prescription drugs, lower your risk of developing life-shortening diseases, and enable the reversal of serious disease; it will also help you control your emotional and addictive overeating, thus helping you to prefer to eat less and to eat more healthfully. It may even enhance the pleasure you get from eating.

UNDERSTANDING NUTRIENT DENSITY

There are two kinds of nutrients: *macronutrients* and *micronutrients*. Macronutrients are protein, carbohydrate, fat, and water. Excluding water, they are the three calorie-containing nutrients. Micronutrients are vitamins, minerals, and phytochemicals, and they are calorie-free. The SAD contains too many macronutrients and not enough micronutrients. A micronutrient-rich diet supplies your body with fourteen different vitamins, twenty-five separate minerals, and thousands of phytochemicals that have a profound effect on human cell function and the immune system. Foods that are naturally rich in these micronutrients are also rich in fiber and water and are naturally low in calories. The ratio of micronutrients to calories in a food is the *nutrient density* of that food.

Given the thousands of fragile phytonutrients in a berry or a sprig of broccoli, nutrient intake is more complex than originally thought. You cannot buy superior nutrition with a series of health-food store supplements; colorful plant food is just too complex and complete with beneficial substances, many of which have not even been identified yet.

The secret to a successful, healthy, and happy life is to eat a diet lower in calories and higher in micronutrients. It's all about nutrient bang per caloric buck. The nutrient density of your body's tissues is proportional to the nutrient density of your diet. My "Health Equation" represents this concept of striving for micronutrient adequacy in fewer calories to improve health and life span:

$$H = N/C$$
Health = Nutrients/Calories

The SAD does the opposite; it contains lots of high-calorie foods that are deficient in micronutrients. To achieve superior health and longevity, we must eat more foods that are micronutrient-rich and have fewer empty calories. Very few people are aware of this simple concept, which explains why oils are NOT healthy. They are rich in calories but are virtually devoid of nutrients and fiber.

In addition, eating fewer calories or moderate caloric restriction in the environment of micronutrient adequacy slows the aging process and advances health and longevity. However, what is also conventionally ignored is that little effort to restrict calories is needed once you consume a diet that is nutritionally superior. When you consume all the high-nutrient produce your body needs, you automatically desire the right amount of calories and no longer feel comfortable eating the amount of food that sustains an unfavorable weight. In other words, it is actually difficult to remain overweight when your diet is excellent.

THE TOP 20 SUPERFOODS

1. Collards, mustard greens, and turnip greens
2. Kale
3. Watercress
4. Bok choy
5. Cabbage (all varieties)
6. Spinach
7. Arugula
8. Lettuce (Boston, romaine, and green leaf)
9. Brussels sprouts
10. Carrots
11. Broccoli
12. Cauliflower
13. Bell peppers (red and green)
14. Mushrooms
15. Tomatoes
16. Berries (all varieties)
17. Pomegranates and cherries
18. Onions (and leeks, scallions, and garlic)
19. Beans (all varieties)
20. Seeds (flax, hemp, chia, sesame, pumpkin, sunflower)

The more high-nutrient food you consume, the less low-nutrient food you desire.

Most traditional dieting concepts have encouraged people to try to juggle macronutrients around—eat more protein and less fat, eat fewer carbs and more protein, eat lots of carbs and no fat, and more variations on this theme. Different camps of thought try to produce studies and reasons why their approach is best. However, long-term diet success and excellent health are rarely achieved with such juggling, because rearranging macronutrient ratios is not very helpful and doesn't address our body's need for micronutrients.

Conventional diet plans all miss the main issue of nutrient density and nutrient completeness, so inevitably they fail. We need to eat less carbs, less protein, and less fat—and that means fewer calories. But there isn't one ratio of fats to carbs to protein that is ideal; in fact, there are various ratios of fat-carbohydrate-protein that are acceptable and even favorable, as long as calories are not overconsumed and micronutrient needs are adequately met.

Eating enough protein is rarely an issue when eating healthfully. Beans, greens, and seeds are particularly high in protein. Many people do not realize that high-nutrient plants contain adequate protein, so even when people eat a totally vegan diet, they get enough protein as long as they don't consume too many calories from oils, sweets, or white flour, which have almost no protein in them at all. Our population is so uninformed that people generally equate protein only with animal products when in fact, almost all plant foods (except fruit) have plenty of protein. Your diet has to be rich in vegetables; otherwise, the nutrients that fuel cellular repair and normal immune function will not be supplied in adequate amounts.

PROTEIN CONTENT OF COMMON FOODS	(GRAMS)
Almonds (3 ounces)	18.0
Lentils, cooked (1 cup)	17.9
Kidney beans, cooked (1 cup)	15.4
Chickpeas, cooked (1 cup)	14.5
Sesame seeds (½ cup)	12.8
Sunflower seeds (½ cup)	11.5
Broccoli, frozen, cooked (2 cups)	11.4
Tofu, extra firm (4 ounces)	11.3
Collards, cooked (2 cups)	10.3
Spinach, frozen (1 cup)	7.6
Peas, frozen (1 cup)	7.0

PROTEIN CONTENT OF COMMON FOODS (*CONT.*)	(GRAMS)
Ground beef, 80% lean, broiled (4 ounces)	29.1
Chicken drumstick, fried	7.2
Whole milk (1 cup)	7.7

MAKING EVERY CALORIE COUNT

Most health authorities agree that we should add more servings of healthy fruits and vegetables to our diet, but I address this issue in a different fashion. Instead of trying to add these foods to your diet, make them the *main focus* of the diet and then consume lesser amounts of foods that are not in this category. The poorer your health, the more your diet has to be vegetable-based. Animal products should be seen as condiments to this plant-predominant diet. Here are my basic guidelines for a healthful diet.

- Eat a large green salad every day.

- Eat at least a ½ cup serving of beans in a soup, salad, burger, or main dish every day.

- Eat at least three fresh fruits a day.

- Eat at least 1 ounce of raw nuts or seeds a day, plus 1 tablespoon of ground flaxseeds or chia seeds daily.

- Eat at least one large serving of cooked or defrosted frozen green vegetables daily.

- Do not eat more than one small serving of animal products per day.

Almost all vitamins and minerals are much higher in a diet of mostly natural foods; the real difference is noted when you measure phytochemicals and especially when you test the antioxidant levels inside the body's tissues, which can be up to one hundred–fold higher, with the toxic elements one hundred–fold lower.

FAST FOOD MENU VS. NUTRITARIAN MENU

FAST FOOD MENU

BREAKFAST
2 glazed doughnuts

Medium (24-ounce) frozen coffee beverage

LUNCH
Fast food hamburger

Medium fast food French fries

Large (32-ounce) cola

DINNER
Canned chicken noodle soup

Frozen macaroni and cheese

Six chicken nuggets (frozen, prepared)

12 ounces sweetened ice tea

Three chocolate chip cookies

PER SERVING: CALORIES 3,493; PROTEIN 81G; CARBOHYDRATES 499G; TOTAL FAT 142G; SATURATED FAT 49G; CHOLESTEROL 286MG; SODIUM 5,680MG; FIBER 18.4G; VITAMIN A 3,477IU; VITAMIN C 10MG; CALCIUM 659MG; IRON 14.7MG; FOLATE 263MCG; MAGNESIUM 191MG; ZINC 8.5MG; SELENIUM 43MCG

PROTEIN 9%; CARBOHYDRATE 55%; FAT 36%

NUTRITARIAN MENU

BREAKFAST
Oatmeal with strawberries and flaxseeds

Chocolate Cherry Smoothie

LUNCH
Taco Salad Wraps

Roasted red pepper over wilted spinach with garlic

Fresh or frozen berries

Water

DINNER
Romaine lettuce salad with tomato, red onion, walnuts, and Walnut Vinaigrette Dressing

Broccoli topped with black beans and Spicy Red Lentil Sauce

Dr. Fuhrman's Vanilla or Chocolate Nice Cream

PER SERVING: CALORIES 1,969; PROTEIN 78G; CARBOHYDRATES 321G; TOTAL FAT 58G; SATURATED FAT 6.7G; CHOLESTEROL 0MG; SODIUM 660MG; FIBER 82G; VITAMIN A 71,162IU; VITAMIN C 641MG; CALCIUM 1,030MG; IRON 34MG; FOLATE 1,704MCG; MAGNESIUM 853MG; ZINC 11.6MG; SELENIUM 30MCG

PROTEIN 15%; CARBOHYDRATE 61%; FAT 24%

The Nutritarian menu has sixty times the amount of vitamin C, but more than one hundred times the amount of disease-fighting antioxidants and phytochemicals—the fast food menu has almost none.

Note that the Nutritarian menu contains about half the calories of the typical fast food menu. Very active larger individuals may require more calories, and smaller, inactive people even fewer calories; but regardless of your optimal caloric needs, this diet style is more filling and satisfying because of all the fiber, bulk, and nutrients. People are satisfied with significantly fewer calories when they eat healthier foods; plus all the nutrients they receive lessen the perception of hunger, thereby naturally normalizing and optimizing weight. Imagine the transformation of health, performance, and emotional well-being in the population if everyone ate a Nutritarian breakfast and a Nutritarian lunch or dinner!

For breakfast, it's so easy to have a cup of steel cut oats or other whole grain soaked in water overnight or cooked in water, with some added almond or soy milk, fresh or frozen fruit, ground flaxseeds, and walnuts—and for lunch, a bowl of vegetable bean soup, a salad with a nut-based vinegar dressing, and some fruit. I encourage people to make a big pot of vegetable bean soup or stew on the weekend and eat it throughout the week.

Eating healthfully does not have to be complicated.

THE SALAD IS THE MAIN DISH

My mantra is to eat salad every day. Raw vegetables, especially raw green vegetables, are linked to a reduced risk of cancer and heart disease and a much longer life.[2] Certain families of raw vegetables are particularly effective in preventing cancer, especially the cruciferous vegetables and the *Allium* (onion) genus. Add raw onions, scallions, arugula, shredded cabbage, or kale to your salad, as well as beans, frozen peas or lentils, and maybe some fresh fruit, such as shredded apple or orange slices. Then coat it with a fantastic dressing.

A nut- or seed-based dressing, usually mixed with vinegar and other flavorful and healthy elements, facilitates the absorption of the fat-soluble phytochemicals and antioxidants in your salad and the meal. Plus the seeds and nuts and even the vinegar have health benefits. I love making delicious salad dressings by blending nuts, seeds, and fruity vinegars with tomato sauce, another liquid, or fruit. Eating delicious and healthy salads is the secret to a long and healthy life.

Everyone should be eating a large salad as a main dish at least once a day. It's not optional; raw vegetables are essential for excellent health.

SEEDS AND NUTS TO THE RESCUE

You can absorb almost ten times as much of the beneficial nutrients from vegetables when you eat nuts or seeds with that same meal. So use them in salad dressings, a dip or sauce or sprinkled on top of a dish. Flaxseeds, hemp seeds, chia seeds, and walnuts are highest in omega-3 fatty acids, though pistachios, pecans, and almonds are very nutritious, too. Flaxseeds and chia seeds also have the anticancer lignans I empha-sized in Chapter 3. I strongly recommend that people eat at least one tablespoon of flax, hemp, or chia every day, as well as a small amount of walnuts. I usually add them every morning to my soaked grain cereal, but you can make all types of dishes, recipes, and desserts that incor-porate these superfoods, as I do in my meals.

Make salads and other dips and dishes with any nut and seed, espe-cially sunflower seeds, which are rich in natural vitamin E fragments and protein. I recommend eating nuts and seeds raw or just lightly toasted because the roasting process alters their beneficial nutrients and produces a carcinogenic compound called acrylamide. Commercially packaged nuts and seeds are also frequently cooked in oil and may be heavily salted.

THE VEGETABLE BEAN SOUP, STEW, OR CHILI IS THE SECRET

It's not hard to eat to live. The trick to making this work without having to shop and cook almost every day is to do one big shopping trip on the weekend, and then that same day, make a big pot of vegetable bean soup or stew for the entire week. You can take that bean soup or chili with you to work or school or when you travel away from home.

Soup is a key menu item in the Nutritarian diet. It's easy to incorporate lots of green leafy vegetables, beans, mushrooms, onions, and tomatoes all in one pot. Nutrients don't get lost in the cooking water when you make a soup. Soups and stews are cooked at 212°F, the boiling point of water. This moisture and the relatively low temperature prevent burning of the food and the resulting nutrient loss and formation of harmful compounds. Soups make great leftovers. Make a big pot, enjoy it for dinner, and then have it for lunch for the next few days.

In my home we usually make in advance both a favorite soup, such as split pea or spicy sweet and sour cabbage and corn, and a dark bean chili for the entire week. We also make at least one of our favorite salad dressings on the weekend, too. Then it's easy during the week to whip up a meal in no time flat, with a thick, hearty soup and some salad, vegetables, fruits, and nuts.

Beans are softer and more digestible if you soak them in water the night before and cook them the next day for a few hours over a low flame. You can also cook dry beans in a pressure cooker to reduce cooking time. If you use canned beans, make sure to select brands that are labeled as "low-sodium" or "no-salt-added."

Remember, soups and other foods don't need salt to be delicious. You can add flavor by using herbs, spices, garlic, onions, and lemon. For example, start your soup or other dish with onions and garlic; then add in your choice of herbs and spices while cooking and finish with a splash of citrus or vinegar. A hint of spiciness from black pepper, cayenne pepper, or red pepper flakes is sometimes just what a soup needs. Stock up on some no-salt seasoning blends, which are a quick and convenient way to add flavor.

And beans aren't just for soups and chili; they have lots of uses. Dried beans are inexpensive, super healthy, rich in protein, low-glycemic, anti-cancer, anti-diabetic, weight-loss favorable, life span extending, filling, and delicious. When you mix beans with some intact whole grains and chopped greens, a bit of spicy peppers and scallions or onions, you have a great main dish.

THE MEAT SPECTRUM: HOW MUCH OR HOW LITTLE?

I hope it's clear that a healthy diet must consist predominantly of whole plant foods that are fresh, frozen, or minimally processed. So the pertinent question is how much animal products such as chicken, fish, and eggs are appropriate in a healthy diet? This question is difficult to answer, and it's difficult for people to accept what's best, especially with so many false and distorted claims circulating. Some people will tell you, for instance, that eating butter (high in saturated fat) and egg yolks (high in cholesterol) is fine.

When you look at the evidence presented by those who make such claims, it's typically from a study comparing two groups that are both eating a relatively unhealthy diet, both with excessive animal products included and then seeing whether high-fat animal products are worse than lower-fat animal products or whether one animal product, such as eggs, makes things worse compared with, say, chicken. In such studies, both study groups have relatively poor outcomes. Too often, researchers don't have enough knowledge about nutrition to design the right studies. The question isn't whether dairy fat is worse than lean meat or oil, or even bread or white rice, since these are all unfavorable food choices.

The real question is this: When you lower or remove some potentially unfavorable option from the diet, what should you replace it with to achieve better health? Are you replacing those calories with a truly healthful option?—because if not, the results of any study will be almost worthless. We don't need to know whether dark meat chicken is worse than light meat chicken if they both increase the risk of heart disease and cancer and the difference is slight. And if white meat turns up to be not as bad as dark meat, it doesn't mean that white meat chicken is good for you. Whenever a study is performed and animal products are removed and replaced with vegetables and beans, the health benefits are dramatic.

Likewise, just because commercial baked goods and high-glycemic carbohydrates such as white bread and white rice may be even more dangerous for your long-term health compared with eggs or poultry doesn't mean that eating eggs and poultry regularly is a good idea or enhances life span. Thousands of studies have already documented the benefits of eating a diet low in animal products and rich in fibrous plant foods. It's hardly worthwhile discussing whether eggs are better or worse than meat, because neither is favorable. The reality is that it is better to eat fewer eggs and less of other animal products and to eat more vegetables, beans, nuts, and seeds.

In fact, when scientists from the World Cancer Research Fund and the American Institute for Cancer Research systematically analyzed more than one thousand studies on this topic, they found that diets low in fibrous plant foods and higher in meat were linked to cancer. As a result, these two organizations recommended that people consume a whole-food, plant-rich diet.[3]

My point is to make it clear that no matter what type of animal product you choose to eat, it should be a minor part of your diet and not the major part. When you eat too many animal products, no matter what type you consume, they decrease the proportion of vegetation you eat and drive growth hormones produced by the body too high, which promotes cell growth and replication, and thus cancer.

Generally, the most respected long-term studies show that the longest-lived Americans are vegans and near-vegans who include in their diets a bit of seafood. A vegetarian diet may include plenty of vegetables, beans, fruits, and nuts that are rich in phytochemicals, anti-oxidants, fiber, magnesium, vitamins C and E, and folate and are low in cholesterol, saturated fatty acids, and sodium. Of course, there are also lots of vegans who eat unhealthy junk foods, so just eating a vegan diet does not define dietary excellence. That is the purpose of the term "Nutritarian"—to identify a diet style that avoids fast food and junk food and emphasizes nutrients. Long-term studies repeatedly demonstrate that death from all causes is significantly lower in vegetarians than in omnivorous populations. Compared with omnivores, the incidence of cancer and type 2 diabetes is also significantly lower. Other than the risks from low vitamin B12 and omega-3 fatty acids, which are easily supplemented, vegans and vegetarians generally live longer than people who eat lots of animal products.[4]

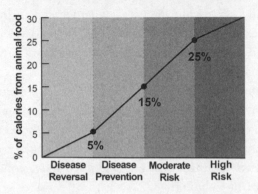

Animal Products and Heart Disease Risk

All animal products are rich in high biological protein, so they all raise IGF-1 levels unfavorably.

Lots of data have already accumulated suggesting that for excellent health, most people need to keep the consumption of animal products at less than 10 percent of total calories. People with known disease, such as diabetes or heart disease, or a high genetic risk of disease, should cut back on animal products even more, most likely to less than 5 percent of total calories to maximize the protective and healing potential of a Nutritarian diet.

When choosing which animal product to eat, keep in mind that red meats have about 100 calories per ounce and white meats, fish, and eggs have about 50 calories per ounce. Especially if you are limiting your animal protein intake to 2–3 ounces, it still can be a relatively minor part of your total caloric intake for the day. And, of course, you should always try to find animal products, even this relatively small amount, that are as close to naturally and wild raised as possible, as opposed, for instance, to being raised in commercial feedlots with higher potential for containing toxins and being contaminated.

The chart above is from my book *The End of Heart Disease,* where I demonstrate through scores of studies that reducing animal products to very low levels facilitates dramatic lowering of blood pressure and cholesterol lowering, and the reversal of advanced heart disease.

Many Nutritarians are vegans and eat no animal products at all; others eat a small amount a few times a week or month; and some eat a small serving once a day. Most Americans eat animal products three times a day, at every single meal. I recommend that you eat no animal products at all for breakfast and lunch, and then if you want to eat some animal products, use only a small amount as a flavoring agent with lots of vegetables with your dinner. For example, make a savory vegetable dish in a wok with mushrooms, onions, cabbage, and broccoli and add just a small amount of shredded chicken or turkey for flavor, instead of eating an entire half chicken as your meal. Many people find that mushrooms and tempeh (fermented soybeans) have the right texture and flavor to become a meat substitute or meat extender, so thus they can use very little animal products in a dish.

In order to get the most profound benefits possible from a Nutritarian diet style, people need to simultaneously cut out fast food and significantly reduce their intake of animal products. Many people reject this advice because they enjoy beef hamburgers and don't want to give up fast food and barbecue. Some tell me, "I'm not giving up meat." Then I show them how they can use only 1 ounce of meat per person, mixing this small amount to add flavor to a patty made from oats, mushrooms, walnuts, and red beans. They are amazed that this healthy burger tastes like a flavorful meat burger even though it contains only 1 ounce of meat.

With proper meal design, even the die-hard meat eater is satisfied with very few animal products in a meal. I want people to eat for both enjoyment and health; therefore, food must be appealing.

WHY SHOULDN'T I EAT FISH EVERY DAY?

Science dictates limits on certain foods, like animal products and oils. And yes, even fish should not be eaten more than a few times a week. Almost all fish, whether it comes from the middle of the ocean, a local lake, or a fish farm, contains methylmercury and other pollutants. These pollutants accumulate in fish as the fish breathe polluted water through their gills. Larger, predatory fish tend to contain more mercury and pollutants than smaller, shorter-lived fish, but all fish contain unfavorable pollutants, including mercury.

Part of the reason mercury is so toxic is because our body tissues accumulate all of the mercury we eat over the years, and it takes a very long time for it to be flushed from our tissues. You might digest a piece of fish in a day or two, but the mercury in the fish will stay with you for years and can continue to accumulate to dangerous levels in your cells if you eat fish too often. If you eat fish too regularly, you are bound to have unsafe levels of mercury and other pollutants from fish in your tissues.

Studies indicate that the more fish a person eats, the higher that person's mercury levels. People who eat fish more than a few times a week have been shown to have blood mercury levels exceeding the maximum suggested by the National Academy of Sciences (less than 5 micrograms). Women who eat fish more than a few times each week have been found to have mercury levels seven times higher than the levels of women who rarely eat fish. And children who regularly eat fish have been found to have mercury levels forty times higher than the national mean.[5]

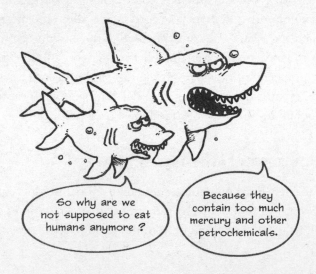

As we age, high body stores of mercury cause brain damage and memory impairment. Eating a lot of fish is also linked to breast cancer, perhaps because of the high levels of mercury and other contaminants in fish or some other factor, (such as excess animal protein) but studies on this subject are clear. In one such study, 23,963 women were followed, and researchers were most surprised by the strong link between high intakes of fish and breast cancer.[6] The women in the study who ate little or no fish had less than half the rates of breast cancer compared with those who ate fish multiple times a week. Moderate amounts of fish may be safe, but too much is a problem. If you eat little or no seafood, you can still get those beneficial fatty acids via a clean supplement.

EATING HEALTHFULLY ON A BUDGET

Dried beans are very inexpensive, and you can buy them, and intact whole grains, in bulk to save money. Plus, they store well. Millet, quinoa, wheat berries, and barley can also be purchased at significant savings in bulk, and families can buy together and share the cost. Root vegetables such as turnips, beets, carrots, parsnips, and rutabaga are not expensive and store well if you buy in quantity. Frequently, the healthiest foods in the world, such as thick green leaves—kale, collards, mustard greens, and different varieties of cabbages—are affordable and also keep for weeks if they are refrigerated or kept in a cool place.

When my wife and I were still students, we would travel to wholesale markets where restaurants and food stores bought their produce, and we would purchase entire cases of fruits and vegetables wholesale and split them up with other families in our apartment building to save money on our food bills. We actually got other health-minded families to food share with us for a minimal fee. My wife even made and sold fruit-containing breads out of intact grains that she coarsely ground herself. Some weeks, with all the produce and breads we sold, our weekly food bill was zero.

When we lived in New York we traveled to Hunts Point in the Bronx to buy food wholesale, and when we lived in South Jersey near Philadelphia, we traveled to the Philadelphia Wholesale Produce Market to buy food in bulk. We also purchased bananas and other fruits that were slightly damaged or a bit too ripe to fetch the usual price, often getting fantastic deals on lots of food that looked imperfect but was perfectly good to eat. We would cut away the bad parts and either freeze or dehydrate the extra food for another day. Certain fresh fruits, such as berries, can be prohibitively expensive, but they are about one-quarter the price if you buy them frozen in big bags. Remember: Frozen produce is still healthful because it retains most of its delicate nutritional value.

So there are ways to save on your food bill: You can strategize about buying bulk and wholesale, coordinate your food purchases with family or friends nearby, or both. The additional benefit of this last option is the support you get from other people for eating healthfully. Develop healthful relationships with your neighbors rather than dysfunctional relationships with people who eat junk food and doctors who peddle drugs and drug paraphernalia (semi-funny joke).

SIMPLE GUIDELINES FOR NUTRITIONAL EXCELLENCE

1. Eat an intact whole grain (such as steel cut oats or quinoa) with seeds and fruit for breakfast.

2. Eat a fresh green salad and veggie bean soup, stew, or chili for lunch, also with a fruit.

3. Eat raw vegetables, with a dip, and a veggie stew or veggies cooked in a wok as a main dish for dinner. Add some root vegetables or squash.

4. End with a fruity dessert, such as one of my "nice creams," or fresh fruit with nuts.

DON'T FRY FOODS OR COOK WITH OIL

Oil is an example of a high-calorie, low-nutrient food. Even though some oils are worse than others, all are fattening and do not contain a significant amount of micronutrients. The more low-nutrient calories you consume in life, the shorter your life. Oil consumption has repeatedly been shown to cause obesity in animals. It is absorbed into the foods, spiking the calories, but unlike eating more fruits or nuts, oil does not make you feel full as it doesn't have any fiber to tell your brain when you are full. In fact, using oil for cooking makes people want to eat even more calories.

Not only does oil have 120 calories per tablespoon and is exceedingly fattening, but when you heat it and fry food in it, it becomes more dangerous. When oils are heated to varying temperatures, aldehydic lipid oxidation products are produced, which are highly mutagenic and carcinogenic.[7] The foods that most link childhood and adolescent diets with adult breast cancer may be cooking oils and French fries. A prospective observational study as part of the Nurses' Health Study II compared women with the lowest quintile of fat intake in their adolescent years with women who had the highest quintile of fat and found a clear increased cancer risk with increasing oil consumption.[8] Similarly, but more ominous, was the link between consumption of French fries between ages 3 and 5 and breast cancer in later life. For each additional serving of fries per week, adult breast cancer risk went up 27 percent.[9] I call them cancer fries.

BASIC COOKING METHODS AND EQUIPMENT

A few cooking techniques and pieces of kitchen equipment will help you make delicious Nutritarian dishes. Let's review them before you begin to enjoy the recipes in the next chapter.

SAUTÉING WITH WATER AND USING A WOK

You can use water or low-sodium vegetable broth instead of oil to sauté onions, garlic, and other vegetables. Simply heat a skillet, pan, or wok on high heat, add 2–3 tablespoons water or broth, and when it's hot, add your vegetables. Covering the pan occasionally will help the food cook faster. Add additional liquid as needed until the vegetables are tender, but don't add too much or the food will be boiled, not sautéed. Let the pan get dry enough for the food to start to brown just a little before you add more liquid. If you are cooking with mushrooms, they give off their own liquid so you may not need to add any more. Coconut water, tomatoes, and wine are also good cooking liquids.

A wok or large skillet is a kitchen essential. Cook up a variety of vegetables with a tasty sauce and you can have dinner on the table in minutes. Cut ingredients into uniform-size pieces and allow plenty of room so they are not crowded and can cook evenly. Give harder vegetables such as carrots, cauliflower, and broccoli a head start before adding any leafy greens since they only need a short amount of time to wilt a bit. For the best nutrient value, flavor, and texture, cook vegetables only until they are crisp tender, meaning that they are softer than raw but still have some firmness to them.

STEAMING

Steaming is a quick and gentle cooking method that allows valuable nutrients to be retained in the food. It's better than boiling, which causes more nutrients to be lost in the cooking water. Steam on the stovetop with a pot containing a small amount of liquid that you bring to a simmer. Place the item to be cooked in a steamer basket above the liquid, and cover the pot. Steam vegetables only until they start to become tender but still retain some firmness. Depending on the vegetable, 8–12 minutes is all it takes. Steamer baskets are very inexpensive and can be used in any pot that has a lid.

BLENDING

I blend up whole food ingredients such as vegetables, nuts, seeds, fruit (fresh, frozen, and dried), and beans to make my salad dressings, sauces, dips, creamy soups, and desserts. A blender is a critical piece of equipment when it comes to making Nutritarian recipes. Invest in a durable, high-powered blender; you won't regret it. It's helpful when the machine has enough power and speed to process your ingredients to the desired smooth consistency.

If you have only a standard, moderately priced blender, add liquid first and then gradually add the other ingredients. You may need to add a bit more water or liquid than the recipe calls for. You may also need to do a bit more chopping before adding fruits or vegetables to the blender. If you are using nuts, soak them in water overnight to soften them before blending. You can also substitute raw cashew or almond butter for whole nuts. You will only need half the amount because the ground nut butter is denser.

EAT INTACT WHOLE GRAINS

Intact grains are whole grains that have been left as close as possible to their unprocessed, natural state. They still contain all the parts of the grain seed—the bran, germ, and endosperm—and have not been milled, ground, or flaked. Intact grains are even better for you than products made with whole grain flour. They have a superior nutritional profile of antioxidants, vitamins, minerals, and fiber and because they are digested slowly, they have a more favorable glycemic index.

Here are some intact whole grains that are easy to incorporate into your meals:

Amaranth: A gluten-free seed that is popular in South America, amaranth maintains a bit of crunch even after cooking. It is higher in the amino acid lysine than most grains, which makes it a good protein source. It can be simmered like other grains or popped in a hot, dry skillet and then used as a crunchy topping for soup, salads, or vegetable dishes.

Barley: One of the first cultivated grains, barley is a good source of both soluble and insoluble fiber. Add it to soups or stews for a rich, substantial consistency. Mushrooms and barley are a classic soup combination. Hulled barley and hulless barley are two different varieties of barley and both are considered whole grains. Quicker cooking pearl barley has been refined and is not a whole grain.

Buckwheat: Despite its name, buckwheat is the seed of a flowering plant that is not related to wheat. It is a good choice for people who are sensitive to gluten. Make a hot morning cereal using buckwheat instead of oats. For a simple lunch or dinner, lightly toast the buckwheat in a skillet, add water or broth, simmer until tender, and then stir in water-sautéed onions, mushrooms, and greens.

Farro: Cultivated in Italy for centuries, farro has a satisfying creamy yet chewy texture and a mild flavor. It can easily be substituted for rice in a variety of recipes. Combine it with kale and white beans for a tasty entrée. Look for whole grain or semi-pearled farro. Pearled farro cooks faster, but the nutritious germ and bran have been removed; semi-pearled farro has more of its germ and bran. Whole grain farro is harder to find. As it is a type of wheat, farro is unsuitable for people with celiac disease, gluten intolerance, or wheat sensitivity or allergy.

Millet: An ancient seed crop, millet is still a staple in many parts of India and Africa. This small seed cooks quickly and has a mild flavor and light texture. Add it to soups or toss it with beans, tomatoes, and other veggies for a warm and tasty salad.

Quinoa: In recent years, quinoa has become a mainstream grain. It's widely available and commonly found in many recipes. Quinoa is a complete protein; it contains all the essential amino acids. Rinse it before cooking to remove the bitter coating of saponin that is on the seeds.

Steel cut oats: To make steel cut oats, the oat kernel, or groat, is cut into several pieces rather than rolled. Steel cut oats have a chewy, substantial texture and are a great choice for a warm and satisfying breakfast. Cook them 10–20 minutes, depending on the texture you prefer. Stir in your choice of nuts, seeds, and fresh or dried fruit.

Wheat berries: The intact whole grain form of wheat, these wheat kernels, or "berries," contain the wheat bran, germ, and endosperm. To cook wheat berries, cover with water and simmer in a covered pot for about 1 hour or until soft. Pair cooked wheat berries with a vegetable stir-fry or toss them with your salad.

Wild rice: Wild rice is brown and has a slender elongated shape. It is not really rice but the seeds of an aquatic grass native to the northern waters of Minnesota, parts of Wisconsin, and adjacent areas of Canada. Wild rice is a good alternative to brown and black rice, which have been shown to absorb high levels of arsenic from the soil and water they are grown in.

Whole grains combine well with other foods and complement beans and greens nicely. You can easily create a complete dinner by mixing a cooked intact grain with your favorite vegetables, beans, and seasonings. The list below will give you some ideas. Many of these items are probably already in your pantry or refrigerator.

Mix intact grains with:

Cooked beans: chickpeas, kidney beans, white beans, split peas, lentils, edamame

Cooked green leafy vegetables: kale, collards, mustard greens, turnip greens, spinach, cabbage

Salad greens: mixed baby greens, romaine lettuce, red leaf lettuce, Boston lettuce, endive, watercress, arugula

Other vegetables: broccoli, cauliflower, asparagus, tomatoes, mushrooms, carrots, fresh or frozen peas, red or green peppers, hot chili peppers, onions, scallions, sweet potatoes, butternut or other squashes

Nuts and fruit: walnuts, raw almonds, raw pumpkin or sunflower seeds, sesame seeds, berries, mango, apples, currants, raisins

Spices and seasonings: basil, parsley, cilantro, garlic, chili powder, cumin, black or cayenne pepper, cinnamon, no-salt seasoning blends, lemon juice, vinegar

(RE)STOCK YOUR PANTRY

Begin this new diet style by cleaning out your refrigerator and cabinets. Get rid of all the foods that trigger your addictive cravings. Review the healthful menus and recipes in the next chapter, begin to stock your pantry and refrigerator, and then start discovering some exciting new recipes. It may be a big leap from your current eating habits to the diet style I'm recommending, but just wait until you see the miraculous results. You might temporarily feel poorly, but after a week the health transformation begins. Even your taste will improve.

To get you started and to demonstrate the Nutritarian pattern of eating, Chapter 8 provides two weeks of sample menus and a variety of delicious recipes. Use these to modify your eating habits gradually, or jump right in and do it to the limit. You can choose to follow the menus exactly or pick and choose the meals and recipes that work for your life-style and preferences. You can switch around the foods and recipes and eat them in different combinations or at different meals. With leftovers, the two weeks of provided menus should give you enough food to last three or even four weeks. Refrigerate and freeze leftovers and use them for other meals. A homemade dressing lasts for several days, and leftover soup or stew makes a perfect lunch or quick dinner.

FRUIT MAKES THE TASTIEST DESSERTS

The most important message of this book is this: No sugar and white flour, no matter what. I want you to retain the thought that sugar and other concentrated sweeteners and white flour products are simply too dangerous to even consider eating. Get those foods out of your house and out of your life. Healthy breads and desserts taste just as good, but even if it takes you a year to accept this, you still need to see these white foods for what they are: addictive drugs, not food.

Dates, raisins, and dried bananas are good replacements for sweetening agents. When you sweeten with dates instead of sugar, an incredible transformation of human biological function occurs. Dates have fiber and phytonutrients, and they are high in sugar. So how does the sugar in dates compare with the sugar in fast food? What is the effect of using dates and raisins to sweeten desserts rather than more conventional sweeteners such as honey, maple syrup, and sugar? The answers have to do with how much calorically dense, high sugar foods such as dates raise blood sugar or triglycerides and create oxidative stress or free radical formation, like sugar does—and these answers are quite shocking.

When scientists used dates instead of sugar in feeding experiments, they found that the blood sugar did not rise like it does with sugar and other sweeteners, triglycerides did not go up, and any increase in oxidative stress was not measurable.[10] Figs, dates, and unsulfured dried apricots do not seem to cause a problem with health, weight, or blood pressure. This is mostly because their sugar is bound to a huge amount of fiber; and combined with all their minerals, trace elements, and phytonutrients and their effect on the bacteria that coat our digestive surfaces, they have a different biological effect as they activate enzyme cofactors in the metabolism of glucose. The extra components in dates make a big difference. The reported glycemic index or glycemic load for dates classifies them as "low to medium"—not even close to the higher range of sugar, white flour, white rice, and white potato.

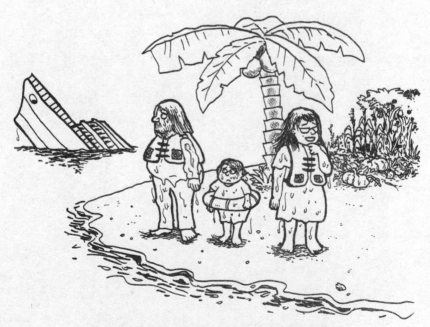

"At least now we'll be able to stick to Dr. Fuhrman's diet."

Certainly, it's easy to eat too much dried fruits and nuts and thereby sabotage your weight-loss goals, but a moderate amount of dried fruits and nuts used in desserts and other recipes is overall favorable, not unfavorable.

You can learn to sweeten and enjoy delicious dishes and desserts with fresh fruit and dried fruit. I share some of my favorites in the next chapter, but hundreds more creative ideas are available in my other books and online to help you make the most delectable healthy desserts ever.

It takes some effort to be super healthy and happy and to have a successful life, but it is so worth it. You can live without fear of disease, you can accomplish what you want to in life, and you can be a good example and leave a favorable legacy for your children and loved ones. Let's all come together and rebuild the health and emotional well-being of Americans by doing whatever we can personally, socially, economically, and politically to establish excellent nutrition all over this beautiful country. Let's stick together and do this.

CHAPTER EIGHT

EATING OUR WAY TO HEALTH

Two Weeks of Sample Menus Followed by
Eighty-Four Great Healthful Recipes

WEEK 1

MONDAY

BREAKFAST
Banana Nut Muffin
Oatmeal*

Fresh or frozen berries

LUNCH
Chili Bean Dip* with
sugar snap peas and
other raw vegetables

Shiitake BLT*

DINNER
Big salad with mixed
greens, tomatoes, red
onion, and shredded
cabbage

Raspberry Dressing*

Easy Lentil and Chickpea
Soup*

Melon or other fruit

TUESDAY

BREAKFAST
Tropical Smoothie*

Sunflower seeds or other
raw nuts or seeds

LUNCH
Big salad with romaine
lettuce, spinach,
tomatoes, and chopped
red onion

Raspberry Dressing*
(leftover) or bottled low-
sodium/no-oil dressing
or flavored vinegar

Easy Lentil and Chickpea
Soup* (leftover)

DINNER
Shredded napa cabbage
tossed with Asian Ginger
Dressing*

Broccoli Stir-Fry with
Tempeh (or chicken or
shrimp)*

Wild Rice

Defrosted frozen
peaches or other fruit

Asterisks indicate recipes that can be found in this chapter.

WEDNESDAY

BREAKFAST
Buckwheat and Berry
Cereal*

LUNCH
Salad-Stuffed Pita
with Creamy Almond
Dressing*

Melon or other fruit

DINNER
Chili Bean Dip* (leftover)
with red bell peppers (or
other raw vegetables)

West African Sweet
Potato Soup*

Steamed fresh or frozen
broccoli or other green
vegetable

Banana Oat Cookies*

THURSDAY

BREAKFAST
Two pieces of fruit

Walnuts or other raw
nuts or seeds

LUNCH
Big salad with mixed
greens, tomatoes,
chopped red onion, and
chopped almonds

Easy Balsamic Almond
Dressing*

West African Sweet
Potato Soup* (leftover)

Grapes or other fruit

DINNER
Tennessee Corn Pone*

Steamed kale or collards

Banana Oat Cookies*
(leftover)

FRIDAY

BREAKFAST
Warm Blueberry
Breakfast*

Homemade Hemp/
Almond Milk*

LUNCH
Kale and Carrot Salad
with Apple Walnut
Dressing*

Melon or other fruit

DINNER
Super Simple Hummus*
with carrots and
cucumbers (or other raw
vegetables)

Black Bean and Avocado
Burgers* or Meat-
Lovers Beef, Bean, and
Mushroom Burgers* on
whole grain rolls with
lettuce, tomato sliced
onion, and low-sugar
ketchup

Vanilla or Chocolate
Nice Cream*

SATURDAY

BREAKFAST
Hot Chai Latte*

Overnight Cinnamon
Apple Oatmeal*

LUNCH
Calypso Salad*

Orange or other fruit

DINNER
Simple Guacamole*
with romaine leaves and
other raw vegetables

Bean Enchiladas*

Fresh or frozen mango
or other fruit

SUNDAY

BREAKFAST
Sweet Beet Carrot Bars*

Fresh or frozen berries

Unsweetened soy,
hemp, or almond milk

LUNCH
Marinated Mushroom
Salad*

Creamy Tomato and
White Bean Soup*

DINNER
New-Style Hash with
Greens and Spicy
Pumpkin Seeds*

Sweet Potato Fries*

Fruit Slushie*

WEEK 2

MONDAY

BREAKFAST
Breakfast Veggie Wraps*

Fresh or frozen berries topped with ground flaxseeds

LUNCH
Millet Salad with Veggies and Black Beans* served over mixed greens

Pineapple or other fruit

DINNER
Succotash Casserole Stew with Cornmeal and Okra Dumplings*

Steamed broccoli

Six-Minute Baked Apple*

TUESDAY

BREAKFAST
Chocolate Smoothie*

LUNCH
Lentil Wraps with Peppers and Onions*

Shredded Brussels Sprouts*

Orange or other fruit

DINNER
Simple Guacamole* with endive leaves (or other raw vegetables)

Dr. Fuhrman's Anticancer Soup*

Sweet Beet Carrot Bars* (leftover)

WEDNESDAY

BREAKFAST
Peach and Berry Breakfast Cobbler*

Unsulfured dried apricots

LUNCH
Big salad with mixed greens, tomato, cucumber, and chopped onion

Easy Balsamic Almond Dressing* or bottled low-sodium/no-oil dressing or flavored vinegar

Dr. Fuhrman's Anticancer Soup* (leftover)

DINNER
Veggie Pizza*

Eggplant Almond Chips*

Strawbeany Ice Cream*

THURSDAY

BREAKFAST
Overnight Cinnamon
Apple Oatmeal*

LUNCH
Big salad with romaine
lettuce, mixed greens,
tomato, black beans,
corn, and pumpkin
seeds (and other
assorted vegetables as
desired)

Simple Guacamole*
(leftover)

Fresh or frozen berries

DINNER
Red Beans with Cajun-
Spiced Zucchini and
Quinoa (with optional
chicken)*

Steamed green beans
with lemon

Defrosted frozen cherries
or other fruit

FRIDAY

BREAKFAST
"Drink Your Breakfast"
Smoothie*

Fresh or frozen berries
with chopped almonds

LUNCH
Chickpea Tuno Salad*
served over chopped
romaine lettuce

Sliced tomatoes

DINNER
Smoky Collard Greens
with Pineapple and
Black-Eyed Peas*

Caribbean-Spiced Baked
Tofu*

Sweet Potato Pie with
Coconut Pecan Crust*

SATURDAY

BREAKFAST
Two pieces of fruit

1 ounce (about ¼ cup)
pumpkin seeds (or other
raw nuts or seeds)

LUNCH
Big salad with romaine
lettuce, spinach,
tomatoes, shredded
cabbage, and choice
of beans (and other
assorted vegetables as
desired)

Nutritarian Ranch
Dressing*

DINNER
Butternut Squash Soup
with Mushrooms*

Stuffed Red Peppers*

Grapes or other fruit

SUNDAY

BREAKFAST

Scrambled Oats* or Weekend Breakfast Frittata*

Fresh or frozen berries

LUNCH

Caribbean-Spiced Baked Tofu* served with mixed greens, tomatoes, and avocado slices

Clementines or other fruit

DINNER

Quinoa Walnut Loaf*

California Creamed Kale*

Sweet Potato Pie with Coconut Pecan Crust* (leftover)

NUTRITARIAN RECIPES

Red Lentil Sauce, 224

Simple Guacamole, 225

Super Simple Hummus, 225

Walnut Cream Vinaigrette, 225

SALADS

Broccoli Raisin Salad, 226

Butternut Squash Salad with Toasted Pumpkin Seeds, 226

Calypso Salad, 227

Chickpea Tuno Salad, 228

Kale and Carrot Salad with Apple Walnut Dressing, 228

Marinated Mushroom Salad, 229

Millet Salad with Veggies and Black Beans, 230

Mixed Greens with Fruits, Nuts, and Roasted Plantains, 231

SOUPS AND STEWS

Broccoli Lentil Soup, 232

Butternut Squash Soup with Mushrooms, 232

Citrusy Black Bean Soup, 233

Corn and Red Pepper Soup with Sweet Potatoes and Kale, 234

Creamy Tomato and White Bean Soup, 234

Dr. Fuhrman's Anticancer Soup, 235

Easy Lentil and Chickpea Soup, 236

Herbed Split Pea Soup, 236

Succotash Casserole Stew with Cornmeal and Okra Dumplings, 237

Tempeh Chili with Sriracha, 238

West African Sweet Potato Soup, 239

MAIN DISHES AND VEGETABLE SIDES

Barbecue Baked Beans, 240

Bean Enchiladas, 240

Broccoli Stir-Fry with Tempeh (or chicken or shrimp), 241

California Creamed Kale, 242

BURGERS, WRAPS, AND QUICK FOOD

DESSERTS

Beverages and Smoothies

Blueberry Orange Smoothie

SERVES 2

1 orange, peeled and seeded

1 banana

1 cup frozen blueberries

1 tablespoon ground flaxseeds

2 cups chopped kale or romaine lettuce

Blend all ingredients together in a high-powered blender until smooth and creamy.

PER SERVING: CALORIES 179; PROTEIN 4G; CARBOHYDRATES 39G; TOTAL FAT 2.7G; SATURATED FAT 0.3G; SODIUM 32MG; FIBER 7.5G; BETA-CAROTENE 6,279MCG; VITAMIN C 129MG; CALCIUM 139MG; IRON 1.7MG; FOLATE 64 MCG; MAGNESIUM 64MG; ZINC 0.6MG; SELENIUM 2.2MCG

Chocolate Smoothie

SERVES 2

2 cups baby spinach

2 cups chopped romaine lettuce

2 cups frozen blueberries or cherries

1/2 cup unsweetened soy, hemp, or almond milk

1 banana

2 regular or 1 Medjool date, pitted

2 tablespoons natural nonalkalized cocoa powder

1 tablespoon ground flaxseeds

Blend all ingredients in a high-powered blender until smooth and creamy.

PER SERVING: CALORIES 230; PROTEIN 6G; CARBOHYDRATES 49G; TOTAL FAT 4.6G; SATURATED FAT 0.9G; SODIUM 55MG; FIBER 11.2G; BETA-CAROTENE 4,213MCG; VITAMIN C 19MG; CALCIUM 161MG; IRON 3.0MG; FOLATE 151MCG; MAGNESIUM 111MG; ZINC 1.3MG; SELENIUM 2.9MCG

"Drink Your Breakfast" Smoothie

SERVES 1

3 cups chopped kale

1/2 avocado

1/4 organic lemon with peel

1/2 banana (frozen works best)

5–6 cherry tomatoes

1 cup water

1 cup ice

Blend all ingredients in a high-powered blender until smooth and creamy.

PER SERVING: CALORIES 287; PROTEIN 10G; CARBOHYDRATES 46G; TOTAL FAT 12.3G; SATURATED FAT 1.7G; SODIUM 107MG; FIBER 12.5G; BETA-CAROTENE 18,989MCG; VITAMIN C 285MG; CALCIUM 315MG; IRON 4.4MG; FOLATE 145MCG; MAGNESIUM 119MG; ZINC 1.6MG; SELENIUM 2.7MCG

Homemade Hemp/Almond Milk

SERVES 5

4 cups water

1/3 cup hemp seeds

1/3 cup raw almonds

2–4 regular or 1–2 Medjool dates, pitted

Blend all ingredients in a high-powered blender until smooth.

PER SERVING: CALORIES 123; PROTEIN 4G; CARBOHYDRATES 10G; TOTAL FAT 8.2G; SATURATED FAT 0.7G; SODIUM 10MG; FIBER 5.4G; BETA-CAROTENE 4MCG; CALCIUM 105MG; IRON 1.3MG; FOLATE 5MCG; MAGNESIUM 68MG; ZINC 0.9MG; SELENIUM 6.5MCG

Hot Chai Latte

SERVES 1

1 teaspoon Chai Spice Mixture

2 regular dates or 1 Medjool date, pitted

1 tablespoon chia seeds

1 1/2 cups unsweetened soy, hemp, or almond milk

For the Chai Spice Mixture

2 teaspoons ground cinnamon

2 teaspoons ground cardamom

1 teaspoon ground ginger

1 teaspoon ground cloves

1 teaspoon ground nutmeg

Blend all ingredients in a high-powered blender on high until smooth and hot (about 4 minutes) or use alternative method of heating.

PER SERVING: CALORIES 180; PROTEIN 5G; CARBOHYDRATES 27G; TOTAL FAT 7.5G; SATURATED FAT 0.3G; SODIUM 281MG; FIBER 6.4G; BETA-CAROTENE 24MCG; CALCIUM 879MG; IRON 2.6MG; FOLATE 8MCG; MAGNESIUM 76MG; ZINC 0.9MG; SELENIUM 5.6MCG

Tropical Smoothie

SERVES 4

2 cups unsweetened soy, hemp, or almond milk

2 bananas

1 cup frozen pineapple

1 cup frozen mango

2–3 cups chopped romaine lettuce or kale

2 tablespoons ground flaxseeds

Blend ingredients together in a high-powered blender.

PER SERVING: CALORIES 140; PROTEIN 3G; CARBOHYDRATES 28G; TOTAL FAT 3.4G; SATURATED FAT 0.2G; SODIUM 97MG; FIBER 4.2G; BETA-CAROTENE 1,522MCG; VITAMIN C 41MG; CALCIUM 287MG; IRON 1.2MG; FOLATE 73MCG; MAGNESIUM 51MG; ZINC 0.5MG; SELENIUM 1.9MCG

Apple Bean Breakfast

SERVES 2

1 apple, cored and chopped
1/4 cup water
1 teaspoon cinnamon
1/2 teaspoon nutmeg
3 whole cloves

1/4 cup frozen chopped kale, spinach, or collards (more if using fresh)
1/4 cup cooked kidney or other beans
1/4 cup raisins
1/4 cup chopped walnuts or other raw nuts

Place the chopped apple in a saucepan with the water. Begin cooking over medium-high heat. Add the remaining ingredients, stir, and cook until the apples are tender, about 5–10 minutes. Remove cloves.

Drain off excess water, if desired.

PER SERVING: CALORIES 237; PROTEIN 6G; CARBOHYDRATES 36G; TOTAL FAT 10.2G; SATURATED FAT 1.1G; SODIUM 23MG; FIBER 7.4G; BETA-CAROTENE 1,400MCG; VITAMIN C 7MG; CALCIUM 72MG; IRON 2.2MG; FOLATE 75MCG; MAGNESIUM 60MG; ZINC 0.9MG; SELENIUM 2.3MCG

Banana Nut Muffin Oatmeal

SERVES 1

2/3 cup water
1/3 cup old-fashioned or steel cut oats (see Note)
1–2 dates, chopped, or 1 tablespoon raisins
1 tablespoon ground flaxseeds

1 banana, cut into chunks
1 tablespoon chopped walnuts
1/4 cup unsweetened soy, almond, or hemp milk

Place water, oats, and dates in a small saucepan and bring to a gentle boil. Reduce heat and simmer 4–5 minutes, or until oats are tender, stirring occasionally to prevent sticking. Place in bowl. Stir in flaxseeds, banana chunks, walnuts, and milk

Note: If using steel cut oats, increase water to 1 1/3 cups and simmer, covered, for 15 minutes, stirring occasionally.

PER SERVING: CALORIES 342; PROTEIN 9G; CARBOHYDRATES 62G; TOTAL FAT 9.1G; SATURATED FAT 1.1G; SODIUM 41MG; FIBER 9.4G; BETA-CAROTENE 33MCG; VITAMIN C 10MG; CALCIUM 53MG; IRON 8MG; FOLATE 47MCG; MAGNESIUM 89MG; ZINC 0.7MG; SELENIUM 6.5MCG

Breakfast Veggie Wraps

SERVES 2

1/2 cup chopped green bell pepper

1/2 cup chopped onion

7 ounces extra firm tofu, drained (half a block)

1 medium tomato, chopped

2 cups firmly packed spinach

1/2 teaspoon garlic powder or no-salt seasoning blend such as Mrs. Dash

1/2 teaspoon turmeric

1 tablespoon nutritional yeast

2 whole grain flour tortillas

1/4 cup low-sodium ketchup or salsa

In a large skillet, heat 2–3 tablespoons water and sauté the green pepper and onion until tender, about 2–3 minutes.

Squeeze as much water as possible from the tofu, then crumble over the peppers and onions. Add tomato, spinach, garlic powder, turmeric, and nutritional yeast and cook until tofu is lightly yellow-browned, about 5–8 minutes, stirring frequently.

Spread the cooked tofu on the tortillas. Top with ketchup or salsa and roll up.

PER SERVING: CALORIES 309; PROTEIN 19G; CARBOHYDRATES 44G; TOTAL FAT 8.3G; SATURATED FAT 1.5G; SODIUM 189MG; FIBER 9.7G; BETA-CAROTENE 2,210MCG; VITAMIN C 55MG; CALCIUM 298MG; IRON 5.4MG; FOLATE 101MCG; MAGNESIUM 87MG; ZINC 2.1MG; SELENIUM 10.6MCG

Buckwheat and Berry Cereal

SERVES 3

1/2 cup raw buckwheat groats, rinsed (see Note)

1 cup unsweetened soy, hemp, or almond milk plus extra if desired

1/2 teaspoon cinnamon

1/2 teaspoon vanilla or almond extract

1 medium apple, diced or grated

1 tablespoon raw almond butter

1 tablespoon chia seeds

1 cup fresh or thawed frozen berries

Place buckwheat, 1 cup of the nondairy milk, cinnamon, and vanilla in a pan. Bring to a boil, reduce heat, cover and simmer for 6 minutes or until groats are soft but not mushy and almost all liquid is absorbed. Stir in apple, almond butter, and chia seeds and simmer for another minute. Stir in berries. Add additional nondairy milk if desired.

May be refrigerated and eaten cold or reheated.

Note: Buckwheat groats are seeds from the buckwheat plant. They are unrelated to wheat and do not contain gluten. Choose raw buckwheat groats, not kasha, which is toasted.

PER SERVING: CALORIES 320; PROTEIN 9G; CARBOHYDRATES 57G; TOTAL FAT 8.9G; SATURATED FAT 0.8G; SODIUM 100MG; FIBER 9.9G; BETA-CAROTENE 38MCG; VITAMIN C 11MG; CALCIUM 339MG; IRON 2.5MG; FOLATE 27MCG; MAGNESIUM 147MG; ZINC 1.7MG; SELENIUM 6.5MCG

Overnight Cinnamon Apple Oatmeal

SERVES 3

1 cup uncooked old-fashioned or steel cut rolled oats

2 1/2 cups unsweetened soy, hemp, or almond milk

1/4 cup raisins or currants

1 apple, peeled, cored, and chopped

1/4 cup chopped walnuts

1 tablespoon ground flaxseeds

1/2 teaspoon cinnamon

Combine oats, nondairy milk, and raisins in a bowl. Refrigerate overnight.

In the morning, mix in the chopped apples, walnuts, ground flaxseeds, and cinnamon. Stir in additional nondairy milk if desired.

PER SERVING: CALORIES 246; PROTEIN 7G; CARBOHYDRATES 31G; TOTAL FAT 12G; SATURATED FAT 1.0G; SODIUM 157MG; FIBER 5G; BETA-CAROTENE 2MCG; VITAMIN C 0.4MG; CALCIUM 456MG; IRON 8.1MG; FOLATE 14MCG; MAGNESIUM 44MG; ZINC 0.6MG; SELENIUM 1.2MCG

Peach and Berry Breakfast Cobbler

SERVES 2

1 cup fresh or frozen sliced peaches

1 cup fresh or frozen strawberries or mixed berries

1/2 cup old-fashioned rolled oats

2 tablespoons raisins

1/8 teaspoon vanilla extract

1/2 cup water (only if using fresh fruit)

2 tablespoons chopped raw walnuts

1/4 teaspoon cinnamon

1/4 teaspoon nutmeg

Combine peaches, berries, oats, raisins, and vanilla in a small saucepan. Add water if using fresh fruit. Cook on medium–high heat until bubbling. Add walnuts, cinnamon, and nutmeg; cover; reduce heat and cook 8–10 minutes on low. Serve warm.

PER SERVING: CALORIES 210; PROTEIN 5G; CARBOHYDRATES 36G; TOTAL FAT 6.9G; SATURATED FAT 0.8G; SODIUM 2MG; FIBER 5.9G; BETA-CAROTENE 132MCG; VITAMIN C 54MG; CALCIUM 33MG; IRON 6MG; FOLATE 31MCG; MAGNESIUM 33MG; ZINC 0.5MG; SELENIUM 0.8MCG

Scrambled Oats

SERVES 4

1 cup steel cut oats (see Note)
2 cups water or low-sodium vegetable broth
1 tablespoon nutritional yeast
1 teaspoon low-sodium miso paste

1/2 teaspoon turmeric
2 cups fresh spinach or other leafy greens
1 cup lightly sautéed sliced mushrooms
Grated red onion for garnish

Combine oats, water or vegetable broth, nutritional yeast, miso, and turmeric in a saucepan and cook, stirring frequently, for about 20 minutes or until oats are tender. Stir in spinach and mushrooms and cook until spinach is wilted.

Garnish with grated onion.

Note: You may also use old-fashioned oats in this recipe. Reduce cooking time to 5 minutes.

PER SERVING: CALORIES 98; PROTEIN 5G; CARBOHYDRATES 17G; TOTAL FAT 1.8G; SATURATED FAT 0.3G; SODIUM 72MG; FIBER 3.2G; BETA-CAROTENE 845MCG; VITAMIN C 5MG; CALCIUM 24MG; IRON 5.7MG; FOLATE 34MCG; MAGNESIUM 19MG; ZINC 0.6MG; SELENIUM 1.9MCG

Sweet Beet Carrot Bars

SERVES 10

1 cup whole wheat flour
1 cup oat flour (see Note)
1 tablespoon low-sodium baking soda
1 cup chopped dates
1 ripe banana, mashed
1 apple, cored, peeled, and chopped

1 cup chopped pineapple
1 cup raw beets, peeled and shredded
1 carrot, peeled and shredded
1 teaspoon vanilla extract
1 cup chopped walnuts
1/2 cup currants or raisins

Preheat oven to 350°F. In a large bowl, combine flour and baking soda. Mix in chopped dates, mashed banana, apple, pineapple, beets, carrots, vanilla, walnuts, and currants.

Spread in a lightly oiled 9-by-9-inch baking pan and bake for 40 minutes or until a toothpick inserted into the center comes out clean. Cool and cut into squares.

Note: You can purchase oat flour in most large supermarkets or health food stores, or make it yourself by processing old-fashioned oats in a food processor until finely ground.

PER SERVING: CALORIES 248; PROTEIN 6G; CARBOHYDRATES 42G; TOTAL FAT 8.7G; SATURATED FAT 1G; SODIUM 142MG; FIBER 6.0G; BETA-CAROTENE 527MCG; VITAMIN C 14MG; CALCIUM 36MG; IRON 3.4MG; FOLATE 43MCG; MAGNESIUM 55MG; ZINC 1MG; SELENIUM 8.7MCG

Warm Blueberry Breakfast

SERVES 2

2 cups frozen blueberries

1/2 cup unsweetened soy, hemp, or almond milk

1/4 cup unsweetened shredded coconut

1/4 cup chopped walnuts

1/4 cup dried currants or raisins

1 banana, sliced

Heat frozen blueberries and nondairy milk until warm. Add remaining ingredients and stir well.

PER SERVING: CALORIES 315; PROTEIN 6G; CARBOHYDRATES 45G; TOTAL FAT 15.1G; SATURATED FAT 4.1G; SODIUM 28MG; FIBER 8.7G; BETA-CAROTENE 65MCG; VITAMIN C 10MG; CALCIUM 117MG; IRON 1.7MG; FOLATE 41MCG; MAGNESIUM 64MG; ZINC 1.1MG; SELENIUM 2.6MCG

Weekend Breakfast Frittata

SERVES 2

1/2 green bell pepper, seeded and chopped

4 green onions, chopped

1 medium portabella mushroom, cut into 1/2-inch slices

2 ounces fresh baby spinach

6 grape tomatoes, halved

2 eggs

1/4 cup unsweetened almond, soy, or hemp milk

1 ounce nondairy cheddar cheese, grated

Wipe a 10-inch oven-proof pan or skillet with a small amount of olive oil. Heat pan over medium heat, add green pepper and sauté until almost tender; add green onions and mushrooms and continue to cook until peppers are tender. Add baby spinach and cook until wilted, then mix in tomatoes. Spread vegetables evenly in pan and reduce heat to low.

In a bowl, mix eggs and nondairy milk. Turn heat up to medium and pour in egg mixture, distributing evenly in the pan. Cook on stove until the sides of the frittata start to brown. Sprinkle grated nondairy cheese evenly over the top. Remove pan from stove and broil on middle rack for about 2 minutes or until cheese is melted and frittata top starts to brown.

PER SERVING: CALORIES 174; PROTEIN 13G; CARBOHYDRATES 9G; TOTAL FAT 10.2G; SATURATED FAT 2.5G; CHOLESTEROL 188.1MG; SODIUM 210MG; FIBER 3G; BETA-CAROTENE 2,069MCG; VITAMIN C 45MG; CALCIUM 225MG; IRON 2.7MG; FOLATE 119MCG; MAGNESIUM 52MG; ZINC 1.7MG; SELENIUM 23.2MCG

Salad Dressings, Dips, and Sauces

Asian Ginger Dressing

SERVES 4

1/2 cup chopped onion

1/4 cup peanut butter

1/2 tablespoon unhulled sesame seeds

6 tablespoons water

5 tablespoons rice vinegar

1–2 tablespoons minced fresh ginger

2 tablespoons chopped celery

2 tablespoons no-salt-added tomato paste (see Note)

1/2 teaspoon Bragg Liquid Aminos or reduced-sodium soy sauce

3 regular or 1 1/2 Medjool dates, pitted and chopped

1 teaspoon lemon juice

1 clove garlic

Ground black pepper, to taste

Blend all ingredients in a high-powered blender until smooth but with texture.

Note: Select tomato products packaged in glass or cartons to avoid BPA.

PER SERVING: CALORIES 146; PROTEIN 5G; CARBOHYDRATES 15G; TOTAL FAT 8.4G; SATURATED FAT 1.2G; SODIUM 52MG; FIBER 3G; BETA-CAROTENE 135MCG; VITAMIN C 5MG; CALCIUM 44MG; IRON 1MG; FOLATE 37MCG; MAGNESIUM 46MG; ZINC 0.8MG; SELENIUM 2.3MCG

Chili Bean Dip

SERVES 6

1 1/2 cups cooked or 1 (15-ounce) can low-sodium kidney beans, drained

1 1/2 cups cooked or 1 (15-ounce) can low-sodium pinto beans, drained

2 tablespoons lemon juice

4 garlic cloves

1 teaspoon Bragg Liquid Aminos or reduced-sodium soy sauce

1/2 cup unhulled sesame seeds or tahini (puréed sesame seeds)

3 regular or 1 1/2 Medjool dates, pitted

1 teaspoon chili powder or to taste

3/4 teaspoon cumin

1/4 teaspoon cayenne pepper, or to taste

1/4 cup chopped cilantro

Place all ingredients except cilantro in food processor or high-powered blender and process until smooth. Stir in cilantro.

PER SERVING: CALORIES 203; PROTEIN 10G; CARBOHYDRATES 28G; TOTAL FAT 6.6G; SATURATED FAT 0.9G; SODIUM 48MG; FIBER 8.7G; BETA-CAROTENE 113MCG; VITAMIN C 4MG; CALCIUM 162MG; IRON 4MG; FOLATE 145MCG; MAGNESIUM 86MG; ZINC 1.9MG; SELENIUM 7.8MCG

Chocobean Butter

SERVES 10

1 cup raw almonds
1 cup walnuts
½ cup cooked black beans
3 tablespoons natural cocoa powder

8 regular or 4 Medjool dates, pitted, chopped
¼ cup unsweetened soy, hemp, or almond milk
1 teaspoon alcohol-free vanilla extract

Roast almonds and walnuts in oven at 350°F, stirring occasionally, until just lightly toasted, about 5 minutes. Place in food processor and process to the consistency of a coarse powder.

Add remaining ingredients and process until smooth and spreadable. Stop the food processor and scrape down the sides as needed. Store refrigerated. It will keep for up to 7 days.

Serving Suggestion: Spread on 100 percent whole grain bread and top with lettuce leaves and sliced bananas.

PER SERVING: CALORIES 196; PROTEIN 6G; CARBOHYDRATES 12G; TOTAL FAT 15.7G; SATURATED FAT 1.4G; SODIUM 6MG; FIBER 4G; BETA-CAROTENE 2MCG; CALCIUM 60MG; IRON 1.3MG; FOLATE 33MCG; MAGNESIUM 75MG; ZINC 1MG; SELENIUM 1.5MCG

Easy Balsamic Almond Dressing

SERVES 1

2 tablespoons water
1 tablespoon raw almond butter
1 ½ tablespoons balsamic vinegar
¼ teaspoon onion powder

¼ teaspoon garlic powder
⅛ teaspoon dried oregano
⅛ teaspoon dried basil

Mash water into almond butter and then whisk in vinegar and other ingredients until smooth.

PER SERVING: CALORIES 127; PROTEIN 4G; CARBOHYDRATES 9G; TOTAL FAT 8.9G; SATURATED FAT 0.7G; SODIUM 10MG; FIBER 2G; BETA-CAROTENE 3MCG; CALCIUM 74MG; IRON 1.1MG; FOLATE 10MCG; MAGNESIUM 51MG; ZINC 0.6MG; SELENIUM 0.7MCG

Nutritarian Ranch Dressing

SERVES 10

1 (12.3-ounce) package firm silken tofu

1/4 cup raw cashews

1 tablespoon ground chia seeds

3 dates, pitted

2 cloves garlic

2 scallions, white and green parts separated and finely chopped

1/4 cup lemon juice

1/2 teaspoon dried basil

1/2 teaspoon dried thyme

1/2 teaspoon dried oregano

1 tablespoon nutritional yeast

1/2 teaspoon Bragg Liquid Aminos or reduced-sodium soy sauce

Freshly ground black pepper or cayenne pepper, to taste

2 tablespoons chopped fresh parsley

2 tablespoons chopped fresh dill

In a high-powered blender, purée the tofu, cashews, chia seeds, dates, garlic, white parts of scallions, lemon juice, basil, thyme, oregano, nutritional yeast, Bragg Liquid Aminos, and pepper. Stir in the parsley, dill, and green parts of scallions and refrigerate until ready to serve. Add water if needed to adjust consistency.

PER SERVING: CALORIES 59; PROTEIN 4G; CARBOHYDRATES 5G; TOTAL FAT 2.8G; SATURATED FAT 0.5G; SODIUM 26MG; FIBER 1.1G; BETA-CAROTENE 67MCG; VITAMIN C 4MG; CALCIUM 32MG; IRON 1.2MG; FOLATE 7MCG; MAGNESIUM 27MG; ZINC 0.7MG; SELENIUM 1.4MCG

Orange Sesame Dressing

SERVES 4

1/4 cup unhulled sesame seeds, divided

1/4 cup raw cashew nuts

2 navel oranges, peeled

2 tablespoons blood orange vinegar or apple cider vinegar

Toast the sesame seeds in a dry skillet over medium-high heat for 3 minutes, mixing with a wooden spoon and shaking the pan frequently. In a high-powered blender, combine 2 tablespoons of the sesame seeds, cashews, oranges, and vinegar. If needed, add orange juice to adjust consistency.

Sprinkle remaining sesame seeds on top of salad.

Serving Suggestion: Toss with mixed greens, tomatoes, red onions, and additional diced oranges, strawberries, or kiwi.

PER SERVING: CALORIES 140; PROTEIN 4G; CARBOHYDRATES 15G; TOTAL FAT 8.3G; SATURATED FAT 1.3G; SODIUM 5MG; FIBER 2.9G; BETA-CAROTENE 61MCG; VITAMIN C 41MG; CALCIUM 123MG; IRON 2.0MG; FOLATE 35MCG; MAGNESIUM 65MG; ZINC 1.3MG; SELENIUM 4.8MCG

Raspberry Dressing

SERVES 4

1 ¼ cups frozen raspberries
(or strawberries)
½ apple, peeled and quartered
4 regular or 2 Medjool dates, pitted
½ clove garlic, chopped

½ teaspoon Dijon mustard
¼ cup water
1 tablespoon balsamic vinegar
1 teaspoon fresh lime juice

Blend ingredients in a high-powered blender until creamy and smooth.

PER SERVING: CALORIES 99; PROTEIN 1G; CARBOHYDRATES 26G; TOTAL FAT 0.2G; SODIUM 10MG;
FIBER 3.2G; BETA-CAROTENE 41MCG; VITAMIN C 21MG; CALCIUM 27MG; IRON 0.6MG; FOLATE 12MCG;
MAGNESIUM 20MG; ZINC 0.2MG; SELENIUM 0.6MCG

Red Lentil Sauce

SERVES 4

½ cup dried red lentils
1 medium onion, chopped
1 clove garlic, chopped
1 ½ cups carrot juice

1 tablespoon MatoZest or other no-salt
seasoning blend, adjusted to taste
1 teaspoon ground cumin
½ teaspoon balsamic vinegar
Pinch cayenne pepper, or to taste

Place the lentils, onions, garlic, and carrot juice in a saucepan. Bring to a boil, cover, and simmer 20–30 minutes until the lentils are soft and pale. Add more carrot juice if needed. Blend the cooked lentil mixture, MatoZest, cumin, vinegar, and cayenne pepper in a food processor or high-powered blender to a smooth purée.

Serve with steamed broccoli, cauliflower, or other vegetables.

PER SERVING: CALORIES 142; PROTEIN 8G; CARBOHYDRATES 27G; TOTAL FAT 0.6G; SATURATED FAT
0.1G; SODIUM 66MG; FIBER 8.9G; BETA-CAROTENE 8,243MCG; VITAMIN C 12MG; CALCIUM 55MG; IRON
2.9MG; FOLATE 131MCG; MAGNESIUM 51MG; ZINC 1.4MG; SELENIUM 2.9MCG

Simple Guacamole

SERVES 4

2 ripe avocados, peeled and pitted
1/2 cup finely chopped onion
1 small tomato, chopped
1 clove garlic, diced

1/4 cup minced fresh cilantro
2 tablespoons fresh lime juice
1/4 teaspoon ground cumin
1/4 teaspoon freshly ground black pepper

Using a fork, mash the avocados in a small bowl. Add the remaining ingredients and stir well.

PER SERVING: CALORIES 130; PROTEIN 2G; CARBOHYDRATES 10G; TOTAL FAT 10.6G; SATURATED FAT 1.5G; SODIUM 8MG; FIBER 5.4G; BETA-CAROTENE 188MCG; VITAMIN C 13MG; CALCIUM 21MG; IRON 0.7MG; FOLATE 69MCG; MAGNESIUM 26MG; ZINC 0.6MG; SELENIUM 0.5MCG

Super Simple Hummus

SERVES 4

1 (15-ounce) can garbanzo beans, no-salt-added or low-sodium
2 tablespoons lemon juice

1/4 cup unhulled sesame seeds
1 clove garlic
1/2 teaspoon ground cumin

Blend all ingredients in a high-powered blender or food processor. Use the garbanzo liquid from the can to adjust consistency. Can be refrigerated in an airtight container for up to 4 days.

PER SERVING: CALORIES 156; PROTEIN 7G; CARBOHYDRATES 20G; TOTAL FAT 6.1G; SATURATED FAT 0.8G; SODIUM 6MG; FIBER 5.8G; BETA-CAROTENE 12MCG; VITAMIN C 4MG; CALCIUM 122MG; IRON 3.3MG; FOLATE 116MCG; MAGNESIUM 63MG; ZINC 1.7MG; SELENIUM 5MCG

Walnut Cream Vinaigrette

SERVES 4

1/4 cup balsamic vinegar
1/2 cup unsweetened soy milk or almond milk
1/4 cup walnuts

1/4 cup raisins
1 teaspoon Dijon mustard
1 clove garlic
1/4 teaspoon dried thyme

Combine all ingredients in a high-powered blender and blend until smooth.

PER SERVING: CALORIES 89; PROTEIN 2G; CARBOHYDRATES 11G; TOTAL FAT 4.5G; SATURATED FAT 0.4G; SODIUM 43MG; FIBER 0.8G; BETA-CAROTENE 3MCG; VITAMIN C 1MG; CALCIUM 83MG; IRON 0.7MG; FOLATE 7MCG; MAGNESIUM 18MG; ZINC 0.3MG; SELENIUM 0.9MCG

Salads

Broccoli Raisin Salad

SERVES 4

1 head broccoli florets cut to bite size

1/4 cup raisins, divided

1 apple, shredded

1/4 cup raw sunflower seeds

3/4 cup unsweetened soy, hemp, or almond milk

1/2 cup raw mixed cashews and almonds

2 tablespoons fresh lemon juice

Combine broccoli, 2 tablespoons of the raisins, shredded apple, and sunflower seeds in a large bowl. In a high-powered blender, blend remaining 2 tablespoons raisins with nondairy milk, nuts, and lemon juice. Pour desired amount of dressing over broccoli mixture and toss to combine. Chill.

PER SERVING: CALORIES 268; PROTEIN 11G; CARBOHYDRATES 32G; TOTAL FAT 13.6G; SATURATED FAT 2G; SODIUM 63MG; FIBER 7.2G; BETA-CAROTENE 564MCG; VITAMIN C 141MG; CALCIUM 90MG; IRON 3.2MG; FOLATE 131MCG; MAGNESIUM 127MG; ZINC 2.1MG; SELENIUM 11.9MCG

Butternut Squash Salad with Toasted Pumpkin Seeds

SERVES 2

4 cups butternut squash, peeled and cubed

Cooking spray or minimal amount of olive oil

1/2 teaspoon black pepper, divided

2 medium shallots, minced

1/4 cup balsamic vinegar

2 tablespoons water

2 teaspoons Dijon mustard

10 cups (about 10 ounces) mixed baby greens

1/4 cup raw pumpkin seeds, lightly toasted (see Note)

Preheat oven to 350°F. Arrange squash in a single layer on a baking pan lightly coated with cooking spray or olive oil. Sprinkle with 1/4 teaspoon black pepper. Bake 35 minutes or until squash is tender and lightly browned, stirring every 15 minutes. Remove from oven, keep warm.

Water-sauté shallots until tender. In a small bowl, whisk together shallots, remaining 1/4 teaspoon pepper, balsamic vinegar, water, and Dijon mustard. Place salad greens in a large bowl. Drizzle vinegar mixture over greens; toss gently to coat. Arrange on serving plates; top with warm butternut squash and pumpkin seeds.

Note: Toast pumpkin seeds in oven at 300°F for 4 minutes or until lightly browned, stirring occasionally.

PER SERVING: CALORIES 295; PROTEIN 11G; CARBOHYDRATES 49G; TOTAL FAT 9.1G; SATURATED FAT 1.6G; SODIUM 108MG; FIBER 10.5G; BETA-CAROTENE 18,918MCG; VITAMIN C 74MG; CALCIUM 270MG; IRON 5.7MG; FOLATE 272MCG; MAGNESIUM 238MG; ZINC 2MG; SELENIUM 5.5MCG

Calypso Salad

SERVES 6

For the Salad

1/2 pound shredded red cabbage

1/2 pound shredded green cabbage

1 cup shredded carrots

1 red bell pepper, seeded and diced

1 jalapeno pepper, seeded and finely chopped (include some seeds if you like it hot)

1 cup corn kernels, fresh or frozen, thawed

1 chopped mango

6 chopped green onions

Chopped fresh cilantro to taste

2 cups cooked black beans

3 tablespoons unhulled sesame seeds, toasted

For the Dressing

1/3 cup unsweetened hemp, soy, or almond milk

1/2 cup fresh or frozen pineapple

1/4 cup fresh orange juice

1/4 cup fresh lime juice

1/4 cup raw cashews

1/4 cup raw almonds

1 tablespoon blood orange vinegar or rice vinegar

1/4 cup currants or raisins

Mix all salad ingredients except sesame seeds together in a large bowl. Combine all dressing ingredients in a high-powered blender and blend until smooth and creamy. Toss the salad with desired amount of dressing and garnish with sesame seeds.

PER SERVING: CALORIES 297; PROTEIN 11G; CARBOHYDRATES 50G; TOTAL FAT 8.4G; SATURATED FAT 1.4G; SODIUM 48MG; FIBER 11G; BETA-CAROTENE 2,810MCG; VITAMIN C 100MG; CALCIUM 156MG; IRON 3.9MG; FOLATE 173MCG; MAGNESIUM 128MG; ZINC 2.2MG; SELENIUM 5.6MCG

Chickpea Tuno Salad

SERVES 5

3 cups cooked or 2 (15-ounce) cans no-salt-added or low-sodium chickpeas

1 cup raw almonds

2 tablespoons lemon juice, or more to taste

1 teaspoon kelp granules

1 (12.3-ounce) package firm silken tofu

3 tablespoons white wine or champagne vinegar

1/2 teaspoon dry mustard powder

2 tablespoons nutritional yeast

3 teaspoons Dijon mustard

2 medium celery stalks, diced

4 green onions, minced

1/3 cup red bell pepper, minced

3/4 cup frozen peas, thawed

Freshly ground black pepper

In a food processor, pulse the chickpeas and almonds until coarsely chopped. Add the lemon juice and kelp granules and pulse a few more times. Transfer to a large mixing bowl.

Place the tofu, vinegar, dry mustard, nutritional yeast, and Dijon mustard in a high-powered blender and blend until smooth. Add to the mixing bowl with the chickpea mixture, along with the celery, green onions, red pepper, peas, and black pepper. Mix thoroughly.

Cover and refrigerate for at least 30 minutes to let the flavors mingle before serving.

PER SERVING: CALORIES 350; PROTEIN 19G; CARBOHYDRATES 34G; TOTAL FAT 16.9G; SATURATED FAT 1.5G; SODIUM 93MG; FIBER 10.8G; BETA-CAROTENE 450MCG; VITAMIN C 19MG; CALCIUM 138MG; IRON 4.4MG; FOLATE 179MCG; MAGNESIUM 135MG; ZINC 3.1MG; SELENIUM 5.5MCG

Kale and Carrot Salad
with Apple Walnut Dressing

SERVES 4

For the Salad

1 lemon, juiced

1/4 cup water

2 apples, cored and diced

3 carrots, thinly sliced

3 celery stalks, thinly sliced

1/4 cup raisins

1 tablespoon fresh mint leaves, finely chopped

5 cups kale, thick stems removed, washed, finely chopped

1/2 cup walnuts, toasted (see Note)

For the Dressing

1 apple, cored and coarsely chopped

1 tablespoon Dijon or stone-ground mustard

3 tablespoons red wine or pomegranate vinegar

3 regular or 1 1/2 Medjool dates, pitted

1/4 cup walnuts, toasted (see Note)

Place the lemon juice and water in the bottom of a large salad bowl. Add the 2 diced apples (for the salad) and toss to coat. Let sit for 10 minutes while preparing the dressing, then drain.

Prepare dressing by placing dressing ingredients in a blender or food processor and blending until creamy. Add a tablespoon or two of water if needed to adjust consistency.

Add carrots, celery, raisins, and mint to the bowl with the drained apples. Add half of the dressing and toss well. Add the kale to the bowl and toss with remaining dressing. Garnish with the remaining ½ cup toasted walnuts.

Note: Toast walnuts for both the dressing and salad (total of ¾ cups) in a small skillet over medium heat for 2–3 minutes until lightly browned.

PER SERVING: CALORIES 329; PROTEIN 8G; CARBOHYDRATES 48G; TOTAL FAT 15.5G; SATURATED FAT 1.5G; SODIUM 142MG; FIBER 9.4G; BETA-CAROTENE 11,639MCG; VITAMIN C 116MG; CALCIUM 180MG; IRON 2.9MG; FOLATE 74MCG; MAGNESIUM 87MG; ZINC 1.3MG; SELENIUM 3.5MCG

Marinated Mushroom Salad

SERVES 4

2 pounds mushrooms, sliced
½ cup water
10 ounces baby spinach
2 ounces arugula

For the Dressing
½ cup water
¼ cup balsamic vinegar
¼ cup walnuts
¼ cup raisins
1 teaspoon Dijon mustard
2 cloves garlic
2 tablespoons chopped shallots
¼ cup chopped red bell pepper
1 tablespoon coarsely chopped fresh thyme or 1 teaspoon dried thyme

Heat a large pan and water-sauté mushrooms for 2–3 minutes until slightly softened. To make the dressing, blend water, vinegar, walnuts, raisins, mustard, and garlic in a food processor or high-powered blender. Remove from blender and mix in shallots, red bell pepper, thyme, and sautéed mushrooms. Serve on top of baby spinach and arugula.

PER SERVING: CALORIES 169; PROTEIN 10G; CARBOHYDRATES 26G; TOTAL FAT 5.5G; SATURATED FAT 0.6G; SODIUM 97MG; FIBER 4.5G; BETA-CAROTENE 4,361MCG; VITAMIN C 36MG; CALCIUM 160MG; IRON 3.8MG; FOLATE 222MCG; MAGNESIUM 105MG; ZINC 3.3MG; SELENIUM 60.8MCG

Millet Salad with
Veggies and Black Beans

SERVES 6

For the Salad

1 1/2 cups dried black beans, soaked overnight, then drained

1 cup millet (see Note)

2 cups water

1 red onion, minced

2 cloves garlic, minced

2 carrots, shredded

2 bell peppers (red and yellow), seeded and cut into thin strips

2 jalapeno peppers, seeded and minced, or to taste

2 cups cherry tomatoes, halved

Fresh parsley, chopped

For the Dressing

3 teaspoons balsamic vinegar

3/4 cup fresh squeezed lemon juice

1/2 teaspoon chili powder

1/2 teaspoon ground cumin

1/4 teaspoon ground allspice

Place the soaked beans in a medium saucepan and cover with water. Bring to a boil, then immediately reduce the heat to low, cover, and let simmer for 1 hour or until tender. Drain.

Combine the millet and water and bring to a boil, then reduce heat to low, cover, and simmer 20 minutes or until tender and the water has been absorbed. Remove from heat, fluff with a fork, and set aside to cool while the beans are cooking. Combine the millet with the cooked beans, onion, garlic, carrots, peppers, tomatoes, and parsley in a large mixing bowl. Whisk the dressing ingredients together and pour desired amount over the salad. Toss gently to blend. Serve warm or cold.

Note: Millet is a tiny seed grain with a delicate, nutty flavor. You may substitute other intact whole grains such as quinoa, farro, or buckwheat groats for the millet.

PER SERVING: CALORIES 342; PROTEIN 16G; CARBOHYDRATES 66G; TOTAL FAT 2.6G; SATURATED FAT 0.5G; SODIUM 29MG; FIBER 12.2G; BETA-CAROTENE 2,678MCG; VITAMIN C 79MG; CALCIUM 91MG; IRON 4.2MG; FOLATE 286MCG; MAGNESIUM 140MG; ZINC 2.7MG; SELENIUM 2.9MCG

Mixed Greens with Fruits, Nuts, and Roasted Plantains

SERVES 3

For the Salad

2 very ripe yellow plantains, peeled, then sliced diagonally into thin 2-inch strips

1 tablespoon chopped pumpkin seeds, toasted (see Note)

1 tablespoon raw sunflower seeds, toasted

1 tablespoon chopped pecans, toasted

1 orange, seeded and sectioned

1 apple or ripe pear, cored and cut into long thin strips

8 ounces arugula or watercress

8 ounces spinach or baby kale

For the Dressing

2 regular dates or 1 Medjool date, pitted

1 tablespoon raw, unhulled sesame seeds

1/2 apple, peeled and cored

3 tablespoons balsamic vinegar

Preheat oven to 350°F. Roast the thinly sliced plantains on a baking sheet for 20 minutes or until lightly browned.

Place the roasted plantain strips in a bowl with the pumpkin seeds, sunflower seeds, pecans, orange, and sliced apple or pear. Blend dressing ingredients in a high-powered blender until smooth, adding water by the tablespoon if needed to adjust consistency. Add dressing and greens to the bowl containing the plantain mixture and toss.

Note: Lightly toast seeds and pecans in a 350°F oven for 3–5 minutes.

PER SERVING: CALORIES 376; PROTEIN 9G; CARBOHYDRATES 78G; TOTAL FAT 7.6G; SATURATED FAT 1G; SODIUM 64MG; FIBER 10.6G; BETA-CAROTENE 8,662MCG; VITAMIN C 156MG; CALCIUM 298MG; IRON 4.3MG; FOLATE 155MCG; MAGNESIUM 159MG; ZINC 1.7MG; SELENIUM 5.7MCG

Soups and Stews

Broccoli Lentil Soup

SERVES 8

8 cups water

2 cups carrot juice, freshly juiced or bottled

1 pound dried lentils

2 pounds plum tomatoes, chopped

4 cups chopped broccoli

2 onions, chopped

3 celery stalks, chopped

2 carrots, chopped

6 cloves garlic, minced

3 small zucchini, chopped

1 tablespoon dried oregano

1 1/2 teaspoons dried basil

1 teaspoon ground coriander

1 teaspoon ground cumin

1 teaspoon dried thyme

1 sweet potato, peeled and chopped

3 tablespoons Riesling Reserve Vinegar or apple cider vinegar

1/2 cup raw cashews

Place all ingredients except vinegar and cashews in a large soup pot. Bring to a simmer and cook for 60 minutes. Remove from heat and add the vinegar. Remove 2 cups or more of soup and purée with the cashews in a food processor or high-powered blender. Stir back into soup.

PER SERVING: CALORIES 337; PROTEIN 19G; CARBOHYDRATES 56G; TOTAL FAT 5.2G; SATURATED FAT 1G; SODIUM 107MG; FIBER 21.8G; BETA-CAROTENE 8,420MCG; VITAMIN C 60MG; CALCIUM 133MG; IRON 6.6MG; FOLATE 337MCG; MAGNESIUM 135MG; ZINC 3.8MG; SELENIUM 7.6MCG

Butternut Squash Soup with Mushrooms

SERVES 4

2 cups water

2 cups unsweetened soy, almond, or hemp milk

1 1/2 cups low-sodium or no-salt-added vegetable broth

6 carrots, sliced

5 celery stalks, cut in 1/2-inch slices

2 onions, chopped

2 medium zucchini, cut in large pieces

2 butternut squash, peeled and cubed

1/4 teaspoon nutmeg

1/4 teaspoon ground cloves

1/4 teaspoon cayenne pepper, or more to taste

10 ounces shiitake, cremini, and/or oyster mushrooms, sliced.

Place all ingredients except mushrooms in soup pot. Bring to a boil, reduce heat, and simmer for 30 minutes.

Place soup in a food processor or blender and blend until smooth. Return to pot, add mushrooms, and simmer for another 30 minutes.

PER SERVING: CALORIES 273; PROTEIN 12G; CARBOHYDRATES 57G; TOTAL FAT 3.3G; SATURATED FAT 0.5G; SODIUM 225MG; FIBER 12.3G; BETA-CAROTENE 19,691MCG; VITAMIN C 89MG; CALCIUM 378MG; IRON 3.9MG; FOLATE 157MCG; MAGNESIUM 162MG; ZINC 2MG; SELENIUM 8.8MCG

Citrusy Black Bean Soup

SERVES 4

1 ½ cups dry black beans, soaked (see Note)

6 cups water

3 cups shredded kale (tough stems removed)

1 medium onion, diced

4 cloves garlic, minced

1 medium green bell pepper, diced

1 ½ cups diced tomatoes

1 tablespoon ground cumin

½ teaspoon chipotle chili powder or to taste

2 tablespoons lime juice

½ cup finely chopped orange

1 teaspoon orange zest (from an organic orange)

¼ cup chopped cilantro

Place soaked, drained beans in a large pot with 6 cups of water. Bring to a boil, reduce heat, and simmer covered for 1 hour. Remove 1 ½ cups of the beans with a slotted spoon and 1 cup of liquid. Blend until smooth and return to the soup pot with the shredded kale.

In a large skillet, heat 2–3 tablespoons water and sauté the onion, garlic, and bell pepper until starting to soften. Add this mixture to the soup pot along with the diced tomatoes, cumin, and chipotle chili powder. Simmer, uncovered, for 15 minutes. Stir in lime juice, chopped orange, orange zest, and cilantro.

Note: Soak beans overnight and then drain, or use the quick soak method: Boil beans 2–3 minutes, cover, let sit for 1 hour, then drain.

PER SERVING: CALORIES 325; PROTEIN 19G; CARBOHYDRATES 62G; TOTAL FAT 2G; SATURATED FAT 0.4G; SODIUM 54MG; FIBER 14.9G; BETA-CAROTENE 5,120MCG; VITAMIN C 110MG; CALCIUM 215MG; IRON 6MG; FOLATE 364MCG; MAGNESIUM 168MG; ZINC 3.3MG; SELENIUM 3.5MCG

Corn and Red Pepper Soup
with Sweet Potatoes and Kale

SERVES 8

6 red bell peppers, diced and divided

1 large onion, finely chopped

2 small mild red chilies (or hotter peppers, depending on taste)

4 sprigs cilantro, finely chopped

4 cups low-sodium or no-salt-added vegetable broth

4 cups water

1 cup raw cashews

1 pound mushrooms (cremini, white button, or portabella), sliced into bite-sized pieces

10 ears sweet corn, kernels removed (or 6 cups frozen), divided

1 pound fresh or frozen finely chopped kale, stems removed

2 large sweet potatoes, peeled and diced

2 small zucchini, cut into half moons

$\frac{1}{4}$ cup parsley, chopped

$\frac{1}{4}$ cup nutritional yeast

Freshly ground pepper, to taste

In a large soup pot, sauté red peppers, onions, and chilies in $\frac{1}{4}$ cup water until onions are translucent or lightly browned. Add the cilantro and sauté for another 2 minutes. Add the broth and water, bring to a boil and simmer for 15 minutes. Cover, shut off the heat, and let sit for 5 minutes. Then purée the cashews in enough of this soup mixture so it blends smoothly, in a high-powered blender and return to the soup pot and stir.

Restart the soup, cooking on a low flame, adding the mushrooms, corn, kale, sweet potatoes, and zucchini. Stir in the parsley, nutritional yeast, and black pepper and cook at least 30 minutes more. Add some unsweetened nondairy milk if necessary to thin the soup to desired consistency.

PER SERVING: CALORIES 321; PROTEIN 13G; CARBOHYDRATES 52G; TOTAL FAT 9.5G; SATURATED FAT 1.6G; SODIUM 137MG; FIBER 9.1G; BETA-CAROTENE 9,697MCG; VITAMIN C 215MG; CALCIUM 136MG; IRON 4.1MG; FOLATE 134MCG; MAGNESIUM 124MG; ZINC 3.2MG; SELENIUM 15.7MCG

Creamy Tomato and White Bean Soup

SERVES 6

1 leek, roots removed and 1 inch discarded at end of top, cut lengthwise and cleaned

$\frac{1}{2}$ small green cabbage, chopped

$\frac{1}{2}$ small onion, chopped

4 cloves garlic, chopped

1 tablespoon tomato paste

$\frac{1}{2}$ tablespoon Bragg Liquid Aminos

2 (15-ounce) cans white beans, any variety, undrained

1 cup water

9 cups fresh or 4 (18-ounce) cartons crushed tomatoes

1 tablespoon no-salt Italian seasoning

2 tablespoons chopped fresh basil

Heat 2–3 tablespoons water in a large soup pot and water-sauté leek, cabbage, onion, and garlic until tender, about 10 minutes. Add tomato paste and Bragg Liquid Aminos and stir in white beans and their liquid, water, crushed tomatoes, and Italian seasoning. Bring to a boil, reduce heat, and simmer 25 minutes.

Remove 4 cups of soup from the pot and blend until smooth and creamy. Return to the pot, stir in basil, and cook 5 more minutes.

PER SERVING: CALORIES 266; PROTEIN 16G; CARBOHYDRATES 55G; TOTAL FAT 1.4G; SATURATED FAT 0.3G; SODIUM 547MG; FIBER 14.9G; BETA-CAROTENE 670MCG; VITAMIN C 57MG; CALCIUM 246MG; IRON 8.7MG; FOLATE 155MCG; MAGNESIUM 140MG; ZINC 2.4MG; SELENIUM 4MCG

Dr. Fuhrman's Anticancer Soup

SERVES 10

½ cup dried split peas

½ cup dried adzuki or red beans

4 cups water or no-salt-added vegetable broth

6–10 medium zucchini

5 pounds large organic carrots, juiced (6 cups juice; see Note)

2 bunches celery, juiced (2 cups juice; see Note)

2 tablespoons VegiZest, Vogue Cuisine VegeBase, or other no-salt seasoning blend, adjusted to taste

1 teaspoon Mrs. Dash or other no-salt seasoning blend that contains pepper

4 medium onions, chopped

3 leeks, roots and 1 inch of top removed, then cut lengthwise and cleaned

2 bunches kale, collard greens, or other greens

½ cup raw cashews

½ cup hemp seeds

2 ½ cups chopped fresh mushrooms (shiitake, cremini, and/or white)

Place the split peas, beans, and water in a very large pot over low heat. Bring to a boil, reduce heat, and simmer. Add whole zucchinis to the pot, and then the carrot juice, celery juice, VegiZest, and Mrs. Dash.

Put the onions, leeks, and kale in a blender and blend with a little bit of the soup liquid. Stir back into the soup pot. Remove the softened zucchini with tongs and blend them in the blender with the cashews and hemp seeds until creamy. Stir this mixture back into the soup pot. Add the mushrooms and continue to simmer until the beans are soft, about 2 hours total cooking time.

Note: Freshly juiced organic carrots and celery will maximize the flavor of this soup. Always clean your juicer after use.

PER SERVING: CALORIES 304; PROTEIN 15G; CARBOHYDRATES 48G; TOTAL FAT 7.9G; SATURATED FAT 1.2G; SODIUM 172MG; FIBER 11G; BETA-CAROTENE 16,410MCG; VITAMIN C 90MG; CALCIUM 180MG; IRON 5.3MG; FOLATE 202MCG; MAGNESIUM 179MG; ZINC 3MG; SELENIUM 8.7MCG

Easy Lentil and Chickpea Soup

SERVES 4

1 medium onion, finely chopped

3 large carrots, finely chopped

4 cups low-sodium or no-salt-added vegetable broth

1 1/2 cups cooked or 1 (15-ounce) can low-sodium or no-salt-added lentils, drained

1 1/2 cups cooked or 1 (15-ounce) can low-sodium or no-salt-added chickpeas, drained

1/4 cup tomato paste

1 teaspoon garlic powder

1 teaspoon thyme

2 teaspoons oregano

1 teaspoon no-salt-added seasoning blend such as Extra Spicy Mrs. Dash, or more to taste

2 cups mushrooms, sliced

2 cups baby kale or spinach, chopped

Sauté onions and carrots in a splash of broth until onions are softened. Add all other ingredients, except kale or spinach, and bring to a boil; then simmer until carrots are desired consistency. Adjust seasonings if you like; then add baby kale or spinach and cook until wilted.

PER SERVING: CALORIES 300; PROTEIN 20G; CARBOHYDRATES 48G; TOTAL FAT 3.8G; SATURATED FAT 0.7G; SODIUM 128MG; FIBER 13.9G; BETA-CAROTENE 6,217MCG; VITAMIN C 48MG; CALCIUM 153MG; IRON 6.9MG; FOLATE 274MCG; MAGNESIUM 89MG; ZINC 2.9MG; SELENIUM 14.9MCG

Herbed Split Pea Soup

SERVES 4

1 3/4 cups dried split peas

4 cups low-sodium or no-salt-added vegetable broth

3 cups water

2 cloves garlic, minced

1/4 teaspoon dried sage

1 teaspoon dried basil

1/2 teaspoon dried thyme

1 tablespoon salt-free poultry seasoning

1/2 cup diced onion

1/2 cup sliced carrots

1/2 cup sliced celery

1 sweet potato, chopped into bite-size pieces

4 packed cups kale or spinach, chopped

Combine split peas, broth, water, garlic, sage, basil, thyme, and poultry seasoning. Cover and simmer 30 minutes, stirring occasionally so the split peas don't stick to the bottom of the pot. Add remaining vegetables. Cover and simmer another 30 minutes.

PER SERVING: CALORIES 304; PROTEIN 20G; CARBOHYDRATES 56G; TOTAL FAT 1.4G; SATURATED FAT 0.2G; SODIUM 175MG; FIBER 20.2G; BETA-CAROTENE 7,251MCG; VITAMIN C 70MG; CALCIUM 171MG; IRON 5.3MG; FOLATE 219MCG; MAGNESIUM 112MG; ZINC 2.5MG; SELENIUM 2.1MCG

Succotash Casserole Stew
with Cornmeal and Okra Dumplings

SERVES 6

For the Succotash Stew

2 cups fresh or frozen butter beans or lima beans

2 cups water

1 large onion, diced

2 cloves garlic, minced

1 sweet red pepper, finely diced

3 cups fresh or frozen corn kernels

1 cup tomatoes, chopped

2 tablespoons nutritional yeast

Ground black pepper

2 tablespoons fresh chopped parsley

For the Cornmeal and Okra Topping

3 green onions, including green tops, finely chopped

1/2 pound fresh or frozen okra, cut into thin slices

1/2 teaspoon cayenne pepper

2 tablespoons ground flaxseed

1 cup coarse yellow cornmeal

4 cups water

1/4 cup currants

Cook beans in 2 cups water in a medium saucepan for about 10 minutes. Drain and set aside, reserving cooking liquid. Water-sauté onions and garlic in a large skillet using a small amount of the bean cooking liquid until onions are translucent, about 10 minutes. Add red pepper and corn kernels, cooking and stirring frequently for about 5 more minutes. Add the beans, tomatoes, nutritional yeast, and black pepper to the skillet. Continue to cook, adding bean liquid until a thick stew consistency is reached.

To prepare the dumplings, add 2 tablespoons of the bean cooking liquid to another skillet and sauté green onions until just wilted. Stir in the okra slices and then the cayenne, flaxseed, and cornmeal.

Slowly add the water and bring to a boil. Reduce heat to low and cook, stirring constantly, until creamy and thoroughly cooked, about 30 minutes. Stir in currants. Drop the cornmeal/okra mixture onto the hot succotash stew by large spoonfuls and cover and cook another 20 minutes.

Alternatively, to make a baked casserole, use a slotted spoon to transfer the stew into a casserole dish, and carefully top with the cornmeal mixture. Bake in a 350°F oven 30–40 minutes until cornmeal is browned and stew is bubbling.

Garnish with chopped parsley.

Note: The Succotash Stew also makes a good stuffing for Stuffed Red Peppers.

PER SERVING: CALORIES 294; PROTEIN 11G; CARBOHYDRATES 60G; TOTAL FAT 2.8G; SATURATED FAT 0.4G; SODIUM 27MG; FIBER 9.1G; BETA-CAROTENE 835MCG; VITAMIN C 57MG; CALCIUM 95MG; IRON 4.2MG; FOLATE 216MCG; MAGNESIUM 96MG; ZINC 1.9MG; SELENIUM 5.4MCG

Tempeh Chili with Sriracha

SERVES 6

8 ounces tempeh, crumbled

1 large onion, chopped

1 medium red bell pepper, chopped

4 cloves garlic, minced

1 medium zucchini, diced

10 ounces mushrooms, sliced

1 1/2 cups frozen corn kernels, thawed

1/2 tablespoon chili powder

1 1/2 tablespoons ground cumin

4 large tomatoes, chopped

3 cups cooked or 2 (15-ounce) cans low-sodium kidney beans, drained

15 ounces low-sodium or no-salt-added tomato sauce

2 cups low-sodium or no-salt-added vegetable broth

2 tablespoons sriracha sauce (see Note)

Preheat oven to 350°F. Bake crumbled tempeh on a silicone baking mat or parchment-lined pan for 25–30 minutes, stirring occasionally. If you are making your own sriracha sauce, you can roast the ingredients at the same time.

Meanwhile, heat 2–3 tablespoons water in a large soup pot and sauté onions, red pepper, and garlic until tender. Add zucchini, mushrooms, and corn and cook until mushrooms release their liquid. Then add chili powder, cumin, tomatoes, beans, tomato sauce, and vegetable broth; stir and bring to a boil. Add baked tempeh and sriracha sauce, reduce heat, cover, and cook on medium low for 20 minutes.

Note: You can make your own healthful, no-salt, no-sugar sriracha sauce. Bake two halved and seeded red bell peppers, 2 serrano peppers, and 3 garlic cloves at 350°F for 25–30 minutes or until soft. Blend all ingredients until smooth.

PER SERVING: CALORIES 321; PROTEIN 21G; CARBOHYDRATES 52G; TOTAL FAT 6G; SATURATED FAT 1.1G; SODIUM 86MG; FIBER 12.1G; BETA-CAROTENE 1,243MCG; VITAMIN C 64MG; CALCIUM 132MG; IRON 6.4MG; FOLATE 194MCG; MAGNESIUM 127MG; ZINC 2.5MG; SELENIUM 6.9MCG

West African Sweet Potato Soup

SERVES 6

1 large onion, chopped

1 cup chopped celery

2 tablespoons minced fresh ginger

1/8 teaspoon hot pepper flakes, or to taste

4 cups peeled chopped sweet potatoes

3 cups water

3 cups low-sodium tomato juice

1 cup low-sodium peanut butter

1/4 cup chopped parsley or cilantro

Heat 2–3 tablespoons water in a soup pot and water-sauté onions and celery until tender. Stir in the ginger and hot pepper flakes and sauté for 1 minute. Add sweet potatoes and water and bring to a boil, cover, reduce heat, and simmer until potatoes are very tender, about 20 minutes. Stir in tomato juice and peanut butter. Working in batches, blend the soup in a high-powered blender. Return to the pot, add the parsley or cilantro, and reheat.

PER SERVING: CALORIES 370; PROTEIN 13G; CARBOHYDRATES 36G; TOTAL FAT 21.6G; SATURATED FAT 3.4G; SODIUM 243MG; FIBER 7.3G; BETA-CAROTENE 8,738MCG; VITAMIN C 42MG; CALCIUM 79MG; IRON 2.1MG; FOLATE 90MCG; MAGNESIUM 111MG; ZINC 1.8MG; SELENIUM 4.6MCG

Barbecue Baked Beans

SERVES 6

2 stalks celery, diced
1/2 red bell pepper, seeded and diced
1/2 green bell pepper, seeded and diced
1 small onion, finely chopped
2 cups coarsely chopped ripe tomatoes
1/2 cup pitted dates, chopped
1/4 cup raisins
1/2 cup water

1/4 cup Dijon mustard
2 tablespoons fresh-squeezed lemon juice
1 tablespoon ground ginger
1 tablespoon garlic powder
1/2 teaspoon chili powder
Pinch cayenne pepper, or to taste
4 1/2 cups cooked or 3 (15-ounce cans) low-sodium or no-salt-added red kidney beans

Heat 2–3 tablespoons water in a large saucepan and water-sauté celery, red and green peppers, and onion over medium-high heat, cooking until vegetables are slightly softened. Add the tomatoes, dates, raisins, and water and continue to cook, reducing the heat to a simmer. Add the mustard, lemon juice, ginger, garlic powder, chili powder, and cayenne. Cover and cook over low heat for about 30 minutes, stirring occasionally. Purée in a blender. Adjust chili powder, cayenne, or other seasonings to taste.

In a casserole dish, combine the kidney beans and blended mixture, reserving about 1/2–1 cup of the barbecue sauce for another use (see Note). Bake until heated through and bubbly, about 25 minutes.

Note: You can brush this barbecue sauce on baked tofu, tempeh, or winter squash or use it as a dipping sauce.

PER SERVING: CALORIES 261; PROTEIN 14G; CARBOHYDRATES 52G; TOTAL FAT 1.5G; SATURATED FAT 0.2G; SODIUM 142MG; FIBER 13.2G; BETA-CAROTENE 533MCG; VITAMIN C 34MG; CALCIUM 71MG; IRON 5.0MG; FOLATE 199MCG; MAGNESIUM 87MG; ZINC 1.8MG; SELENIUM 6.5MCG

Bean Enchiladas

SERVES 6

1 medium green bell pepper, seeded and chopped
1/2 cup sliced onion
8 ounces no-salt-added or low-sodium tomato sauce, divided
2 cups cooked pinto or black beans or canned no-salt-added or low-sodium beans

1 cup frozen corn kernels
1 tablespoon chili powder
1 teaspoon ground cumin
1 teaspoon onion powder
1 tablespoon chopped fresh cilantro
1/8 teaspoon cayenne pepper, or to taste
6 corn or (100% whole grain) flour tortillas

Sauté the green pepper and onion in 2 tablespoons of the tomato sauce until tender. Stir in the remaining tomato sauce, beans, corn, chili powder, cumin, onion powder, cilantro, and cayenne. Simmer 5 minutes. Spoon about ¼ cup of the bean mixture on each tortilla and roll up. Serve as is or bake for 15 minutes in a 375°F oven.

PER SERVING: CALORIES 267; PROTEIN 13G; CARBOHYDRATES 47G; TOTAL FAT 4.3G; SATURATED FAT 0.7G; SODIUM 166MG; FIBER 11.8G; BETA-CAROTENE 259MCG; VITAMIN C 19MG; CALCIUM 70MG; IRON 4MG; FOLATE 101MCG; MAGNESIUM 56MG; ZINC 1MG; SELENIUM 1.3MCG

Broccoli Stir-Fry with Tempeh (or chicken or shrimp)

SERVES 4

1 (8-ounce) package tempeh, cut into small cubes (see Note) (or 8 ounces sliced chicken breast or 8 ounces peeled and deveined shrimp)

½ cup water

1 tablespoon Bragg Liquid Aminos or reduced-sodium soy sauce

2 tablespoons rice vinegar

⅓ cup crushed tomatoes

1 cup fresh or frozen pineapple, finely chopped

2 teaspoons cornstarch

¼ cup no-salt-added or low-sodium vegetable broth

2 heads broccoli, cut into florets

1 large onion, sliced

2 red bell peppers, seeded and sliced

1 cup sliced mushrooms

2 carrots, thinly sliced

4 cloves garlic, sliced

1 tablespoon ginger, chopped

2 cups wild rice, cooked in 5 cups water for 30 minutes

2 tablespoons unhulled sesame seeds, toasted

2 tablespoons basil, sliced

Place cubed tempeh in a small saucepan and simmer in water 8–10 minutes. Add Bragg Liquid Aminos, vinegar, crushed tomatoes, pineapple, and cornstarch; mix well.

Heat vegetable broth in a large skillet or wok and add tempeh mixture, broccoli, onion, peppers, mushrooms, carrots, garlic, and ginger and stir-fry until veggies are tender but still crisp and tempeh is lightly browned, about 5 minutes. If needed, add additional water or stock to prevent sticking.

You can substitute small cubes of chicken breast, shrimp, or tofu for the tempeh. Serve over wild rice garnished with sesame seeds and basil.

Note: Tempeh is made from fermented soybeans and sometimes added grains. It is formed in the shape of a patty or cake. It has a nutty taste but easily absorbs the flavors of the foods it is cooked with. You can also use tofu in this recipe. Cube the tofu after draining and squeezing out as much excess water as possible. Do not simmer; add to the wok and stir-fry with the vegetables. Freezing the tofu in advance, defrosting, and cubing offers a chewier texture.

PER SERVING: CALORIES 258; PROTEIN 12G; CARBOHYDRATES 48G; TOTAL FAT 4.3G; SATURATED FAT 0.6G; SODIUM 263MG; FIBER 9.7G; BETA-CAROTENE 4,187MCG; VITAMIN C 239MG; CALCIUM 170MG; IRON 3.2MG; FOLATE 177MCG; MAGNESIUM 105MG; ZINC 2.6MG; SELENIUM 6.8MCG

California Creamed Kale

SERVES 4

2 bunches kale, leaves removed from tough stems and chopped coarsely

½ cup raw cashews

⅓ cup hemp seeds

¾ cup unsweetened soy, hemp, or almond milk

4 tablespoons onion flakes

1 tablespoon nonfortified nutritional yeast or other no-salt seasoning blend

Place kale in a large steamer pot and steam 10 minutes. Place remaining ingredients in a high-powered blender and blend until smooth. Place kale in a colander and press to remove excess water. In a wooden bowl, coarsely chop and mix kale with the cream sauce.

Note: You can also use this sauce with broccoli, spinach, and other steamed vegetables.

PER SERVING: CALORIES 244; PROTEIN 12G; CARBOHYDRATES 20G; TOTAL FAT 14.5G; SATURATED FAT 2.1G; SODIUM 54MG; FIBER 4.3G; BETA-CAROTENE 6,539MCG; VITAMIN C 90MG; CALCIUM 189MG; IRON 4.5MG; FOLATE 41MCG; MAGNESIUM 169MG; ZINC 2.9MG; SELENIUM 4.4MCG

Caribbean Greens and Sweet Potatoes (with optional fish)

SERVES 6

1 cup dried, unsweetened shredded coconut

1 ½–2 cups water

1 onion, chopped

3 garlic cloves, minced

1 hot pepper, such as habanera or jalapeno, seeded and diced

1 red bell pepper, seeded and diced

1 carrot, diced

2 sweet potatoes, cut into 1-inch chunks

Pinch allspice or to taste

1 tablespoon fresh thyme or 1 teaspoon crushed dried thyme

1 pound mixed greens (for instance, collards, kale, turnip greens, cabbage), at least 2 varieties, cut into small ribbons

2–3 green onions, chopped for garnish

Optional: 8 ounces salmon or a white fish such as halibut or sea bass, with 1 tablespoon lime juice

In a high-powered blender, mix coconut and water to make coconut "milk." Combine blended coconut milk, onion, garlic, peppers, carrot, sweet potatoes, allspice, and thyme in a heavy-bottomed pot. Bring to a boil on medium-high heat, then reduce to simmer. Cook about 10 minutes, then add the mixed greens. Continue to cook down until all vegetables are tender and sweet potatoes have started to break apart to help thicken the stew, about 20 minutes.

If desired, plate the dish and season top with flaked, baked fish. To bake fish, preheat oven to 375°F. Lightly wipe bottom of a rectangular pan with olive oil. Place fish in the pan, folding thin ends under if necessary for even thickness. If fish has skin, place it skin-side down. Drizzle lime juice over fish. Bake uncovered 15–20 minutes or until fish flakes easily with a fork.

PER SERVING: CALORIES 176; PROTEIN 4G; CARBOHYDRATES 23G; TOTAL FAT 9.1G; SATURATED FAT 7.7G; SODIUM 65MG; FIBER 6.5G; BETA-CAROTENE 8,524MCG; VITAMIN C 92MG; CALCIUM 102MG; IRON 1.8MG; FOLATE 50MCG; MAGNESIUM 49MG; ZINC 0.8MG; SELENIUM 3.6MCG

Caribbean-Spiced Baked Tofu

SERVES 4

1 tablespoon paprika

1 teaspoon ground cumin

1 teaspoon ground ginger

1 teaspoon ground chili powder or cayenne pepper

1/2 teaspoon ground thyme

1/2 teaspoon garlic powder

1/4 teaspoon turmeric

1/4 teaspoon allspice

Pinch of any of the following, depending on taste: mace, cinnamon, nutmeg, coriander, cardamom, cloves

1 pound extra-firm tofu

Mix all the spices together. This will make about 1/4 cup, which is enough for about 3–4 pounds tofu. Store the mixture in an airtight container for other uses or to make more baked tofu.

Preheat oven to 350°F. Slice tofu into 8 slices about 1/3-inch thick. Press and drain all liquid from tofu between layers of paper towels until dry. Gently rub each slice of tofu, front and back, with approximately 1/2 teaspoon of the spice mixture. Line a baking sheet with parchment paper or use a silicone baking mat. Place tofu slices on the baking sheet and bake for 30 minutes, turning after 15 minutes. It can also be baked on a wire rack without turning.

PER SERVING: CALORIES 116; PROTEIN 12G; CARBOHYDRATES 5G; TOTAL FAT 7.1G; SATURATED FAT 0.7G; SODIUM 23MG; FIBER 1.5G; BETA-CAROTENE 554MCG; VITAMIN C 1MG; CALCIUM 215MG; IRON 3.3MG; FOLATE 21MCG; MAGNESIUM 68MG; ZINC 1.4MG; SELENIUM 15.4MCG

Cauliflower Steaks with Garbanzo Purée

SERVES 2

1 large head cauliflower
1/2 teaspoon ground turmeric
1 teaspoon MatoZest or another no-salt Italian seasoning
Ground pepper, to taste
1/4 cup pine nuts or chopped walnuts

1 large shallot, chopped
1/2 cup no-salt-added or low-sodium vegetable broth or more as needed
1/4 cup raisins
1/2 cup cooked garbanzo beans
1/4 cup chopped parsley

Preheat the oven to 350°F. Cut cauliflower vertically into 1/2-inch-thick steaks. You should end up with 2–3 steaks and some extra pieces. Rinse lightly with water and season on both sides with turmeric, no-salt seasoning, and pepper. Place steaks and small pieces on a lightly oiled baking dish, cover with foil, and bake 25–30 minutes or until lightly browned and tender, turning after 15 minutes. Remove small pieces of cauliflower and return steaks to the oven with the heat turned off to keep warm.

Meanwhile, sauté pine nuts or walnuts in a dry pan until lightly toasted. Remove from pan and set aside. Sauté shallots in the pan with 2 tablespoons vegetable broth for a few minutes, until translucent. Add raisins and cook until raisins become plump, adding broth as needed to keep them moist.

In a high-powered blender, blend the small cauliflower pieces, half of the pine nuts or walnuts, half of the raisin mixture, the garbanzo beans, half of the parsley, and enough broth to provide a smooth purée.

Transfer purée to a serving platter, place cauliflower steaks on top of purée, and garnish with the remaining nuts, raisin mixture, and parsley.

PER SERVING: CALORIES 361; PROTEIN 15G; CARBOHYDRATES 53G; TOTAL FAT 14.1G; SATURATED FAT 1.2G; SODIUM 173MG; FIBER 13.7G; BETA-CAROTENE 389MCG; VITAMIN C 215MG; CALCIUM 151MG; IRON 5.3MG; FOLATE 337MCG; MAGNESIUM 141MG; ZINC 3.1MG; SELENIUM 4.5MCG

Creamy Garlicky Grits

SERVES 6

1/2 cup raw cashews

1 cup water

2 cups water or no-salt-added or low-sodium vegetable broth

1 cup stone-ground cornmeal

3 cloves garlic, finely minced or crushed in a garlic press

1/3 red onion, finely chopped

1 jalapeno, seeded and finely chopped

1/2 cup frozen or fresh off-the-cob corn kernels

1 cup unsweetened soy, hemp, or almond milk

1 tablespoon nutritional yeast

1 teaspoon ground cumin

1/4 cup chopped cilantro

1 tablespoon toasted unhulled sesame seeds

Place cashews and 1 cup water in a high-powered blender and process until smooth and creamy. Set aside. Meanwhile, boil 2 cups water or vegetable stock in a medium saucepan and whisk in cornmeal until all lumps are gone. Reduce heat to low, cover, and cook 10–12 minutes, until all the water is absorbed, stirring occasionally to prevent sticking.

In a separate skillet, water-sauté garlic, onion, jalapeno, and corn in a small amount of water 10–12 minutes. Add corn mixture to cornmeal mixture along with nondairy milk, blended cashews, nutritional yeast, and cumin; stir well. Cover and cook on low 30–40 minutes, checking and stirring occasionally to prevent sticking. Garnish with cilantro and sesame seeds.

PER SERVING: CALORIES 202; PROTEIN 6G; CARBOHYDRATES 30G; TOTAL FAT 6.8G; SATURATED FAT 1.1G; SODIUM 84MG; FIBER 2.5G; BETA-CAROTENE 68MCG; VITAMIN C 5MG; CALCIUM 112MG; IRON 1.8MG; FOLATE 20MCG; MAGNESIUM 57MG; ZINC 1.4MG; SELENIUM 5.8MCG

Crustless Spinach Quiche

SERVES 4

2 cups chopped onion

2 teaspoons chopped garlic

3 cups chopped spinach

1 teaspoon Bragg Liquid Aminos or reduced-sodium soy sauce

1/2 cup chopped fresh mint

1/2 teaspoon black pepper or to taste

1 (14-ounce) package firm tofu

1/4 cup raisins or unsweetened, unsulfured dried cherries or blueberries

Preheat oven to 350°F. Sauté the chopped onions and garlic in 2–3 tablespoons of water. Cook a few minutes, until softened. Remove from stove. Place in food processor along with spinach, Bragg Liquid Aminos, mint, pepper, and tofu and mix thoroughly. Stir in dried fruit. Transfer mixture to a casserole dish or pie pan. Bake 30 minutes, or until mixture is thickened.

PER SERVING: CALORIES 164; PROTEIN 12G; CARBOHYDRATES 19G; TOTAL FAT 6.1G; SATURATED FAT 0.6G; SODIUM 88MG; FIBER 3.5G; BETA-CAROTENE 1,268MCG; VITAMIN C 17MG; CALCIUM 241MG; IRON 4MG; FOLATE 88MCG; MAGNESIUM 86MG; ZINC 1.5MG; SELENIUM 13.7MCG

New-Style Hash with Greens and Spicy Pumpkin Seeds

SERVES 4

For the Hash

2 teaspoons brown mustard seeds

1 teaspoon ground cumin

1 medium onion, diced

1 1/2 cups no-salt-added or low-sodium vegetable broth

1/2 cup millet, rinsed and drained

3–4 fresh hot green serrano chilies, seeded and minced, or to taste

2 red bell peppers, seeded and diced

1 large zucchini, diced

1/2 cup quinoa, rinsed and drained

2 tablespoons fresh parsley, chopped

Ground black pepper, to taste

For the Greens

1/4 cup raw pumpkin seeds

1 teaspoon coriander seeds, crushed

1 teaspoon Bragg Liquid Aminos or reduced-sodium soy sauce

1/4 teaspoon cayenne pepper

2 cloves garlic, minced

2 pounds leafy greens, (such as turnip greens, collards, mustard greens, spinach, chard, or kale)

1/2 lemon, juiced

1/4 teaspoon ground black pepper

Heat a medium saucepan over medium-high heat. When hot, add the mustard seeds. When they begin to pop, add the cumin, then the onions, and cook until translucent. Stir in the vegetable broth and millet, cover, and cook for 15 minutes. Add the chilies, peppers, zucchini, and quinoa to the pot and cook another 20 minutes, or until all liquid is absorbed. Serve over greens, as described below.

To prepare the greens, toast the pumpkin seeds and coriander seeds in a large skillet until they begin to pop or darken, tossing in pan to prevent burning. When cool, stir in the Bragg Liquid Aminos, cayenne pepper, and garlic and set aside. Coarsely chop the greens and add to the pan and stir in batches—they will wilt while they cook, making more room in the pan—until all greens are in the pan. Keep the pan covered when not adding greens or stirring to help with wilting and maintaining moisture. Add a few drops of water if needed to prevent sticking. Remove from heat, stir in lemon juice, and add black pepper to taste.

Serve "hash" on a bed of the wilted greens. Garnish with the parsley and toasted spicy pumpkin seeds.

PER SERVING: CALORIES 351; PROTEIN 17G; CARBOHYDRATES 58G; TOTAL FAT 8.1G; SATURATED FAT 1.2G; SODIUM 178MG; FIBER 15G; BETA-CAROTENE 15,668MCG; VITAMIN C 333MG; CALCIUM 303MG; IRON 7.6MG; FOLATE 549MCG; MAGNESIUM 230MG; ZINC 2.8MG; SELENIUM 10MCG

Pan-Roasted Vegetables

SERVES 6

12 ounces Brussels sprouts

2 large stalks broccoli, cut into florets

1/2 head cauliflower, cut into florets

8 ounces baby carrots, cut in half

1 bunch asparagus, hard ends removed and cut into 2-inch pieces

6 cloves garlic, minced

2 tablespoons black fig vinegar or balsamic vinegar

1 teaspoon Bragg Liquid Aminos or reduced-sodium soy sauce

1 tablespoon olive oil

Preheat oven to 375°F. To prepare Brussels sprouts, cut off stem base and remove outer leaves if not fresh looking. Toss all ingredients in a large bowl and lightly rub with olive oil. Pour into a large baking pan and spread evenly. Cover and bake for 30 minutes. Remove the cover, stir, and bake for an additional 20 minutes or until vegetables are tender and just lightly browned, stirring occasionally.

PER SERVING: CALORIES 84; PROTEIN 5G; CARBOHYDRATES 16G; TOTAL FAT 1.3G; SATURATED FAT 0.2G; SODIUM 106MG; FIBER 5.9G; BETA-CAROTENE 3,032MCG; VITAMIN C 108MG; CALCIUM 81MG; IRON 2.5MG; FOLATE 110MCG; MAGNESIUM 38MG; ZINC 0.8MG; SELENIUM 4MCG

Quick Greens and Beans

SERVES 2

1 large onion, sliced

3 cloves garlic, thinly sliced

1 bunch collard greens, stems removed and cut into $\frac{1}{2}$-inch strips

$\frac{1}{4}$ teaspoon red pepper flakes or more to taste

$\frac{1}{2}$ cup low-sodium or no-salt-added vegetable broth

1 $\frac{1}{2}$ cups cooked or 1 (15-ounce) can cannellini beans, drained

1 $\frac{1}{2}$ cups chopped tomato

2 tablespoons lemon juice

Heat 2–3 tablespoons water in a large sauté pan or wok and water-sauté onion and garlic until tender. Add collards, red pepper flakes, and vegetable broth; cover and cook 5 minutes. Add beans, tomatoes, and lemon juice; cover and continue cooking an additional 5 minutes or until collards are wilted and tender. Add additional vegetable broth if needed to prevent sticking.

PER SERVING: CALORIES 276; PROTEIN 17G; CARBOHYDRATES 53G; TOTAL FAT 1.2G; SATURATED FAT 0.2G; SODIUM 67MG; FIBER 14.9G; BETA-CAROTENE 3,379MCG; VITAMIN C 57MG; CALCIUM 270MG; IRON 5.8MG; FOLATE 264MCG; MAGNESIUM 116MG; ZINC 2.4MG; SELENIUM 3.7MCG

Quinoa Walnut Loaf

SERVES 6

1 cup quinoa, rinsed well

2 cups no-salt-added or low-sodium vegetable broth

1 cup chopped onions

3 tablespoons tomato paste, plus extra reserved for top of loaf

$\frac{1}{2}$ cup diced red bell pepper

$\frac{1}{2}$ cup chopped mushrooms

$\frac{1}{2}$ cup diced celery

1 cup chopped walnuts

2 tablespoons chopped parsley

1 teaspoon no-salt-added Italian seasoning

$\frac{1}{2}$ teaspoon garlic powder

In a medium saucepan, bring quinoa, vegetable broth, and onions to a boil; reduce heat to low, cover, and simmer 15–20 minutes or until quinoa is tender and broth has been absorbed. In a bowl, combine the tomato paste, bell pepper, mushrooms, celery, walnuts, parsley, Italian seasoning, and garlic powder. Add to the cooked quinoa/onion mixture and mix well. Lightly rub a loaf pan with a minimal amount of oil. Fill pan with mixture and press down evenly. Spread a $\frac{1}{8}$-inch layer of reserved tomato paste over top. Bake at 200°F for 30 minutes.

Delicious served on a bed of steamed or sautéed spinach, kale, or Swiss chard.

PER SERVING: CALORIES 269; PROTEIN 8G; CARBOHYDRATES 27G; TOTAL FAT 15.9G; SATURATED FAT 1.4G; SODIUM 17MG; FIBER 4.5G; BETA-CAROTENE 373MCG; VITAMIN C 22MG; CALCIUM 47MG; IRON 2.8MG; FOLATE 85MCG; MAGNESIUM 110MG; ZINC 2.1MG; SELENIUM 5.2MCG

Red Beans with Cajun-Spiced Zucchini and Quinoa (with optional chicken)

SERVES 6

2 cups dried red kidney beans, soaked overnight

6 cups water

2 bay leaves

1 large onion, chopped

1 cup mushrooms, sliced

2 carrots, chopped

3 stalks celery, diagonally sliced

3 cloves garlic, chopped

2 medium zucchini, halved and sliced

1 teaspoon oregano

1 teaspoon thyme

1 teaspoon cayenne pepper

1 tablespoon no-salt-added Cajun or Creole seasoning

3 cups cooked quinoa or other intact whole grain

Optional: 6 ounces shredded cooked chicken breast

Drain and rinse soaked beans. Combine beans, 6 cups of water, and bay leaves in a heavy pot and bring to boil on high heat. Reduce heat and simmer, covered, for about 2 hours or until beans are tender. In another large pot or skillet, sauté onions, mushrooms, carrots, and celery until onion is translucent, about 5 minutes, then add garlic and cook another minute, making sure the garlic does not burn. Add a tablespoon or two of water if needed to prevent sticking.

Toss zucchini slices with oregano, thyme, cayenne, and Cajun seasoning and add to the onion mixture. Reduce heat and cook 10–12 minutes or until vegetables are tender. Add the cooked beans to onion and zucchini mixture and stir.

Serve over cooked quinoa, steel cut oats, or other intact whole grain. If desired, top each serving with shredded chicken.

PER SERVING: CALORIES 356; PROTEIN 21G; CARBOHYDRATES 65G; TOTAL FAT 2.5G; SATURATED FAT 0.2G; SODIUM 61MG; FIBER 20.6G; BETA-CAROTENE 2,186MCG; VITAMIN C 19MG; CALCIUM 187MG; IRON 8.2MG; FOLATE 316MCG; MAGNESIUM 184MG; ZINC 3.1MG; SELENIUM 6.3MCG

Shredded Brussels Sprouts

SERVES 4

2 cloves garlic, chopped

3/4 pound Brussels sprouts, very thinly sliced

1/4 cup toasted walnuts, chopped (see Note)

2 tablespoons raisins or currants

1 tablespoon nutritional yeast

Freshly ground black pepper

Heat 2 tablespoons water in a large skillet and sauté garlic for 1 minute, then add Brussels sprouts and cook 2–3 minutes, until warm and slightly wilted. Add a small amount of additional water if needed to prevent sticking. Remove from heat and toss with chopped toasted walnuts, raisins, and nutritional yeast. Season with black pepper. Serve hot or cold.

Note: Toast walnuts in a small skillet over medium heat for 2–3 minutes until lightly browned.

PER SERVING: CALORIES 100; PROTEIN 5G; CARBOHYDRATES 13G; TOTAL FAT 4.4G; SATURATED FAT 0.5G; SODIUM 23MG; FIBER 4.4G; BETA-CAROTENE 386MCG; VITAMIN C 73MG; CALCIUM 50MG; IRON 1.6MG; FOLATE 59MCG; MAGNESIUM 34MG; ZINC 1MG; SELENIUM 1.9MCG

Slow Cooker Refried Beans

SERVES 9

3 cups dry pinto or other beans, rinsed

1 medium onion, coarsely chopped

1 jalapeno pepper, seeded and chopped

2 tablespoons minced garlic

2 teaspoons chili powder, or more to taste

1 teaspoon cumin

1/2 teaspoon black pepper

9 cups low-sodium or no-salt-added vegetable broth

Place all ingredients in a slow cooker and stir to combine. Cook on high 6–8 hours or until beans are soft and mash easily, adding more water if needed. Strain the beans and reserve the cooking liquid. Mash the beans with a potato masher, adding the reserved liquid as needed to reach desired consistency.

Use as a side dish or dip, or as a filling in vegetable burritos or enchiladas. For tasty tostadas, spread a layer of refried beans on toasted corn tortillas and then top with shredded lettuce or other greens, diced tomatoes, sliced avocado, and chopped red onion.

You can freeze leftovers in individual portions to enjoy later.

PER SERVING: CALORIES 248; PROTEIN 14G; CARBOHYDRATES 45G; TOTAL FAT 1G; SATURATED FAT 0.2G; SODIUM 155MG; FIBER 10.5G; BETA-CAROTENE 101MCG; VITAMIN C 7MG; CALCIUM 107MG; IRON 4MG; FOLATE 341MCG; MAGNESIUM 117MG; ZINC 1.6MG; SELENIUM 18.4MCG

Smoky Collard Greens with Pineapple and Black-Eyed Peas

SERVES 4

1 large onion, sliced

2 cloves garlic, chopped

1/2 pound chopped collard greens

1/2 cup fresh or frozen pineapple, finely chopped

2 cups cooked or low-sodium or no-salt-added canned or frozen black-eyed peas

1 cup no-salt-added or low-sodium vegetable broth or water

1/4 teaspoon chipotle chili powder

1/4 teaspoon red pepper flakes

Preheat a large skillet or pot with a lid, on high heat. Add onion slices and cook, stirring frequently, until the onions are lightly browned, adding a small amount of vegetable broth or water if needed to unstick the browned or caramelized bits. Add garlic and cook for another minute. Stir in collards and pineapple. Cover pot, reduce heat to medium, and cook for 5 minutes. Stir in cooked black-eyed peas, vegetable broth, chipotle chili powder, and red pepper flakes and heat through. Adjust chili powder and red pepper to taste.

PER SERVING: CALORIES 145; PROTEIN 9G; CARBOHYDRATES 28G; TOTAL FAT 0.8G; SATURATED FAT 0.2G; SODIUM 51MG; FIBER 8.3G; BETA-CAROTENE 2,255MCG; VITAMIN C 27MG; CALCIUM 121MG; IRON 2.5MG; FOLATE 280MCG; MAGNESIUM 57MG; ZINC 1.3MG; SELENIUM 3.1MCG

Stuffed Red Peppers

SERVES 4

1 red onion, finely chopped

4 cloves garlic, minced

1 carrot, diced

4 large mushrooms, diced

1 small cherry pepper or jalapeno pepper, diced

2 small zucchini or yellow squash, diced

1 small eggplant, peeled if desired, diced

2 medium tomatoes, diced

⅓ cup bulgur wheat

1 tablespoon nutritional yeast

1 teaspoon Bragg Liquid Aminos or reduced-sodium soy sauce

2 teaspoons no-salt Italian seasoning blend

4 large red bell peppers

Heat 2–3 tablespoons of water in a large pot and sauté the onions and garlic for 2 minutes. Add the carrots, mushrooms, pepper, zucchini, eggplant, and tomato and cook for 5 minutes. Add the bulgur wheat, nutritional yeast, Bragg Liquid Aminos, and seasoning blend. Stir and continue to simmer about 10 more minutes, or until vegetables are tender.

Preheat oven to 325°F. Cut off the tops of the red bell peppers and remove all seeds and ribs. Spoon the vegetable mixture into the cavities, packing lightly. Stand on a baking tray and bake for 30 minutes.

PER SERVING: CALORIES 180; PROTEIN 8G; CARBOHYDRATES 38G; TOTAL FAT 1.4G; SATURATED FAT 0.2G; SODIUM 91MG; FIBER 12.7G; BETA-CAROTENE 4,586MCG; VITAMIN C 251MG; CALCIUM 74MG; IRON 2.3MG; FOLATE 145MCG; MAGNESIUM 86MG; ZINC 1.9MG; SELENIUM 6.8MCG

Tennessee Corn Pone

SERVES 4

¾ cup unsweetened, soy, hemp, or almond milk

2 teaspoons apple cider vinegar

2 tablespoons ground flaxseed

½ cup yellow cornmeal

½ teaspoon baking soda

1 ½ cups cooked or 1 (15-ounce) can low-sodium or no-salt-added black-eyed peas, drained

1 cup frozen corn, thawed

Preheat oven to 400°F. Whisk together milk, vinegar, and flaxseed. In separate bowl, whisk together cornmeal and baking soda. Combine milk mixture with the cornmeal mixture. Combine black-eyed peas and corn and place in an 8-by-8-inch baking dish. Pour cornmeal mixture over the top. Bake 25–30 minutes, until set and golden brown.

PER SERVING: CALORIES 207; PROTEIN 10G; CARBOHYDRATES 35G; TOTAL FAT 3.8G; SATURATED FAT 0.5G; SODIUM 180MG; FIBER 7.9G; BETA-CAROTENE 6MCG; VITAMIN C 3MG; CALCIUM 85MG; IRON 2.7MG; FOLATE 157MCG; MAGNESIUM 80MG; ZINC 1.8MG; SELENIUM 3.8MCG

Burgers, Wraps, and Quick Food

Avocado Toast with
Grilled Onion and Tomatoes

SERVES 2

1/2 red onion, sliced very thinly

1 ripe avocado, mashed

2 (100% whole grain) pitas, lightly toasted

1 medium tomato, sliced

2 tablespoons raw sesame or pumpkin seeds, lightly toasted

Black pepper or crushed red pepper flakes, to taste

Preheat a dry frying pan until hot, and sizzle-cook the sliced onion on the heated dry pan for 3 minutes until glistening with just a touch of brown. (When you throw sliced onions on a hot dry pan, they will sizzle.) Spread the mashed avocado on top of the toasted pita. Add tomato slices and grilled onion and sprinkle with toasted seeds. Season with your choice of ground black pepper or red pepper flakes.

PER SERVING: CALORIES 266; PROTEIN 8G; CARBOHYDRATES 30G; TOTAL FAT 15G; SATURATED FAT 2G; SODIUM 120MG; FIBER 9.2G; BETA-CAROTENE 1,570MCG; VITAMIN C 16MG; CALCIUM 23MG; IRON 2.4MG; FOLATE 78MCG; MAGNESIUM 76MG; ZINC 1.2MG; SELENIUM 1.2MCG

Black Bean and Avocado Burgers

SERVES 4

1 tablespoon ground flaxseeds

2 1/2 tablespoons water

1 1/2 cups cooked or 1 (15-ounce) can no-salt-added or low-sodium black beans, drained

1/2 ripe avocado

3/4 cup oat flour (see Note)

1/4 cup finely diced onion

1/2 cup finely diced red pepper

2 tablespoons low-sodium ketchup

1/4 teaspoon black pepper

Preheat oven to 350°F. Combine flaxseed and water in a small bowl and let sit for 5 minutes. Add beans and avocado to a bowl and mash with the back of a fork, leaving some beans whole. Add the flaxseed mixture, oat flour, onion, red pepper, ketchup, and black pepper and combine well. Form into four burgers. Place on a lightly greased or parchment-lined baking sheet and bake for 30 minutes. Turn burgers over carefully after the first 15 minutes, reshaping if necessary.

Serve on a 100% whole grain bun with tomato, sliced red onion, and lettuce or on a bed of leafy greens.

Note: You can buy oat flour in many markets or health food stores. To make your own, process old-fashioned oats in a food processor or high-powered blender until ground.

PER SERVING: CALORIES 197; PROTEIN 9G; CARBOHYDRATES 31G; TOTAL FAT 4.9G; SATURATED FAT 0.7G; SODIUM 5MG; FIBER 9.5G; BETA-CAROTENE 356MCG; VITAMIN C 27MG; CALCIUM 30MG; IRON 5.5MG; FOLATE 124MCG; MAGNESIUM 62MG; ZINC 1MG; SELENIUM 1.4MCG

Eggplant Almond Chips

SERVES 2

1 eggplant, peeled

1/4 cup almond meal (ground almonds)

2 tablespoons nutritional yeast

2 teaspoons garlic powder

1 teaspoon onion powder

Dash black pepper

1–2 teaspoons olive oil or small amount of olive oil spray

Cut eggplant into thin (1/4-inch-thick) bite-size pieces. In a mixing bowl, combine almond meal, nutritional yeast, garlic powder, onion powder, and black pepper. Lightly brush or spray eggplant pieces with olive oil and coat with almond mixture. Bake at 375°F for 15 minutes, flip, then bake for an additional 10–15 minutes or until crisp and lightly browned.

PER SERVING: CALORIES 188; PROTEIN 9G; CARBOHYDRATES 21G; TOTAL FAT 8.9G; SATURATED FAT 0.9G; SODIUM 10MG; FIBER 11.3G; BETA-CAROTENE 37MCG; VITAMIN C 5MG; CALCIUM 65MG; IRON 1.6MG; FOLATE 59MCG; MAGNESIUM 78MG; ZINC 2.5MG; SELENIUM 1.9MCG

Lentil Wraps with Peppers and Onions

SERVES 4

1 cup uncooked brown or green lentils

2 cups water

1 bay leaf

1 tablespoon Dijon mustard

1 teaspoon Bragg Liquid Aminos or reduced-sodium soy sauce

¼ cup walnuts, toasted and ground

1 medium onion, sliced

2 cloves garlic, sliced

1 medium green bell pepper, seeded and sliced

1 medium red bell pepper, seeded and sliced

½ cup sliced mushrooms

4 whole grain flour tortillas (see Note)

Combine lentils, water, and bay leaf and cook until tender, about 45 minutes. Drain lentils and remove bay leaf. Add mustard, Bragg Liquid Aminos, and ground walnuts to lentils. Set aside. Heat 1–2 tablespoons water in a large pan and sauté the onion until tender, about 5 minutes, then add garlic, bell peppers, and mushrooms and cook for an additional 5 minutes or until just tender. Lightly toast the tortillas; spread with lentil mixture; top with peppers, mushrooms, and onions; and roll up.

Note: You can substitute cabbage for the flour tortillas. Use the large outer leaves and cook in boiling water for 4 minutes or until just limp. Drain and trim thick rib from the center of each leaf before making wraps.

PER SERVING: CALORIES 393; PROTEIN 22G; CARBOHYDRATES 62G; TOTAL FAT 7.7G; SATURATED FAT 1G; SODIUM 253MG; FIBER 22G; BETA-CAROTENE 558MCG; VITAMIN C 68MG; CALCIUM 94MG; IRON 6.5MG; FOLATE 264MCG; MAGNESIUM 83MG; ZINC 2.9MG; SELENIUM 10.1MCG

Meat-Lovers Beef, Bean, and Mushroom Burgers

SERVES 6

1 small onion, chopped

1 clove garlic, minced

2 cups mushrooms, chopped

1/4 cup unhulled sesame seeds

1 1/2 cups cooked or 1 (15-ounce) can no-salt-added or low-sodium kidney beans, drained

1 teaspoon dry basil

1/2 teaspoon dry oregano

1/8 teaspoon black pepper

1/4 cup whole grain bread crumbs

6 ounces (about 1 cup) organic ground beef (see Note for meatless option)

Preheat oven to 300°F. Water-sauté onions and garlic until beginning to soften, about 2 minutes. Add mushrooms and cook for about 5 minutes, until all liquid is evaporated. Grind sesame seeds in food processor. Add mushroom mixture, beans, and spices and process until well combined. Spoon into a bowl and mix in bread crumbs and beef.

Form into 6 medium-size patties. Place burgers on a baking sheet lined with parchment paper or lightly wiped with olive oil. Bake for 40 minutes, turning after 20 minutes.

Note: To make without ground beef, add an additional 1 1/2 cups cooked beans.

PER SERVING: CALORIES 208; PROTEIN 14G; CARBOHYDRATES 23G; TOTAL FAT 7G; SATURATED FAT 2.1G; CHOLESTEROL 17.6MG; SODIUM 56MG; FIBER 6.7G; BETA-CAROTENE 3MCG; VITAMIN C 2MG; CALCIUM 106MG; IRON 4.1MG; FOLATE 116MCG; MAGNESIUM 66MG; ZINC 2.9MG; SELENIUM 14.5MCG

Salad-Stuffed Pita with Creamy Almond Dressing

SERVES 4

For the Dressing

1 cup unsweetened soy, hemp, or almond milk

1 cup raw almonds

1/4 cup balsamic vinegar

2 tablespoons fresh lemon juice

1/4 cup raisins

2 teaspoons Dijon mustard

For the Sandwich

2 cups shredded lettuce

2 cups shredded spinach

1 tomato, chopped

1 avocado, peeled and chopped

1/2 cup thinly sliced red onion.

4 (100% whole grain) pitas or flour tortillas

Blend dressing ingredients in a high-powered blender until smooth and creamy.

Combine lettuce, spinach, tomato, avocado, and onion. Toss with desired amount of dressing. (Reserve leftover dressing for another use.) Stuff into whole grain pitas. If making wraps, place on wrap, roll up tightly, and cut in half.

PER SERVING: CALORIES 309; PROTEIN 9G; CARBOHYDRATES 38G; TOTAL FAT 15.3G; SATURATED FAT 1.5G; SODIUM 179MG; FIBER 8.8G; BETA-CAROTENE 3,483MCG; VITAMIN C 17MG; CALCIUM 104MG; IRON 3MG; FOLATE 114MCG; MAGNESIUM 86MG; ZINC 1MG; SELENIUM 3.2MCG

Shiitake BLT

SERVES 3

For the Shiitake Bacon

4 regular or 2 Medjool dates, pitted and chopped

1 teaspoon Bragg Liquid Aminos or low-sodium soy sauce

1 teaspoon garlic powder

1/2 teaspoon chili powder

1/4 teaspoon ground cumin

1/4 cup water

7 ounces shiitake mushroom tops, halved

For the Avocado Mayonnaise

1 ripe avocado, peeled and pitted

1 tablespoon apple cider vinegar

1 teaspoon nutritional yeast

1/2 teaspoon chopped rosemary

6 slices (100% whole wheat) bread or 3 (100% whole wheat) pitas or wraps

Lettuce, sliced tomato, sliced onion

Preheat oven to 375°F. To make the shiitake bacon, mash together dates, Bragg Liquid Aminos, garlic powder, chili powder, cumin, and water in a medium bowl. Add the sliced mushrooms and toss until mushrooms are well-coated with date mixture. Spread evenly on a baking sheet lined with parchment paper. Bake until mushrooms are dried and browned, about 1 hour.

To make the avocado mayonnaise, mash together the avocado, vinegar, nutritional yeast, and rosemary in a small bowl.

Toast bread or pita, spread with avocado mayonnaise, and add shiitake bacon, lettuce, sliced tomato, and sliced onion. If making a wrap, add ingredients and roll up.

PER SERVING: CALORIES 310; PROTEIN 12G; CARBOHYDRATES 49G; TOTAL FAT 9.6G; SATURATED FAT 1.5G; SODIUM 363MG; FIBER 11.7G; BETA-CAROTENE 2,673MCG; VITAMIN C 11MG; CALCIUM 107MG; IRON 3MG; FOLATE 142MCG; MAGNESIUM 96MG; ZINC 2.5MG; SELENIUM 27.1MCG

Sweet Potato Fries

SERVES 4

4 sweet potatoes
1 tablespoon garlic powder
1 tablespoon onion powder

Preheat oven to 400°F. Peel sweet potatoes if not organic. Cut into strips. Lay on a nonstick baking sheet. Sprinkle garlic powder and onion powder on potatoes. Bake for 45 minutes, turning every 15 minutes, until tender and lightly browned.

PER SERVING: CALORIES 126; PROTEIN 3G; CARBOHYDRATES 29G; TOTAL FAT 0.1G; SODIUM 74MG; FIBER 4.4G; BETA-CAROTENE 11,062MCG; VITAMIN C 4MG; CALCIUM 48MG; IRON 1MG; FOLATE 17MCG; MAGNESIUM 36MG; ZINC 0.5MG; SELENIUM 1.6MCG

Taco Salad Wraps

SERVES 4

For the Dressing

2 ripe avocados
2 tablespoons nutritional yeast
1/4 cup unsweetened soy, hemp, or almond milk
2 tablespoons lime juice
1/2 teaspoon cumin
1/2 teaspoon chili powder, regular or chipotle

For the Wraps

1 cup cooked red kidney or black beans or low-sodium canned beans, drained
4 (100% whole grain) flour tortillas
1 cup frozen corn kernels, thawed
4 plum tomatoes, chopped
2 cups shredded romaine lettuce

Blend dressing ingredients in a blender until smooth and creamy. With a fork or potato masher, mash beans, leaving slightly chunky. Spread desired amount of dressing on each tortilla and then top with bean mixture, corn, chopped tomato, and lettuce. Fold up the bottom edge of the tortilla until it partially covers the filling, then fold in the left and right sides of the tortilla and roll up. Slice in half diagonally.

Refrigerate leftover dressing for another use.

PER SERVING: CALORIES 335; PROTEIN 15G; CARBOHYDRATES 50G; TOTAL FAT 9.9G; SATURATED FAT 1.4G; SODIUM 165MG; FIBER 13.6G; BETA-CAROTENE 1,600MCG; VITAMIN C 17MG; CALCIUM 83MG; IRON 4.6MG; FOLATE 145MCG; MAGNESIUM 57MG; ZINC 1.8MG; SELENIUM 1.8MCG

Veggie Pizza

SERVES 4

1 cup chopped broccoli

1 cup chopped cauliflower

1/2 red bell pepper, chopped

3 slices onion, chopped

1/2 pound mushrooms, chopped

1 teaspoon Bragg Liquid Aminos or reduced-sodium soy sauce

3 tablespoons balsamic vinegar

1 teaspoon MatoZest or other no-salt seasoning, adjusted to taste

1/4 teaspoon garlic powder (or to taste)

4 (100% whole grain) flour tortillas

1 cup low-sodium or no-salt-added tomato sauce

2 tablespoons shredded nondairy mozzarella cheese

Preheat oven to 350°F. In large bowl, mix all ingredients except for tortillas, tomato sauce, and nondairy cheese. Spread on a large cookie sheet with edges and bake for 30 minutes or until vegetables are tender, stirring occasionally.

Remove toppings from oven and increase temperature to 400°F. Place tortillas on cookie sheet and spread sauce on tortillas, coating thinly all the way to the edges. Evenly distribute the veggies on top and sprinkle with nondairy cheese. Bake 7–10 minutes or until the edges turn golden brown.

Remove from oven, allow to cool, then slice and serve. May be refrigerated and reheated in the oven the next day.

PER SERVING: CALORIES 257; PROTEIN 12G; CARBOHYDRATES 39G; TOTAL FAT 6.6G; SATURATED FAT 1.0G; SODIUM 282MG; FIBER 8.4G; BETA-CAROTENE 519MCG; VITAMIN C 61MG; CALCIUM 133MG; IRON 3.3MG; FOLATE 63MCG; MAGNESIUM 29MG; ZINC 0.9MG; SELENIUM 13.0MCG

Desserts

Apple Surprise

SERVES 6

1 cup raisins

1/4 cup water

8 apples, peeled, cored, and diced

1/2 cup chopped walnuts

4 tablespoons ground flaxseeds

1 tablespoon cinnamon

Place raisins in bottom of pot and cover with 1/4 cup water. Place diced apples on top. Cover and steam over very low heat for 7 minutes, or until apples are tender. Transfer apple/raisin mixture to a bowl and mix well with remaining ingredients.

This recipe keeps well in the refrigerator for several days.

PER SERVING: CALORIES 267; PROTEIN 4G; CARBOHYDRATES 50G; TOTAL FAT 8.7G; SATURATED FAT 0.8G; SODIUM 5MG; FIBER 6.3G; BETA-CAROTENE 39MCG; VITAMIN C 9MG; CALCIUM 58MG; IRON 1.3MG; FOLATE 15MCG; MAGNESIUM 51MG; ZINC 0.7MG; SELENIUM 1.8MCG

Banana Oat Cookies

SERVES 7

1/2 cup raisins or chopped dates

2 ripe bananas, mashed

1 1/2 cups old-fashioned oats

1/3 cup chopped walnuts or raw almonds

1/4 cup unsweetened, shredded coconut

1 teaspoon vanilla extract or powdered vanilla bean

1/8 teaspoon cinnamon

1/4 cup 100% all-fruit preserves, any flavor, if desired

Add 2 tablespoons of water to raisins or dates and soak for 30 minutes. Preheat oven to 325°F. Combine the mashed bananas and oats. Add the nuts, coconut, vanilla, cinnamon, and soaked dates or raisins. Mix well. Drop by tablespoons onto a nonstick cookie sheet. If desired, flatten a little, make an indentation in the center of the cookie, and add a small dollop of fruit spread. Bake for 13 minutes or until golden brown. Makes 14 cookies.

PER SERVING: CALORIES 179; PROTEIN 4G; CARBOHYDRATES 29G; TOTAL FAT 6.7G; SATURATED FAT 2G; SODIUM 2MG; FIBER 4.2G; BETA-CAROTENE 10MCG; VITAMIN C 3MG; CALCIUM 12MG; IRON 4.7MG; FOLATE 14MCG; MAGNESIUM 25MG; ZINC 0.3MG; SELENIUM 1.4MCG

Creamy Beany Chocolate Mousse

SERVES 3

1 1/2 cups cooked or 1 (15-ounce) can no-salt-added or low-sodium black beans, drained

1 small apple, peeled and cored

1 ripe banana

1/2 cup natural, nonalkalized cocoa powder

6 regular or 3 Medjool dates, pitted

1/4 cup soy, hemp, or almond milk

2 tablespoons ground flaxseeds

2 teaspoons vanilla extract

1/2 teaspoon cinnamon

1/4 cup unsweetened, shredded coconut for garnish, if desired

Add all ingredients except coconut to a high-powered blender and blend thoroughly until smooth. Add more nondairy milk by the tablespoon if needed to blend, being careful not to add too much. Mixture should be thick. Place in bowls, cover, and chill well in refrigerator before serving. Garnish with coconut if desired.

PER SERVING: CALORIES 357; PROTEIN 13G; CARBOHYDRATES 66G; TOTAL FAT 9.9G; SATURATED FAT 5.9G; SODIUM 19MG; FIBER 18.3G; BETA-CAROTENE 40MCG; VITAMIN C 5MG; CALCIUM 84MG; IRON 4.8MG; FOLATE 153MCG; MAGNESIUM 188MG; ZINC 2.5MG; SELENIUM 7.1MCG

Fruit Slushie

SERVES 4

5 cups fresh fruit chunks (such as watermelon, cantaloupe, mango, or peaches)

2 tablespoons fresh-squeezed lime juice

6 regular or 3 Medjool dates, pitted

1 teaspoon lime zest

1 cup ice cubes

Blend all ingredients in a high-powered blender until smooth. Freeze 15–20 minutes or until just partially frozen. Stir and serve.

PER SERVING: CALORIES 90; PROTEIN 2G; CARBOHYDRATES 23G; TOTAL FAT 0.3G; {SATURATED FAT?} SODIUM 2MG; FIBER 1.8G; BETA-CAROTENE 580MCG; VITAMIN C 19MG; CALCIUM 20MG; IRON 0.6MG; FOLATE 9MCG; MAGNESIUM 24MG; ZINC 0.2MG; SELENIUM 1.1MCG

Fudgy Black Bean Brownies

SERVES 12

2 cups cooked or canned no-salt-added or low-sodium black beans, drained

1 ¼ cups regular dates or 10 Medjool dates, pitted

2 tablespoons raw almond butter

1 teaspoon vanilla

½ cup natural, nonalkalized cocoa powder

1 tablespoon ground chia seeds

Optional Chocolate Topping

1 ripe avocado

½ cup water

4 tablespoons natural, nonalkalized unsweetened cocoa powder

10 regular or 5 Medjool dates, pitted

Splash vanilla extract

Preheat oven to 200°F. Combine the black beans, dates, almond butter, and vanilla in a food processor or high-powered blender. Blend until smooth. Add the remaining ingredients and blend again. Spread into a very lightly oiled 8-by-8-inch baking pan. Bake for 1 ½ hours. Cool completely and apply topping if desired. Cut into small squares. Store in a covered container in the refrigerator up to 1 week.

To make topping, blend all ingredients in a high-powered blender.

PER SERVING: CALORIES 123; PROTEIN 4G; CARBOHYDRATES 25G; TOTAL FAT 2.4G; SATURATED FAT 0.5G; SODIUM 2MG; FIBER 5.6G; BETA-CAROTENE 18MCG; CALCIUM 40MG; IRON 1.4MG; FOLATE 48MCG; MAGNESIUM 59MG; ZINC 0.8MG; SELENIUM 1.4MCG

Six-Minute Baked Apple

SERVES 2

2 apples, halved and cored

1 teaspoon cinnamon

⅛ cup raisins

2 regular dates or 1 Medjool date, pitted and chopped

½ lemon, zest only

2 tablespoons finely ground or chopped raw almonds

Put 1 tablespoon water in a small microwaveable baking dish with no lid. Place the four apple halves in the baking dish, cut sides up. Cover the exposed apple sides with the cinnamon. Press the raisins into the holes where the apple cores were removed. Microwave for 5 minutes. (You can also bake apples in a conventional oven at 350°F for 25 minutes or until soft.)

Meanwhile, mash together the dates, lemon zest, and ground almonds with a fork. When the apples are done cooking, place on a serving dish and reserve cooking liquid. Mash the cooking liquid into the date mixture and spread over the top of the apples.

PER SERVING: CALORIES 165; PROTEIN 2G; CARBOHYDRATES 39G; TOTAL FAT 2.3G; SATURATED FAT 0.2G; SODIUM 1MG; FIBER 4.6G; BETA-CAROTENE 40MCG; VITAMIN C 9MG; CALCIUM 46MG; IRON 1MG; FOLATE 5MCG; MAGNESIUM 28MG; ZINC 0.3MG; SELENIUM 0.2MCG

Strawbeany Ice Cream

SERVES 4

2 cups fresh or 1 (10-ounce) bag frozen strawberries

¾ cup cooked pinto beans (or canned, unsalted)

1 cup unsweetened soy or almond milk

8 regular dates or 4 Medjool dates, pitted

½ cup raw cashews

1 teaspoon nonalcohol vanilla extract

Blend all ingredients in a high-powered blender until smooth. Freeze until almost set, about 2 hours.

PER SERVING: CALORIES 242; PROTEIN 7G; CARBOHYDRATES 38G; TOTAL FAT 8.5G; SATURATED FAT 1.4G; SODIUM 50MG; FIBER 6.5G; BETA-CAROTENE 40MCG; VITAMIN C 30MG; CALCIUM 177MG; IRON 2.8MG; FOLATE 76MCG; MAGNESIUM 91MG; ZINC 1.5MG; SELENIUM 5.9MCG

Sweet Potato Pie with
Coconut Pecan Crust

SERVES 8

For the Crust

1 cup pecans

1/2 cup rolled oats

1/2 cup unsweetened hemp or almond milk

8 regular or 4 Medjool dates, pitted

2 tablespoons unsweetened coconut flakes

1/8 teaspoon vanilla bean shreds or nonalcohol vanilla extract

For the Filling

1 teaspoon agar flakes

2 oranges, 1 juiced and 1 peeled and chopped

2 cups cooked sweet potatoes, mashed

12 ounces silken tofu, drained (see Note)

2 regular or 1 Medjool date, pitted

2 teaspoons pumpkin pie spice (see Note)

1/2 cup pecans, chopped

Preheat oven to 350°F. Combine crust ingredients in a food processor and pulse until well-combined. Press mixture into a 9-inch pie pan.

To make the filling, dissolve the agar flakes in the orange juice. Place in a high-powered blender or food processor along with the sweet potato, chopped orange, tofu, dates, and pumpkin pie spice and blend until smooth. Spoon sweet potato mixture onto piecrust. Garnish with chopped pecans and bake for 40 minutes. Let pie cool and then refrigerate for at least 2 hours before serving.

Note: Silken tofu (also called Japanese-style tofu) has a softer consistency than regular tofu. Unlike regular tofu, silken tofu is sometimes packaged in aseptic boxes that do not require refrigeration. Because of this, silken tofu is sometimes sold in a different section of the grocery store than regular tofu, which is packed in water and requires refrigeration.

Note: You can make your own pumpkin pie spice by mixing 1 1/4 teaspoons cinnamon and 1/4 teaspoon each of ginger, nutmeg, and cloves.

PER SERVING: CALORIES 310; PROTEIN 6G; CARBOHYDRATES 37G; TOTAL FAT 17G; SATURATED FAT 2.3G; SODIUM 24MG; FIBER 6.3G; BETA-CAROTENE 7,784MCG; VITAMIN C 29MG; CALCIUM 91MG; IRON 3.1MG; FOLATE 23MCG; MAGNESIUM 53MG; ZINC 1.2MG; SELENIUM 1.3MCG

Vanilla or Chocolate Nice Cream

SERVES 4

1/4 cup raw walnuts

2 ripe bananas, frozen (see Note)

1/3 cup soy, hemp, or almond milk (frozen ahead of time)

4 regular or 2 Medjool dates, pitted

1 teaspoon nonalcoholic vanilla extract or 2 tablespoons natural nonalkalized cocoa powder

Using a high-powered blender, blend walnuts to a fine powder. Add remaining ingredients and blend on high speed until smooth and creamy. Serve immediately or store in freezer for later use.

Note: Freeze ripe bananas at least 8 hours in advance. Peel bananas and seal in a plastic bag before freezing.

PER SERVING: CALORIES 141; PROTEIN 2G; CARBOHYDRATES 25G; TOTAL FAT 4.6G; SATURATED FAT 0.5G; SODIUM 11MG; FIBER 2.9G; BETA-CAROTENE 27MCG; VITAMIN C 5MG; CALCIUM 22MG; IRON 0.6MG; FOLATE 23MCG; MAGNESIUM 38MG; ZINC 0.4MG; SELENIUM 1.9MCG

CHAPTER NINE

FREQUENTLY ASKED QUESTIONS

1. I KNOW LOTS OF PEOPLE WHO EAT FAST FOOD AND JUNK FOOD ALL THE TIME, AND THEY ARE PERFECTLY HEALTHY AND PLENTY SMART. WHAT ABOUT THAT?

We all have different genetic weaknesses and tendencies. Some people are more sensitive to nutritional insults than others. Some of us can resist apparent signs of early life damage even when eating suboptimally. However, damage still accumulates over the years, and it almost always catches up with us, resulting in serious disease in midlife or later. Nobody escapes the cumulative damage from a diet heavy in fast foods, even if the damage can't be seen when we're younger.

The United States has the most overweight and diabetic population ever recorded in the history of the world. The amount of suffering experienced today by so many people with serious medical conditions that can be avoided is simply heartbreaking. We have to expect that those people who are eating the unhealthiest and are the most addicted to food will be the ones who most resist change. They often propose irrational excuses why they should not change their bad habits. Lots of people still smoke cigarettes; everyone is not going to quit, despite the overwhelming evidence of danger. All we can hope for is that everyone is properly informed and educated. My hope and goal are to make the tools available for those who want to protect their health and the health

Age of Death: SAD vs. Nutritarian Diet

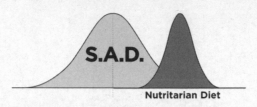

of their loved ones, and that those who want to, can get professional help to change when they need it.

LIFE SPAN PROBABILITIES: A BELL-SHAPED CURVE

Let's look at age of death. If you plot age of death among people on a similar diet, you get a bell-shaped curve of possibilities, where the center of the curve represents the average age of death for a particular population. If there is a great difference between the ages at which people die, the width of the curve is greater. If there is less difference, the width is narrower. For people eating the SAD, the curve is wide, meaning that people eating this diet die at a wide variety of ages. Some live much longer, which is balanced with others who die very young.

If we look at populations eating heavily from natural plants and avoiding processed foods (the "Nutritarian diet" on the figure), such as in the Blue Zones around the world, the curve not only shifts to the right by ten to fifteen years (that is, people live longer generally), but it also narrows considerably. Without poor nutrition, people are much less likely to die prematurely (except for accidents). My experience as a physician over the past twenty-five years caring for thousands of people adhering to my nutritional guidance (Nutritarians) has indicated that thriving well into one's 90s is not just possible, but most probable.

The vast majority of adults older than 65 in the United States take medications for their heart and high blood pressure. Many also take diabetes medications and antidepressants. Almost all Americans die of diseases related to nutritional ignorance. But premature death is not the only problem; all the morbidity, suffering, and physical, emotional, and intellectual deficits that occur as people age make their lives very difficult and even tragic. The fast food eaters don't just die fifteen to twenty years prematurely; they suffer greatly (and needlessly) during the last two decades of their lives.

I believe that many millions of people would be willing to make more substantial dietary improvements if they knew about and understood the true risks involved with taking medications for high blood pressure, high cholesterol, and high blood sugar levels. Medications are not very effective at mitigating the morbidity and mortality associated with these chronic diseases of dietary folly. Dramatic protection against heart disease, stroke, dementia, and cancer cannot and does not occur from access to medical care; it can only happen when people eat very healthfully—and when they have the information they need to take charge of their health destiny. The problem is that too many millions of people do not have this information. Nor do many of them have access to healthy foods, as we have seen. They are not given the opportunity to even make the choice to live healthfully.

But with that information and available healthy food, and with effort and time spent learning new recipes, we can all find that a healthy diet becomes more and more enjoyable as our taste and food preferences

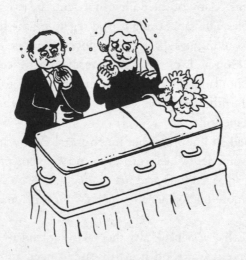

"I heard the food doesn't taste so good once you're in the coffin."

change the more we eat healthy food. Healthy food can taste great! You don't enjoy living more when you eat dangerously.

2. WHY CAN'T A MULTIVITAMIN MAKE UP FOR WHAT PROCESSED FOODS LACK?

Real food contains too many important factors that have never seen the inside of a vitamin pill. An important message of this book is that we need to eat real food to be healthy: We cannot expect supplements to do the job for us.

Many delicate, valuable phytonutrients are lost through processing and cooking food. These nutrients number in the thousands, and eating a variety of plants is the only way to get them. Important phytochemicals form during chewing, as plant enzymes are released and activated. Some of these enzymes are heat-sensitive, so the more the plant food is cooked, the more nutrients are lost.

For example, eating a salad every day made up of mostly raw vegetables is a critical centerpiece of a health-supporting, life span—enhancing diet. The reason is because heat inactivates the enzyme myrosinase, which is needed for the production of cell-supporting and cancer-fighting nutrients. Many of these phytonutrients are not as available in cooked vegetables. The same thing is true regarding the health benefits of raw scallions, onions, and shallots, to maintain function of the enzyme called alliinase. Hundreds of other delicate, supportive compounds are found in colorful plants that interact with each other to improve and safeguard our health, and these compounds and enzymes cannot be found in supplements.

I want to add an important but much more radical and universally unappreciated point here. The fortification and supplementation of foods with petroleum-derived folic acid may actually increase the risk of disease, and even more tragic, increase the risk of cancer and a premature death.

Many studies have evaluated whether taking a standard multivitamin-mineral supplement wards off heart disease, cancer, and dementia or extends life span. Overall, the results of the majority of such studies show very little benefit, if any. A meta-analysis conducted for the U.S. Preventive Services Task Force assessed the evidence from twenty-seven studies on vitamin and mineral supplementation that included more than 450,000 people and found no evidence of benefit for preventing heart disease and only a minimal benefit for reducing cancer risk.[1] A significant number of studies also show that the commonly included nutrients in multivitamins can cause harm. These data are a bit complicated and need to be explained and understood further.

Any study looking at the risks and benefits of long-term multivitamin use is by its nature poor science. That's because multivitamins have too many variables and mix together some potentially useful elements

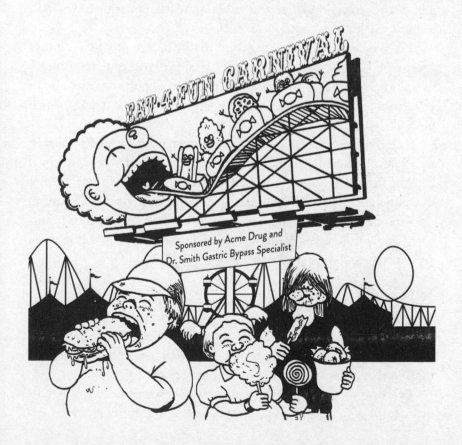

with other potentially harmful ones. Studying multivitamin use is as illogical as studying the Mediterranean diet: Is it the fish that is good or bad for you? Or the tomato sauce, walnuts, and olive oil? Or did the oil cause more weight gain and death? Does the white pasta and cheese in the Mediterranean diet promote a longer life span, or the pizza crust? You can see the point: Too many variables are lumped together to be able to get any useful information about which elements are good or bad when they are included all together in one study.

We need to evaluate one intervention at a time to really learn which are the most favorable or unfavorable components of a diet. When we do that with the Mediterranean diet, we invariably find out that the white flour pasta and the pizza crust are unfavorable. Clearly, a Mediterranean diet is far from an ideal diet, and just because it is better than the SAD, it is not scientific to position it as such.

Likewise, a study evaluating the benefits of a multivitamin lumps together elements such as vitamin D, vitamin B12, and zinc supplementation, which may have benefits in certain populations, with other elements such as beta-carotene, folic acid, vitamin A, and copper, which most likely have overall harmful effects.

These studies are examples of poor science and wasted resources; they tell us almost nothing. Therefore, the inconsistent and marginal benefits shown by these studies on whole multivitamins do not offer us any insights on which elements, if any, aid health or are effective in reducing cancer or extending life span. We have to study each micronutrient individually to ascertain its risks and value. I explain this in more detail below and offer suggestions.

FOLIC ACID IS NOT FOLATE

Let's consider the practice of supplementing flours and foods with folic acid and vitamin A and look at the benefits and risks. If you understand the complexity of this issue, you will be able to better understand why supplements cannot take the place of eating right.

Folate is a B vitamin that is universally present in plants. A synthetic form of folate called **folic acid** is used in dietary supplements and fortified foods. Folic acid is derived from petroleum and is not the same compound as the real folate that is found in fruits, vegetables, and beans.

Synthetic folic acid is highly absorbable, but then the body has to modify it so it can behave like real folate. The body can convert only a limited amount of folic acid into folate, so most people ingesting folic acid have unmodified folic acid circulating in their bloodstream and in the tissues of their body. Remember: Folic acid is a manufactured chemical substitute for folate, and throughout human history, folate has been the protective vitamin ingested from eating real food. Only in our recent fast food era have people been encouraged to supplement with folic acid because they no longer eat sufficient vegetation, which is naturally high in folate.

The problem begins with folic acid competing for absorption into the body, thus decreasing the absorption of the folate in fruits, beans, and vegetables. Once inside our body's cells, the real competition begins where folic acid binds to folate-dependent enzymes, creating potential hazards in their function. DNA synthesis is affected, leading to more DNA errors in dividing and replicating cells, which potentially can increase the risk of developing cancer.

Almost every obstetrician today prescribes a folic acid–containing supplement to pregnant women to protect the growing fetus from neural tube defects. The neural tube is the embryo's precursor to the central nervous system, which comprises the brain and spinal cord. Neural tube defects occur during early fetal development because modern women are not eating vegetables—not because they require a petroleum-derived chemical to have a normal child. Modern health authorities repeatedly try to solve health issues with pills instead of fixing the real problem, in this case, the lack of green vegetables in the diet.

Instead of encouraging women to eat more vegetables and beans to give birth to normal children, we give them folic acid pills. Instead of encouraging people to eat more vegetables and lose weight to reverse type 2 diabetes, we give them pills. Instead of encouraging people to eat more vegetables so they can lower their cholesterol and prevent heart disease, we give them statin drugs. The problem with these "pill solutions" is that they have unintended side effects. It is more effective and safer to lower your blood pressure and reverse your diabetes through an excellent diet and exercise, not medication. It is more effective and safer to maintain a normal level of folate in your body by eating properly, not by taking a supplement containing folic acid.

When people ingest folic acid routinely in multivitamins and fortified foods, their bodies get overloaded with the stuff, and unintended consequences result. For instance, we know from animal studies that the presence of artificial folic acid promotes the progression of precancerous lesions to cancer and the spread of cancer, including breast cancer.[2] In addition, taking folic acid during pregnancy to prevent neural tube defects may actually damage the child. Let's look at some of the evidence, but remember, it can take thirty to fifty years to see increases in cancer occurrence from ingesting folic acid.

- A study compared breast cancer death rates between women who took folic acid during their pregnancies and those who did not. Thirty years later, those women who took a hefty dose of folic acid were twice as likely to have died from breast cancer.[3]

- A ten-year study on more than thirty-five thousand women taking multivitamins showed that women who took a multivitamin containing folic acid had a 20 percent increased occurrence of breast cancer compared with women not supplementing with folic acid.[4] (Note that ten years would underestimate the increased cancers that could have been created.)

- Researchers looking to find a benefit from using folic acid to prevent breast cancer followed more than twenty-five thousand women and were shocked to find the opposite—folic acid supplement use was associated with a higher incidence of breast cancer.[5]

- A 2011 meta-analysis of folic acid supplementation and colon cancer found people taking the supplement for three years or longer increased their risk of developing advanced adenoma by 50 percent.

A 2012 meta-analysis of folic acid supplementation found a 21 percent increase incidence of cancers at all sites.[6]

- One randomized controlled trial of folic acid supplementation reported that men who took folic acid had triple the prostate cancer risk compared with men who took a placebo.[7]

Some studies looking at this issue have not shown an increase in breast cancer incidence in women supplementing with folic acid. This is most likely because the studies are not well-controlled and do not follow the study populations long enough. When atomic bombs exploded in Hiroshima and Nagasaki in Japan to end World War II, cancer deaths began to appear about ten years later, and the rates were still climbing after forty years. We cannot look at studies performed for fewer than ten years to ascertain the potential cancer-promoting effects of an intervention.

Today, even people who do not take a supplement containing folic acid still have a large exposure to supplemental folic acid in fortified foods, so this is a difficult subject to study when our entire population is exposed to folic acid from multiple sources every day. A systematic review and meta-analysis of nineteen studies discussing this issue was published in 2012 and showed an increase in prostate cancer in men taking folic acid in supplements and a borderline increase in overall cancer.[8] Remember, even a negative study does not mean folic acid is safe; it just means that the study could not detect the harm. Given that our modern population ingests multiple carcinogenic substances, it is nearly impossible to isolate every contributor to determine individual effects.

When people eat commercial baked goods, they don't just ingest cancer-causing additives, such as bromate and sodium phosphate, and bleaching and softening agents, such as benzoyl peroxide and azodicarbonamide; they also consume a load of folic acid because all of these things are added to the fortified white flour used in commercial baking. Add the underlying risks of the high-glycemic flour as well as the synthetic folic acid in a multivitamin, and you have a witches' brew for cancer promotion.

Unlike supplemental folic acid, we know that eating real food with real folate offers significant protection against cancer. Folate is abundant in all green vegetables, and folate-containing foods include hundreds of protective nutrients. We do not need synthetic folic acid supplements to meet our daily folate requirements. Here are a few examples of folate-rich foods (as a reference point, the U.S. recommended daily allowance for folate is 400 micrograms).

	MICROGRAMS OF FOLATE
Asparagus (1.5 cups cooked)	402
Edamame (1 cup cooked)	358
Lentils (1 cup cooked)	358
Broccoli (2 cups cooked)	337
Chickpeas (1 cup cooked)	282
Adzuki beans (1 cup cooked)	278
Romaine lettuce (3 cups raw)	192
Brussels sprouts (2 cups cooked)	187
Spinach (3 cups raw)	175

When you eat produce to get your folate, you radically improve your nutritional status in many ways, as these are all micronutrient-rich foods in general, containing many antioxidants and phytochemicals.

However, it is not healthy to be deficient in folate, and certainly for people who can't or won't eat vegetables, taking some folic acid is better than nothing. But everyone should be informed that ingesting an excessive amount of folic acid from a combination of fortified foods and supplements can be dangerous. Too much exposure to folic acid during pregnancy may increase respiratory problems in children such as asthma and pneumonia.[9] There is even evidence that excessive blood levels of folate (which likely is from excessive exposure to folic acid) at childbirth is associated with doubling the risk of autism in children.[10]

One thing we know for sure: If women ate more green vegetables and beans throughout their lives, they would get plenty of folate, and their offspring not only would be protected against neural tube defects but also would get hundreds of other beneficial compounds that offer protection against childhood cancers. It has been known for years that a lack of green vegetables in mothers' diets increases the risk of childhood cancers in their offspring.[11] The diet before conception also affects these risks. If the public were fully informed on all these issues, maybe more people would eat right and we would have many fewer children with autism, brain tumors, and leukemia. Now is the time for public health authorities to promote a diet with adequate folate from plant foods.

Future studies may indicate that some people metabolize folic acid and vitamin B12 differently and are at higher risk than others from excesses. However, this would not be an issue if women got their needed folate from a healthy diet. We can't stop the folic acid recommendations across the board yet, because so many women still don't eat healthfully, but at least we can start to reeducate our population about the necessity of getting these nutrients from their natural sources, and the profound benefits from doing so.

This is a complicated issue, and most people are in the dark about it. But it has important implications because excluding accidents, cancer is the leading cause of death in children younger than 15. This missed opportunity to educate young women about the critical importance of a healthy diet that contains adequate folate to have a normal and healthy child leads to many subtle medical issues in children that can affect them throughout their lives—including allergies and autoimmune diseases. Advocating folic acid supplements, instead of sufficient vegetables and beans to obtain folate, likely harms and even kills thousands of children every year.

SUPPLEMENTS AND FORTIFICATION OF FOODS IS
PART OF THE PROBLEM, NOT THE SOLUTION

When you eat a healthy diet, you are exposed to a huge amount of carotenoids, such as beta-carotene, a precursor to vitamin A in the body. The body converts beta-carotene (as well as alpha-carotene and beta-cryptoxanthin) into vitamin A, so if people eat enough colorful vegetables, there would be no need for vitamin A supplementation. People are exposed to preformed vitamin A in supplements and in fortified foods, and it has been shown that even in ranges not normally considered toxic, it can be harmful. A review of sixty-eight randomized trials of vitamin A supplementation, with a mean dose of 20,000 IU, showed an average 16 percent increased mortality over an average of three years.[12] Since this analysis was not over decades, it likely underestimates the damage from excess vitamin A intake.

The amount of vitamin A in typical multivitamins has been shown to increase the risk of osteoporosis and hip fractures, and excess vitamin A in fortified foods makes these effects even worse. One study showed a doubling of the hip fracture rate with more vitamin A, comparing an intake of 1,500 IU vitamin A with 4,500 IU, the latter being the typical amount found in vitamin supplements.[13] High doses of vitamin A during pregnancy have also been linked to birth defects.[14]

A more recent evaluation of all relevant trials carried out around the world showed that taking vitamin A, beta-carotene, and vitamin E supplements increased mortality—that is, the risk of sudden death was higher for those who took such supplements. Some skeptics doubted these findings, claiming that people taking supplements likely had worse diets because they believed that the supplements would improve their health. These doubts were rejected in later randomized trials, which means that study participants were randomly assigned to take the supplements or a placebo. The results showed the same dangers from the supplements as the earlier studies had shown. This new study carried out in 2011 was based on eleven new trials and used ordinary dosages typically found in vitamin pills that were linked to the increased death rate.[15] The researchers tested both single vitamins and multivitamins, and they found increased mortality in both cases.

The full spectrum of natural vitamin forms that is found in natural foods, such as eight separate vitamin E fragments or hundreds of carotenoids, behaves much differently from the vitamins we take as supplements or get from fortified foods in our diet. As the saying goes, "You can't fool Mother Nature."

Supplements cannot take the place of a healthy diet and should be avoided—especially the widely available inexpensive varieties. This does not mean that the judicious use of supplements to cover nutritional gaps in a person's diet is not important; it just means we have to review the data carefully regarding each ingredient and the precise form of supplement being used, and assure that the dosage used is not excessive.

3. WHAT ABOUT THOSE WHO DON'T EAT RIGHT? AND, DO PEOPLE WHO EAT HEALTHFULLY NEED ANY SUPPLEMENTS AT ALL?

Unquestionably, people who eat fast food, commercial baked goods, processed meats, fried foods, and soft drinks are dangerously deficient in micronutrients, especially antioxidants and phytochemicals. We have to recognize that despite the potential dangers of certain supplemental ingredients, this group is more likely to be better off with a carefully chosen assortment of supplements, including powdered whole food extracts, phytochemical isolates, and a full spectrum of low-dose antioxidants.

Of course, supplementation will not grant them optimal health, but it is better than being severely deficient in micronutrients. However, it is important to remember that individual nutrients and isolated nutrient extracts and synthetics can still be potentially harmful. Take care not to overdose on any micronutrient that could have negative effects, especially in excess amounts.

A large number of Americans eat what they consider a "healthy" diet, but so often that diet still does not include sufficient vegetables, beans, onions, mushrooms, berries, and seeds and still is too close to the SAD (meaning they eat too many processed foods and animal products). These people are not exposed to enough micronutrients and phytochemicals. For these people, a supplement with a dehydrated vegetable-based formula with dozens of phytochemical extracts from superfoods is likely beneficial, though not as valuable as eating an excellent diet. There are other groups of people who may benefit from supplementing their diets with certain vitamins and minerals:

1. **The elderly:** Vitamin B12 absorption decreases with age, and elderly people may also need higher amounts of calcium and vitamin D. Zinc is also important for the elderly, as the body's ability to absorb zinc can decrease and immunity wanes in later life, increasing the risk of a person developing influenza and pneumonia. A significant amount of research indicates that such supplementation is particularly important in the aging population to decrease the risk of infections, especially life-threatening pneumonia.[16]

   Calcium can also be an issue for the elderly, as bones age and grow brittle. Green vegetables, beans, and seeds are generally rich in calcium, and a diet including these foods is healthful for the bones. Taking too much supplemental calcium in a concentrated form can lead to increased blood vessel calcification and may increase heart disease risk.[17] So even in postmenopausal women, the right diet and the moderate use of food-derived calcium in small amounts (such as 150–250 milligrams) with meals is a better choice than a high dose (500–1000 milligrams) of calcium taken at once, which may have detrimental health effects.[18]

2. **Vegans and vegetarians:** Vitamin B12 is found only in animal foods. Depending on food choices and the care taken to cover insufficiencies, vegans and vegetarians may also have suboptimal levels of vitamin K2, zinc, iron, vitamin D, and omega-3 fatty acids (see page 283).

3. **Children who are picky eaters:** Children who do not eat a varied diet may benefit from the regular use of a carefully designed supplement

that contains a variety of powdered superfood extracts and micro-nutrients. Children's developing brains also benefit from a DHA-EPA supplement, since reliance on seafood in today's world can expose children to too much mercury and petrochemicals, both of which are found in fish.

Others who may benefit from taking multivitamins include people who have had weight-loss surgery, people who are on very low-calorie diets, people who have a poor appetite, and people who don't get enough nutrients from food alone because of a medical or genetic reason.

Many people think that a healthy diet should supply all the nutrients we need for optimal health; this is pretty close to being true, but there are exceptions. The first exception is vitamin D, known as the "sunshine vitamin," because the only way to obtain enough vitamin D naturally is from the rays of the sun. These days, however, most people work indoors, and many live in more northern climates with less daily sunshine. Also, with our mixed backgrounds, our skin has differing abilities to produce vitamin D from the sun—not only because of skin pigmentation but also because of genetic factors.

Sure, if we lived most of our lives outdoors, with not much cloth-ing on—aging and wrinkling our skin in the process and in some cases creating a higher risk of developing skin cancer—then we wouldn't need vitamin D supplements. The bottom line is that supplementing with vitamin D3 is important for many people to maintain an optimally healthy level in their bodies. Being severely deficient in any nutrient, even when arising from a desire to stay "natural," is not healthful for anyone and gets many individuals into trouble, as I've frequently seen in my medical practice. A vitamin D deficiency does not just increase one's risk of getting osteoporosis; it also can increase the risk of cancer.[19]

On the other hand, too high a dose of supplemental vitamin D can also have untoward effects.[20] A 25-hydroxy vitamin D blood test can assure that people are not taking too much or too little, aiming for blood levels between 30 and 50 ng/dL. For most people who do not get enough sun exposure, a daily dose of 2,000 IU vitamin D3 (the preferred form) assures they will reach a favorable blood level without the risk of taking too much. Occasionally, people need more or less.

There is another important concept to grasp here: A growing segment of our health-seeking population restricts or omits animal products in order to protect against chronic diseases. As animal product consumption becomes more infrequent, the risk of vitamin B12 deficiency looms larger. So as we strive for more healthy produce and fewer animal products, we need to have a reliable source of B12. If you are elderly or completely vegan, your need for B12 can be significantly higher than the recommended daily intake because only a small percentage of a B12 supplement is absorbed at one time, and the supplements are generally taken only once a day.

Zinc, vitamin K2, and iodine are also nutrients that could be suboptimal depending on your choice of foods, and many very healthy eaters can still be low in one of these nutrients if they don't consume animal products for zinc or seaweeds, seafood, or iodinated salt for iodine. Plant foods do contain adequate zinc, but because of the binding of zinc to plant phytates, the bioavailability is lower.[21] This means that despite adequate zinc in the diet, many vegans may require a bit more for optimal immune function. Zinc needs can vary, and zinc absorption can decrease with aging.[22]

Just because some supplements are potentially dangerous doesn't mean that all supplemental ingredients are harmful or not beneficial. In fact, when extensively studied, many have been shown to be life span favorable in general populations.

YOUR SUPPLEMENT SHOULD NOT CONTAIN	YOUR SUPPLEMENT SHOULD CONTAIN
Folic acid	Vitamin B12
Vitamin A	Vitamin D
Beta-carotene	Iodine
Vitamin E	Zinc
Copper	Vitamin K2

Vitamin K2 is another example of a supplement that may benefit the general population as well as those people eating an excellent diet. There are two natural forms of vitamin K: the K1 found in plants, especially green vegetables, and the lesser-known K2, which is more difficult to obtain from modern diets. Several studies have found that vitamin K2 reduces the risk of hip and spine fractures and reduces bone loss with aging.[23] Vitamin K2 is found in some animal products, such as fish eggs and organ meats or natto, a fermented soy product, so supplemental K2 likely has significant benefits.

Supplements of the omega-3 fatty acids EPA and DHA can also have important health benefits for those people who don't eat seafood regularly. As discussed in Chapter 2, EPA and DHA are important for brain development and health, affecting intelligence and even emotional stability. Omega-3 fatty acids are also important nutrients for protection against depression, dementia, and neurological disorders.

The study results diagramed below tested fatty acid levels in 167 vegans of various ages who were eating a natural diet and avoided processed foods. Results showed that 64 percent had insufficiencies and that 27 percent had more severe deficiencies. These deficiencies were easily corrected with a low-dose vegan DHA/EPA supplement. There was no correlation with DHA insufficiency and ALA levels, the short-chain

Omega-3 Index in Vegans[24]

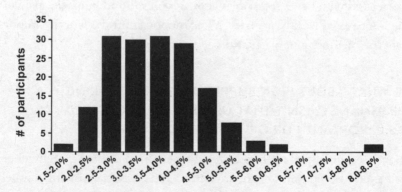

Omega-3 index measures levels of EPA and DHA in red blood cell membranes and represents long-term exposure to these beneficial fatty acids. Levels less than 3.5 percent are particularly alarming, because once your brain shrinks, no supplemental regimen can enlarge it again.

omega-3 fat found in leafy greens, walnuts, and flaxseeds from which the body can make EPA and DHA. There was also no correlation with the amount of omega-6 oil consumption. This means that the differences were largely due to a wide genetic variability in the conversion of ALA to DHA, since the problem was not solved by higher ALA intake and lower omega-6 intake. The important learning point here is that vegans and people who don't eat fish may be placing themselves at needless risk of later life memory loss and dementia if they don't take supplements. If a person is uncertain regarding their needs, thankfully, blood tests are easily available to check for adequacy.

More than a dozen epidemiological studies have reported that reduced levels of omega-3 fatty acids were associated with an increased risk for age-related cognitive decline or dementia, such as Alzheimer's disease. In the Women's Health Initiative Memory Study of more than eleven hundred postmenopausal women, a higher omega-3 index was correlated with larger total normal brain volume and hippocampal volume measured eight years later.[25] The hippocampus is critically important for memory and orientation.

4. WHAT ABOUT IRON SUPPLEMENTATION DURING PREGNANCY? ISN'T THAT UNIVERSALLY ACCEPTED AS IMPORTANT FOR OFFSPRING INTELLIGENCE?

Iron is essential for a baby's developing brain and future intelligence, but excess iron promotes oxidative stress and is associated with elevated blood pressure in pregnancy and low birth weight.[26] It's important to understand that some additional nutrients from supplements may be useful during pregnancy and breastfeeding, but others (like vitamin A) can cause birth defects. Levels of DHA and vitamin D and iron status are important, but the amount needed may be different from person to person. Iron is particularly critical because both too much and too little can cause problems for the unborn child.

For a subset of women with adequate iron stores, taking supplemental iron can harm their child. It is wise for pregnant women to learn their iron status via a ferritin blood test, starting early in pregnancy, and then use this information to decide the appropriate level of supplementation (if any) to complement a health-promoting diet because absorption of iron varies so much among people.

During pregnancy, a woman's iron needs increase, and it is estimated that 18 percent of pregnant women are iron deficient.[27] Each woman needs to be evaluated to determine her own iron needs. Adequate iron stores are essential for early infant brain development and are needed to support the large increase in blood volume that occurs during pregnancy. Iron adequacy is also important for the mother-child bonding during infancy.[28] Most importantly, iron deficiency in the mother can lead to iron deficiency in her breast-fed infant, which may impair health and future intelligence.[29]

Iron is more readily absorbed from animal than from plant food sources. For this reason, it is important for pregnant women (and those planning to becoming pregnant), especially those eating a vegan, vegetarian, or flexitarian diet, to maintain adequate iron stores.[30] In recent years, researchers have begun to support the idea of making individualized iron supplementation recommendations, rather than providing blanket guidelines for all pregnant women. Research scientists studying this issue have concluded that recommending a fixed dose of iron to avert deficiencies in all women does not result in optimal outcomes. It is safest to use the minimum effective dose. Substantial evidence shows that those women who have plenty of iron stores (documented by blood tests) to support a healthy pregnancy should not take any supplemental iron.

To be consistent with the current science, and to make the best decision to maximize the health of both mother and child, my iron recommendations for pregnant women are more intricate than standard recommendations. The goal of iron supplementation should be to achieve the "sweet spot" of adequacy for the baby's development without excess.

I recommend that when a pregnant woman's iron stores are low, with a ferritin level less than 30 ng/mL or hemoglobin less than 11 g/dL she should supplement with a low dose (such as 15–30 milligrams) of iron two to three times daily. When the ferritin level is in the middle range of 31–80 ng/mL and hemoglobin greater than 11 g/dL, supplementation with the standard dose of 9–27 milligrams iron (once daily) is reasonable, depending on the test results within that range. However, with ferritin levels greater than 80 ng/mL and hemoglobin greater than 12.5 g/dL, I do not recommend any iron supplements. Of course, women should discuss these recommendations with their personal physicians.

5. HOW BAD FOR YOU ARE ALCOHOLIC BEVERAGES?

Most people believe what they want to hear, and this is particularly true with how alcohol intake is related to health. We latch onto information which tells us that red wine is good for the heart or that drinking alcohol is okay in moderation. However, scientific evidence on this subject says otherwise. After declaring alcohol a carcinogen in 1988, the International Agency for Research on Cancer went further in 2014 and concluded that there is no safe amount of alcohol when it comes to cancer risk.[31] In its "14th Report on Carcinogens," the National Toxicology Program of the U.S. Department of Health and Human Services lists "alcoholic beverage consumption" as a known human carcinogen.[32] The research evidence indicates that the more alcohol a person drinks—particularly the more alcohol a person drinks regularly over time—the higher his or her risk of developing an alcohol-associated cancer. Based on data from 2009, an estimated 3.5 percent of all cancer deaths in the United States each year can be attributed to alcohol intake.[33]

The risks of drinking a small amount of alcohol, such as a few drinks a week, is certainly minimal, but health authorities should not encourage it because even light drinking is somewhat risky. Most people are under the impression that "social drinking" is harmless. But in a meta-analysis of 222 studies comprising ninety-two thousand light drinkers and sixty thousand nondrinkers with cancer, it was estimated that light drinking could have contributed to five thousand deaths each from oropharyngeal cancer and breast cancer, and twenty-four thousand from esophageal squamous cell carcinoma yearly.[34]

Alcohol consumption also elevates your risk of developing other cancers. A 2016 review article noted strong evidence that alcohol causes cancer at seven sites: the mouth/pharynx, larynx, esophagus, colon, rectum, breast, and liver.[35] Links have also been found between alcohol consumption and leukemia; multiple myeloma; and cancers of the head and neck, stomach, cervix, vulva, vagina, and skin.[36] The evidence suggests that the relationship between alcohol consumption and cancer is dose-dependent; that is, light drinking increases cancer risk lightly, and heavy drinking escalates that risk into danger zones.

More than one hundred epidemiological studies have looked at the association between alcohol consumption and the risk of breast cancer in women. These studies have consistently found an increased risk of breast cancer associated with increasing alcohol intake. A meta-analysis of fifty-three of these studies (which included a total of fifty-eight thousand women with breast cancer) showed that women who drank more than 45 grams of alcohol per day (approximately three drinks) had 1.5 times the risk of developing breast cancer as nondrinkers. The risk of breast cancer was higher across all levels of alcohol intake: For every 10 grams of alcohol consumed per day (slightly less than one drink), researchers observed a small (7 percent) increase in the risk of breast cancer. The Million Women Study in the United Kingdom (which included more than twenty-eight thousand women with breast cancer) provided a more recent, and slightly higher, estimate of breast cancer risk at low to moderate levels of alcohol consumption: Every 10 grams of alcohol consumed per day was associated with a 12 percent increase in the risk of breast cancer.[37] If you want to live as long as possible, the safest choice is to not drink alcohol at all.

Scientists think that acetaldehyde, a compound formed during the digestion of alcohol, may be responsible for the development of these types of cancers. In addition, alcoholic beverages also contain other carcinogenic substances, such as arsenic, benzene, cadmium, formaldehyde, lead, ethyl carbamate, acrylamide, and aflatoxins.[38]

Some people say that red wine is good for the heart. The link between alcohol and a reduced risk for coronary heart disease is thought to primarily be due to the fact that alcohol interferes with blood clotting. But this effect is valuable only in a person who consumes a dangerous, heart-disease–promoting diet, which increases the propensity of clot formation to abnormal levels. For someone who eats a healthful diet rich in unrefined plant foods, a high level of protection against heart disease will already exist, and then one would not want to abnormally thin the blood with alcohol because it could cause bleeding, increasing the risk of hemorrhagic stroke.[39]

An added risk of light drinking is that it can lead to occasional binge drinking or heavy drinking—consuming three or more drinks a day—which is dangerous and associated with cardiomyopathy, hypertension, and potentially life-threatening arrhythmias.[40] Younger people who have higher rates of excessive or binge drinking more frequently suffer the adverse consequences of acute intoxication (accidents, violence, and social problems). In fact, among males 15–59 years of age in the United States, alcohol abuse is the leading risk factor for premature death.[41]

Red wine contains a widely studied beneficial compound from grape skins called *resveratrol*. This compound has been shown to have several anti-inflammatory and antioxidant effects that may contribute to cardiovascular protection.[42] However, at this point, we don't know whether resveratrol in red wine contributes additional protection beyond the blood-thinning effects of alcohol, and it is unlikely that the resveratrol benefit would outweigh the carcinogenic risk of the alcohol.

Regardless of those possible benefits, it doesn't make sense to consume a carcinogenic substance just to get resveratrol, because resveratrol can also be found in grapes, raisins, blueberries, cranberries, peanuts, and other plant foods.

6. HOW DO YOU GET YOUR KIDS TO EAT HEALTHFULLY, ONCE THEY HAVE BECOME PICKY EATERS AND WON'T EAT FRUITS AND VEGETABLES AND ONLY WANT JUNK FOOD?

There are two important approaches to the secret of getting children to eat healthfully. The first one is relatively simple: Only keep healthy food in the house. Children's environments should not expose them to dangerous choices, such as drug use, alcohol, cigarettes, and junk food, and they should understand the reasons why. The second approach is to model the behavior and eating you want your children to follow. Children will frequently copy their parents' behavior, especially when that behavior makes logical sense and can be explained to them.

Once children have been exposed to highly sweetened, artificial foods, it becomes more difficult to change their behavior because they frequently no longer desire healthy fruits and vegetables. Family meetings can be important—to discuss the problem of unhealthy food consumption and changes that the family agrees are important. In a family meeting, every person has input and can make suggestions. Children can help motivate parents to eat better, and parents can help motivate children to eat better.

One great way to start this conversation with your children is to enlist their help in your efforts to eat better. Explain why you are no longer eating sweets and white flour and processed foods, and how they can help you stick to a healthy diet. Kids love their parents and want them to live a long life. Focusing on you gets the focus off the children so they don't feel criticized for their eating choices. They will also want to learn this information. When they learn how much food can affect life span and health, they will easily grasp why it is important not to be tempted with unhealthy foods around the house. Then, as a consequence, they will understand that family members can all help and support each other in retraining the taste buds, learning to cook healthier, and removing unhealthful temptations from the home.

My mission is to help people recognize that learning about optimal nutrition for a better life is essential, basic knowledge—like reading and writing. It should be a part of our education from early in life.

In today's unhealthy world with fast food and junk food all over the place, we need regularly scheduled family meetings to plan the week's shopping and menus, enlist everybody in helping out, and discuss and share why it is so important for everyone to eat healthfully. And in family meetings, you can "show them the evidence." This doesn't have to be all or nothing, especially at the beginning. By working as a family unit, and properly supporting each other, you all can improve your health habits. Use this as an opportunity to bring your family together with a common goal. Your children can understand the concept of Frankenfoods being designed by the fake food industry to make people like them better than real food made by nature.

They can also understand that it takes time to develop a liking for natural foods, but the more they eat them, the more they will like them. The only way to remove food addiction to junk food is to abstain from

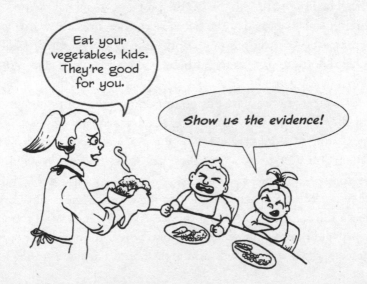

eating junk food. Fortunately, your family can have fun together trying the great-tasting, healthful recipes and desserts in this book, and in my cookbooks; making these tasty and healthy alternatives to what the family is eating now is a great family project. Achieving better health, fitness, and intellectual accomplishment via excellent nutrition is exciting, and having this as a family goal is a form of love. I have occasionally asked my children, "What would you do if you were the father and you loved your child as much as I love you?" They get it.

7. IF A PERSON ALREADY IS SUFFERING FROM CHRONIC DIETARY-INDUCED ILLNESS, SUCH AS DEPRESSION, AGITATION, POOR SLEEP, FATIGUE, OBESITY, DIABETES, OR HIGH BLOOD PRESSURE, WHAT CAN HE OR SHE DO TO GET WELL WITHOUT DRUGS?

The most rewarding part of my career as a physician has been enabling the transformation of people's lives and watching them recover their health. My experience and the experience of many other physicians specializing in lifestyle medicine is that nutritional excellence is far more powerful than drugs. This story is not merely about prevention; it is about the fact that targeted nutrition has amazing therapeutic potential to revolutionize health care, to help people, and to save our economy from the staggering costs of caring for such a sickly society. It not only enables people to normalize their weight, blood pressure, and cholesterol and reverse diabetes, but also enables complete recoveries from asthma, depression, and autoimmune diseases such as psoriasis, lupus, and rheumatoid arthritis. People suffering from severe chronic ailments can return to normal, healthy lives. I have a unique perspective among primary care physicians because I have used nutritional excellence therapeutically for more than twenty-five years and have observed the miraculous healing power of the well-nourished body, which in most cases can heal itself.

In 2016, I published a study in the *American Journal of Lifestyle Medicine* documenting an average drop in systolic blood pressure of 26 mm/Hg in 443 people following a Nutritarian diet.[43] I included numerous cases of advanced obstructive coronary artery disease that resolved. I am not the only physician who has observed, and published studies regarding dramatic reversal of even advanced heart disease as a result of excellent nutrition. This is already well-established in the scientific literature. In 2012, I published a study in the *Open Journal of Preventive Medicine* which demonstrated that 90 percent of patients with type 2 diabetes following a high-nutrient, low-glycemic diet were able to stop taking all of their medications for diabetes; their mean HbA1c after one year was 5.8 percent, which is within the normal, nondiabetic range.[44]

Nutrition is powerful medicine, and most conventional physicians in the United States today underuse it. I remember that first pharmacology lecture in medical school when the professor told us to never forget that all drugs are toxic and should be used only as a last resort. The problem was, we never learned about other options, such as changing a person's diet sufficiently. I am proud to say that my life's work is a testament to the effectiveness of nutritional and lifestyle medicine for most chronic diseases. Tens of thousands of people have recovered from chronic illnesses for which conventional medicine has no cure. There will always be some advanced and severe illnesses that are beyond the help of nutritional and lifestyle modifications, but even in such cases, excellent nutrition can reduce the need for medications and thereby medication side effects.

8. HOW MUCH SALT IS ACCEPTABLE IN ONE'S DIET?

Salt is sodium chloride, and sodium is an important mineral that is essential for proper functioning of the human body. However, the SAD contains dangerously high amounts of sodium, almost 80 percent of which comes from processed foods and foods we get at restaurants and fast food joints. For millions of years the human diet didn't contain any added salt—only the sodium present in natural foods, which usually adds up to less than 1,000 milligrams of sodium per day. The dietary intake of sodium in the United States today is about 3,500 milligrams per day.

Numerous observational studies and randomized controlled trials document the fact that high sodium intake increases blood pressure.[45]

The evidence implicating excess sodium intake as a major cause of high blood pressure levels has been called "overwhelming."[46] A recently published large long-term lifestyle intervention study showed that a 25–35 percent reduction in dietary sodium over ten to fifteen years results in a 25–30 percent lower risk of cardiovascular disease outcomes.[47] It is estimated that a 50 percent decrease in sodium consumption in the United States could prevent at least 150,000 deaths annually.[48] According to a meta-analysis of sixty-one studies, the lower an individual's blood pressure, at least down to $1^{15}/_{75}$ mm Hg, the lower the risk of stroke or heart attack.[49] There was no "threshold" below which the risk did not decrease; of course, that is assuming the lower blood pressure is "earned" through healthy eating, exercise, and salt avoidance and is not just medicated downward.

But the effects of salt intake are not all about blood pressure. The interesting finding from many different studies is that high salt intake is linked to increases in all-cause mortality and that its death-hastening effects occur in those people who are not "salt sensitive" to its blood pressure effects.[50] In other words, significant amounts of sodium in the diet predicts overall mortality and risk of coronary heart disease, independent of other cardiovascular risk factors, including blood pressure.[51]

The most compelling evidence is from long-term trials following individuals over decades. A 2016 study followed the lives and deaths of participants over many years, clarifying and giving substance to the undeniable reality that higher salt intake kills. The study included multiple twenty-four-hour urine samples collected from adults between the ages of 30 and 54 who were then followed for an average of twenty-four years. The results showed a direct linear association between average sodium intake and total mortality (death from all causes). The more sodium consumed, the higher the death rate. And just the opposite was found as well—fewer deaths occurred in people with the lowest intake of sodium.[52]

Natural foods such as fruits and vegetables all contain sodium. The amount of sodium humans and other animals need is contained in the natural foods we eat. If we just ate natural foods without added salt, we would most likely consume about 500–750 milligrams of sodium a day. Real food supplies the perfect amount of minerals people need to maximize their health. The human body was designed to function on food, and early humans did not consume extra salt. Our Stone Age ancestors consumed a diet consisting of mainly fruits, vegetables, nuts, seeds, fish, insects, and wild game and obtained all the sodium they required, as well as the other minerals. This eat-what-you-can-find diet continued for approximately one hundred thousand generations, during which time salt was not added to food.

Today, people in most areas of the world consume ten times as much sodium as is found in a natural "unsalted" diet. Our species developed agriculture around three hundred generations ago, and the Industrial Age again changed our diet over a span of five to ten generations until now. As we have already seen, the "Processed Food Era" started after World War I, two to three generations ago. This means we live with "thrifty genes" that were selected over a long period during which our ancestors had to deal with low salt intake, periods of starvation, and caloric inadequacy.[53] These genes were selected to conserve sodium in the body, not get rid of it.

Since almost all Americans and modern industrialized societies consume so much salt, we have to look at isolated or primitive populations to really see the long-term result of low salt intake. It is still possible to find pockets of people living on mostly natural food diets, without added salt. Tribes in New Guinea, the Amazon Basin, the highlands of Malaysia, and rural Uganda all eat very little salt. Hypertension is unheard of in these regions, and blood pressure does not rise steadily with age as it does in the United States and other countries with high salt intakes. The most elderly members of these populations have blood pressure readings like those we see in children. When salt is introduced into these salt-free cultures, however, blood pressure climbs.[54] In all human populations studied by medical anthropologists, it is known that people in all salt-free cultures (that is, those cultures not using salt as a condiment) experience almost no increase in blood pressure even into old age. By contrast, blood pressure rises significantly over many years in all human populations in which salt is added to food in significant quantities, resulting in most people sooner or later ending up with high blood pressure.

High-sodium diets ultimately lead to high blood pressure, which causes an estimated two-thirds of strokes and almost half of all heart attacks. According to the NIH, consuming less sodium is one of the single most important ways to prevent cardiovascular disease.[55] Certainly, not smoking, maintaining a healthy body weight, eating a nutrient-dense diet rich in vegetables and fruits, and limiting the intake of *trans* and saturated fats are critical; but too much sodium in our diets ranks right up there as a primary killer in our modern toxic food environment, and most people overlook this until it is too late.

Salt is also the strongest factor related to stomach cancer. Sodium intake data from twenty-four countries were significantly correlated to stomach cancer mortality rates. Additional studies have found positive correlations between salt consumption and the incidence of gastric cancer.[56] A high salt diet also increases growth of the ulcer-promoting bacteria *H. pylori* in the stomach, which is also a risk factor for gastric cancer.[57]

Reducing dietary salt is not only important for people who already have elevated blood pressure, but limiting added salt is essential for all of us to remain in good health. Since natural foods supply us with 600–800 milligrams of sodium a day, it is wise to limit any additional sodium, over and above what is in natural food, to just a few hundred milligrams. Even the CDC reports that salt kills far more Americans than tobacco (or anything else) and that almost 90 percent of all Americans, including everyone over the age of 40, should cut their salt intake by nearly two-thirds, to 1,500 milligrams per day.[58] Medications cannot do nearly what diet improvement and salt reduction can do, and more and more physicians and scientists recognize this. Just cutting out excess salt from the diet can return blood pressure to normal, which can reduce the risk of heart disease by at least 70 percent.

It is also important to note that expensive and exotic sea salts are still just salt. All salt originates from the sea—and sea salts are still more than 98 percent sodium chloride and therefore contribute to your diet the same amount of sodium per teaspoon as regular salt. Sea salts may contain small amounts of trace minerals, but the amounts are insignificant compared with those in natural plant foods, and the excess sodium doesn't magically become less harmful.

Salt also deadens taste buds, meaning that when you avoid highly salted and processed foods, you will regain your ability to detect and enjoy the subtle flavors in natural foods and experience heightened pleasure from natural, unsalted foods. Your taste buds will get stronger when you stay away from highly salted foods. Of course, this takes time to occur.

9. IF I'VE EATEN ALL THE WRONG FOODS MOST OF MY LIFE, IS IT TOO LATE FOR ME TO CHANGE NOW? HOW MUCH IS MY GOOSE COOKED?

Your goose is never fully cooked. Heart attacks and strokes are the leading cause of death in the modern world, and cardiovascular disease kills more individuals than all cancers added together. But, you can make a decision *right now* to never have a heart attack or stroke and make the necessary changes in your eating habits to almost guarantee this never happens.

For instance, you can always reduce your risk of developing lung cancer by quitting smoking at any point before cancer begins. Likewise, you can reduce your risk of a variety of cancers with nutritional excellence, even if it is too late to maximally protect yourself against cancer at an advanced age. Even people who have cancer have been shown to live longer eating the healthful, anticancer dietary suggestions discussed in this book. Many studies have already been referenced here on G-BOMBS demonstrating this fact.

Nutritional excellence can do what drugs can't do; drugs lower risk maybe 10–15 percent, while superior nutrition has the potential to lower risk 100 times that. In my twenty-five years of medical practice offering nutritional advice, I have not heard of anyone who has followed my program strictly for years who has ever had a heart attack or died from heart disease. I have cared for thousands of individuals with heart disease, many of them with very advanced heart disease, and I have seen miraculous healing happen, including improvement of ejection fraction and resolution of atrial fibrillation. It has been exciting and rewarding to see people earn back excellent health and celebrate their health recoveries.

I don't know about you, but it's not enough for me to lower my risk of experiencing sudden cardiac death by a mere 30–40 percent. I want that risk to be zero, if possible. With the dietary advice in this book, and my other books on these subjects, I present the medical evidence which shows that you can achieve dramatic reduction in weight, cholesterol levels, triglyceride levels, and cardiac risk that simply cannot be accomplished through medication. In other words, nutrition trumps standard pharmacology.

Cancer is a bit different because the years that you eat an unhealthful diet, including fast food and commercial meats, take their toll on the body and can cumulatively damage DNA. After sixty years of very poor eating habits, the change to an excellent diet cannot reduce risk by 99 percent, like it can with heart disease. My guess is that it will reduce risk of cancer by 50–75 percent. I base that estimate on studies that show reductions in cancer deaths after nutritional interventions. For example, one study followed for ten years women already diagnosed with breast cancer and found the death rate from breast cancer was 71 percent lower over those ten years for women who ate higher amounts of lignans (found particularly in flaxseed and chia seeds).[59] But, we are not talking just about flaxseeds here. When we put together a synergistic portfolio of foods, fresh herbs, and spices that have anticancer benefits and avoid unhealthy foods, we can restore immune system functioning and enhance the ability of the body to fight the initiation, development, and spread of cancer. It may not have the extreme benefits we see for heart disease, but the benefits are still remarkable.

Of course, the anticancer benefits are more profound the earlier in life one adopts a healthy diet, and the more advanced the cancer, the less likelihood we will observe such positive effects. Still, one never knows what benefits will accrue and what the body can accomplish when fed right. It is never too late to try to protect your health.

You can slow the aging process now, maintain a healthy weight, lower your blood pressure, prevent or reverse diabetes, protect yourself against a stroke and the so-common mental decline seen with aging, and overall live a better-quality, healthier, and longer life from making these improvements in your eating habits.

Too many people suffer and die needlessly, and I'm sure millions of people of all ages would adopt a healthier diet style if they learned about the profound benefits they would receive. I hope you join me on this quest to inform and motivate others to take better care of their health and to protect all of our children, enabling them to reach their full potentials for health and happiness. Let's bond together in our mutual desire to spread kindness and goodwill and to value every person's human potential for health and happiness. I wish you and your family a rewarding and pleasurable experience in your quest for excellent health.

ACKNOWLEDGMENTS

I want to thank and recognize many people who assisted me with this book. First of all, Robert (Bob) Phillips has been and continues to be dedicated to helping me and many others for years; his contribution to this book is invaluable. I want to thank Reggie Thomas, who had a vision years ago, and encouraged this project right from the start. I appreciate his assistance setting up events in urban areas to reach people in need with life-saving nutritional information. I appreciate my skilled supportive team at DrFuhrman.com, specifically Deana Ferrari, PhD, who assists me with research collection and interpretation; Linda Popescu, RD, who assists with recipes, nutritional analysis, and menus; Lauren Russell and Tim Shay, who assisted with diagrams and graphs; and Doris Walfield, who proofread and made edits. Mimi McGee contributed many fantastic recipes used in this book. Mary Becker also helped with the recipes, preparing, testing, and tweaking them to my liking. Colin Goh's art brought my cartoon concepts to life. Lisa Fuhrman spent many invaluable hours reading, giving me important feedback and editing. I am also appreciative of the wonderful team at Harper, especially Gideon Weil, who has been a strong supporter of my work and his early vision for my series of books to spearhead nutrition-based healthcare, and Production Editor Lisa Zuniga and Director of Publicity Melinda Mullin.

NOTES

INTRODUCTION: PARTICIPANTS IN OUR OWN DESTRUCTION

1 Lane M, Robker RL, Robertson SA. Parenting from before conception. *Science.* 2014;345:756–60; Dominguez-Salas P, Moore SE, Baker MS, et al. Maternal nutrition at conception modulates DNA methylation of human metastable epialleles. *Nat Commun.* 2014;5:3746; Lane M, Zander-Fox DL, Robker RL, McPherson NO. Peri-conception parental obesity, reproductive health, and transgenerational impacts. *Trends Endocrinol Metab.* 2015;26:84–90; Marques AH, Bjorke-Monsen AL, Teixeira AL, Silverman MN. Maternal stress, nutrition and physical activity: impact on immune function, CNS development and psychopathology. *Brain Res.* 2015;1617:28–46; Prado EL, Dewey KG. Nutrition and brain development in early life. *Nutr Rev.* 2014;72:267–84.

2 Heckman JJ, Lafontaine PA. The American high school graduation rate: trends and levels. *The Review of Economics and Statistics.* 2010;92(2):244–62; U.S. Department of Education. U.S. high school graduation rate hits new record high. http://www.ed.gov/news/press-releases/us-high-school-graduation-rate-hits-new-record-high-0.

3 Fuchs FD. Why do black Americans have higher prevalence of hypertension? An enigma still unsolved. *Hypertension.* 2011;57(3):379–80.

4 Howard G, Lackland DT, Kleindorfer DO, et al. Racial differences in the impact of elevated systolic blood pressure on stroke risk. *JAMA Int Med.* 2013;173(1):46–51.

5 Mozaffarian D, Benjamin EJ, Go AS, et al. Heart disease and stroke statistics—2016 update: a report from the American Heart Association. *Circulation.* 2016;133:e38–e360.

6 U.S. Department of Health and Human Services, Office of Minority Health. Diabetes and African Americans. http://minorityhealth.hhs.gov/omh/browse.aspx?lvl=4&lvlID=18.

7 Mozaffarian D, Benjamin EJ, Go AS, et al. Heart disease and stroke statistics—2016 update: a report from the American Heart Association. *Circulation.* 2016;133:e38–e360.

8 Albain KS, Unger JM, Crowley JJ, et al. Racial disparities in cancer survival among randomized clinical trials. *JNCI J National Cancer Institute.* 2009;101(14):984–92; National Cancer Institute. Cancer health disparities. https://www.cancer.gov/about-nci/organization/crchd/cancer-health-disparities-fact-sheet.

9 U.S. Department of Health and Human Services. Racial and ethnic disparities in Alzheimer's disease: a literature review. 1 February 2014. https://aspe.hhs.gov/report/racial-and-ethnic-disparities-alzheimers-disease-literature-review.

10 Aune D, Sen A, Prasad M, et al. BMI and all cause mortality: systematic review and non-linear dose-response meta-analysis of 230 cohort studies with 3.74 million deaths among 30.3 million participants. *BMJ.* 2016;353:i2156; Fryar CD, Gu Q, Ogden CL. Anthropometric reference data for children and adults: United States, 2007–2010. *Vital Health Stat.* 2012;11:1–48.

11 Ayyad C, Andersen T. Long-term efficacy of dietary treatment of obesity: a systematic review of studies published between 1931 and 1999. *Obes Rev*. 2000;1:113–19.

CHAPTER ONE: FAST FOOD AND DISEASE

1   Flegal KM, Kruszon-Moran D, Carroll MD, et al. Trends in obesity among adults in the United States, 2005 to 2014. *JAMA*. 2016;315:2284–91.

2   Murray CJ, Atkinson C, Bhalla K, et al. The state of US health, 1990–2010: burden of diseases, injuries, and risk factors. *JAMA*. 2013;310:591–608.

3   Gallup. Tobacco and smoking, 2016. http://www.gallup.com/poll/1717/tobacco-smoking .aspx.

4   Gallup. Fast food still major part of U.S. diet, 2013. 6 August 2013. http://www.gallup.com /poll/163868/fast-food-major-part-diet.aspx.

5   Shikany JM, Safford MM, Newby PK, et al. Southern dietary pattern is associated with hazard of acute coronary heart disease in the Reasons for Geographic and Racial Differences in Stroke (REGARDS) study. *Circulation*. 2015;132:804–14.

6   Chiuve SE, McCullough ML, Sacks FM, Rimm EB. Healthy lifestyle factors in the primary prevention of coronary heart disease among men: benefits among users and nonusers of lipid-lowering and antihypertensive medications. *Circulation*. 2006;114(2):160–67; Chomistek AK, Chiuve SE, Eliassen AH, et al. Healthy lifestyle in the primordial prevention of cardiovascular disease among young women. *J Am Coll Cardiol*. 2015;65:43–51.

7   Xu J, Murphy SL, Kochanek KD, Bastian BA. Deaths: final data for 2013. *Natl Vital Stat Rep*. 2016;64:1–119.

8   Odegaard AO, Koh WP, Yuan JM, et al. Western-style fast food intake and cardiometabolic risk in an Eastern country. *Circulation*. 2012;126:182–88.

9   Mattes RD, Dreher ML. Nuts and healthy body weight maintenance mechanisms. *Asia Pac J Clin Nutr*. 2010;19:137–41.

10 Atkinson FS, Foster-Powell K, Brand-Miller JC. International tables of glycemic index and glycemic load values: 2008. *Diabetes Care*. 2008;31:2281–83.

11 Hu J, La Vecchia C, Augustin LS, et al. Glycemic index, glycemic load and cancer risk. *Ann Oncol*. 2013;24:245–51; Mullie P, Koechlin A, Boniol M, et al. Relation between breast cancer and high glycemic index or glycemic load: a meta-analysis of prospective cohort studies. *Crit Rev Food Sci Nutr*. 2016;56:152–59; Nagle CM, Olsen CM, Ibiebele TI, et al. Glycemic index, glycemic load and endometrial cancer risk: results from the Australian National Endometrial Cancer study and an updated systematic review and meta-analysis. *Eur J Nutr*. 2013;52:705–15; Melkonian SC, Daniel CR, Ye Y, et al. Glycemic index, glycemic load, and lung cancer risk in non-Hispanic whites. *Cancer Epidemiol Biomarkers Prev*. 2016;25:532–39.

12 Fraser GE1, Shavlik DJ. Risk factors for all-cause and coronary heart disease mortality in the oldest-old: The Adventist Health Study. *Arch Intern Med*. 1997;157(19):2249–58.

13 Meule A, Gearhardt AN. Food addiction in the light of DSM-5. *Nutrients*. 2014;6:3653–71.

14 Gearhardt AN, Yokum S, Orr PT, et al. Neural correlates of food addiction. *Arch Gen Psychiatry*. 2011;68:808–16.

15 Taylor VH, Curtis CM, Davis C. The obesity epidemic: the role of addiction. *Can Med Assoc J*. 2009;182:327–28.

16 Burger KS, Stice E. Frequent ice cream consumption is associated with reduced striatal response to receipt of an ice cream–based milkshake. *Am J Clin Nutr*. 2012;95:810–17; Stice E, Yokum S, Blum K, Bohon C. Weight gain is associated with reduced striatal response to palatable food. *J Neurosci*. 2010;30:13105–9.

17 Devaraj S, Wang-Polagruto J, Polagruto J, et al. High-fat, energy-dense, fast-food-style breakfast results in an increase in oxidative stress in metabolic syndrome. *Metabolism*. 2008;57:867–70.

18 Patel C, Ghanim H, Ravishankar S, et al. Prolonged reactive oxygen species generation and nuclear factor-kappaB activation after a high-fat, high-carbohydrate meal in the obese. *J Clin Endo Metabol.* 2007;92:4476–79; Khansari N, Shakiba Y, Mahmoudi M, et al. Chronic inflammation and oxidative stress as a major cause of age-related diseases and cancer. *Recent Pat Inflamm Allergy Drug Discov.* 2009;3:73–80; Federico A, Morgillo F, Tuccillo C, et al. Chronic inflammation and oxidative stress in human carcinogenesis. *International J Cancer.* 2007;121:2381–86; Vives-Bauza C, Anand M, Shirazi AK, et al. The age lipid A2E and mitochondrial dysfunction synergistically impair phagocytosis by retinal pigment epithelial cells. *J Biol Chem.* 2008;283:24770–80; Egger G, Dixon J. Inflammatory effects of nutritional stimuli: further support for the need for a big picture approach to tackling obesity and chronic disease. *Obes Rev.* 2010; 11:137–49; Bhosale P, Serban B, Bernstein PS. Retinal carotenoids can attenuate formation of A2E in the retinal pigment epithelium. *Arch Biochem Biophys.* 2009;483:175–81; Zota AR, Phillips CA, Mitro SD. Recent fast food consumption and bisphenol A and phthalates exposures among the U.S. population in NHANES, 2003–2010. *Environ Health Perspect;* doi:10.1289/ehp.1510803.

19 Kurokawa Y, Maekawa A, Takahashi M, et al. Toxicity and carcinogenicity of potassium bromate: a new renal carcinogen. *Environ Health Perspect.* 1990;87:309–35.

20 León JB, Sullivan CM, Sehgal AR. The prevalence of phosphorus containing food additives in top selling foods in grocery stores. *J Ren Nutr.* 2013;23(4):265–70.

21 Trasande L, Zoeller RT, Hass U, et al. Estimating burden and disease costs of exposure to endocrine-disrupting chemicals in the European union. *J Clin Endocrinol Metab.* 2015;100(4):1245–55; Lerner A, Matthias T. Changes in intestinal tight junction permeability associated with industrial food additives explain the rising incidence of autoimmune disease. *Autoimmun Rev.* 2015;14(6):479–89; Northstone K, Joinson C, Emmett P, et al. Are dietary patterns in childhood associated with IQ at 8 years of age? A population-based cohort study. *J Epidemiol Community Health.* 2011;66(7):624–28; doi:10.1136/jech.2010.111955.

22 Fuhrman J, Sarter B, Glaser D, Acocella S. Changing perceptions of hunger on a high nutrient density diet. *Nutr J.* 2010;9:51.

23 Franz MJ, Van Wormer JJ, Crain AL, et al. Weight-loss outcomes: a systematic review and meta-analysis of weight-loss clinical trials with a minimum 1-year follow-up. *J Am Diet Assoc.* 2007;107:1755–67.

24 Fuhrman J, Singer M. Improved cardiovascular parameter with a nutrient-dense, plant-rich diet-style: a patient survey with illustrative cases. *Am J Lifestyle Med.* 15 October 2015.

25 Fulgoni VL, Keast DR, Bailey RL, Dwyer J. Foods, fortificants, and supplements: where do Americans get their nutrients? *J Nutr.* 2011;141:1847–54; Cogswell ME, Zhang Z, Carriquiry AL, et al. Sodium and potassium intakes among US adults: NHANES 2003–2008. *Am J Clin Nutr.* 2012;96:647–57.

26 Kearns CE, Schmidt LA, Glantz SA. Sugar industry and coronary heart disease research: a historical analysis of internal industry documents. *JAMA Intern Med.* 12 September 2016; doi:10.1001/jamainternmed.2016.5394; quotation from O'Connor, A. "How the Sugar Industry Shifted Blame from Fat." *New York Times,* 12 September 2016.

27 De Natale C, Annuzzi G, Bozzetto L, et al. Effects of a plant-based high-carbohydrate/high-fiber diet versus high–monounsaturated fat/low-carbohydrate diet on postprandial lipids in type 2 diabetic patients. *Diabetes Care.* 2009;32(12):2168–73.

28 Lustig RH. Fructose: it's "alcohol without the buzz." *Adv Nutr.* 2013;4(2):226–35.

29 Gross LS, Li L, Ford ES, et al. Increased consumption of refined carbohydrates and the epidemic of type 2 diabetes in the United States: an ecological assessment. *Am J Clin Nutr.* 2004;79(5):774–79.

30 Bray GA, Nielsen SJ, Popkin BM. Consumption of high-fructose corn syrup in beverages may play a role in the epidemic of obesity. *Am J Clin Nutr.* 2004;79:537–43.

31 Akar F, Uludag O, Aydin A, et al. High-fructose corn syrup causes vascular dysfunction associated with metabolic disturbance in rats: protective effect of resveratrol. *Food Chem Toxicol.* 2012;50:2135–41.

32 DiNicolantonio JJ, O'Keefe JH, Lucan SC. Added fructose: a principal driver of type 2 diabetes mellitus and its consequences. *Mayo Clin Proc.* 2015;90(3):372–81; Stephan BC, Wells JC, Brayne C, et al. Increased fructose intake as a risk factor for dementia. *J Gerontol A Biol Sci Med Sci.* 2010;65(8):809–14.

33 Dufault R, LeBlanc B, Schnoll R, et al. Mercury from chlor-alkali plants: measured concentrations in food product sugar. *Environ Health.* 26 January 2009;8:2.

34 Uribarri J, Woodruff S, Goodman S, et al. Advanced glycation end products in foods and a practical guide to their reduction in the diet. *J Am Diet Assoc.* 2010;110(6):911–16.

35 Vitek MP, Bhattacharya K, Glendening JM, et al. Advanced glycation end products contribute to amyloidosis in Alzheimer disease. *Proc Natl Acad Sci USA.* 1994;91:4766–70; Cai W, Uribarri J, Zhu L, et al. Oral glycotoxins are a modifiable cause of dementia and the metabolic syndrome in mice and humans. *Proc Natl Acad Sci USA.* 2014;111:4940–45.

36 Kaushik S, Wang JJ, Wong TY, et al. Glycemic index, retinal vascular caliber, and stroke mortality. *Stroke.* 2009;40(1):206–12.

37 George MG, Tong X, Kuklina EV, Labarthe DR. Trends in stroke hospitalizations and associated risk factors among children and young adults, 1995–2008. *Ann Neurol.* 2011;70:713–21; Smith SE, Fox C. Ischemic stroke in children and young adults: etiology and clinical features. UpToDate. http://www.uptodate.com/contents/ischemic-stroke-in-children-and-young-adults-etiology-and-clinical-features.

38 Griffiths D, Sturm J. Epidemiology and Etiology of Young Stroke. Stroke Res Treat 2011; doi: 10.4061/2011/209370. Smailovic D. Strokes in young adults: epidemiology and prevention Vasc Health Risk Manag. 2015;11:157–164.

39 Cawley J, Meyerhoefer C. The medical care costs of obesity: an instrumental variables approach. *J Health Econ.* 2012;31:219–30.

40 Song M, Fung TT, Hu FB, et al. Association of animal and plant protein intake with all-cause and cause-specific mortality. *JAMA Intern Med.* 2016;176(10):1453–63; Sinha R, Cross AJ, Graubard BI, et al. Meat intake and mortality: a prospective study of over half a million people. *Arch Intern Med* 2009;169:562–71.

41 National Cancer Institute. Chemicals in meat cooked at high temperatures and cancer risk. https://www.cancer.gov/about-cancer/causes-prevention/risk/diet/cooked-meats-fact-sheet; Niedernhofer LJ, Daniels JS, Rouzer CA, et al. Malondialdehyde, a product of lipid peroxidation, is mutagenic in human cells. *J Biol Chem* 2003;278:31426–33.

42 Gilsing AMJ, Fransen F, de Kok TM, et al. Dietary heme iron and the risk of colorectal cancer with specific mutations in KRAS and APC. *Carcinogenesis.* 2013;34:2757–66; Gilsing AMJ, Berndt SI, Ruder EH, et al. Meat-related mutagen exposure, xenobiotic metabolizing gene polymorphisms and the risk of advanced colorectal adenoma and cancer. *Carcinogenesis.* 2012;33:1332–39; Mourouti N, Kontogianni MD, Papavagelis C, et al. Meat consumption and breast cancer: a case-control study in women. *Meat Sci.* 2015;100:195–201; Inoue-Choi M, Sinha R, Gierach GL, Ward MH. Red and processed meat, nitrite, and heme iron intakes and postmenopausal breast cancer risk in the NIH-AARP Diet and Health Study. *Int J Cancer.* 2016;138(7):1609–18; Aykan NF. Red meat and colorectal cancer. *Oncol Rev.* 2015;9:288.

43 Chan DS, Lau R, Aune D, et al. Red and processed meat and colorectal cancer incidence: meta-analysis of prospective studies. *PloS One.* 2011;6:e20456; Inoue-Choi M, Sinha R, Gierach GL, Ward MH. Red and processed meat, nitrite, and heme iron intakes and postmenopausal breast cancer risk in the NIH-AARP Diet and Health Study. *Int J Cancer.* 2016;138:1609–18; Larsson SC, Wolk A. Red and processed meat consumption and risk of

pancreatic cancer: meta-analysis of prospective studies. *Br J Cancer*. 2012;106:603–7; Bylsma LC, Alexander DD. A review and meta-analysis of prospective studies of red and processed meat, meat cooking methods, heme iron, heterocyclic amines and prostate cancer. *Nutr J*. 2015;14:125.

44 Vasan RS, Beiser A, Seshadri S, et al. Residual lifetime risk for developing hypertension in middle-aged women and men: the Framingham Heart Study. *JAMA*. 2002;287:1003–10.

45 Frohlich ED, Varagic J. The role of sodium in hypertension is more complex than simply elevating arterial pressure. *Nat Clin Pract Cardiovasc Med*. 2004;1(1):24–30.

46 Sanders PW. Vascular consequences of dietary salt intake. *Am J Physiol Renal Physiol*. 2009;297:F237–43.

47 De Wardener HE, MacGregor GA. Harmful effects of dietary salt in addition to hypertension. *J Hum Hypertens*. 2002;16:213–23; Harmon K. Salt linked to autoimmune diseases: nanowires show sodium chloride may cause harmful T-cell growth. 6 March 2013. *Nature*. http://www.nature.com/news/salt-linked-to-autoimmune-diseases-1.12555; Tsugane S, Sasazuki S. Diet and the risk of gastric cancer: review of epidemiological evidence. *Gastric Cancer*. 2007;10:75–83; Teucher B, Dainty JR, Spinks CA, et al. Sodium and bone health: impact of moderately high and low salt intakes on calcium metabolism in postmenopausal women. *J Bone Miner Res*. 2008;23:1477–85.

48 McDonald's Nutrition Calculator, https://www.mcdonalds.com/us/en-us/about-our-food/nutrition-calculator.html.

49 Calculated on two pieces original recipe chicken, baked beans, coleslaw, and mashed potatoes and gravy, Kentucky Fried Chicken Interactive Nutrition Menu, https://www.kfc.com/nutrition/full-nutrition-guide. Last updated 18 April 2016.

50 Bolhuis DP, Costanzo A, Newman LP, Keast RSJ. Salt promotes passive overconsumption of dietary fat in humans. *J Nutr*. 2016; doi:10.3945/ jn.115.226365.

51 Ma Y, He FJ, MacGregor GA. High salt intake: independent risk factor for obesity? *Hypertension*. 2015;66:843–49.

52 Carvalho JJ, Baruzzi RG, Howard PF, et al. Blood pressure in four remote populations in the INTERSALT study. *Hypertension*. 1989;14:238–46; Ulijaszek SJ, Koziel S, Hermanussen M. Village distance from urban centre as the prime modernization variable in differences in blood pressure and body mass index of adults of the Purari delta of the Gulf Province, Papua New Guinea. *Ann Hum Biol*. 2005;32:326–38; Gurven M, Blackwell AD, Rodriguez DE, et al. Does blood pressure inevitably rise with age?: longitudinal evidence among forager-horticulturalists. *Hypertension*. 2012;60:25–33.

53 Bibbins-Domingo K, Chertow GM, Coxson PG, et al. Projected effect of dietary salt reductions on future cardiovascular disease. *N Engl J Med*. 2010;362:590–99.

54 Wong K. *Monterey County Herald*. School lunches: fast food for thought? Cafeterias face challenge of offering balanced diet and a balanced budget. 24 February 2000. https://www.nasw.org/users/Katwong/publications/mocoherald/fastfood.html.

55 Chen G. Why fast food is "healthier" than school lunches: the shocking USDA truth. Public School Review. Updated June 21, 2016. https://www.publicschoolreview.com/blog/why-fast-food-is-healthier-than-school-lunches-the-shocking-usda-truth.

56 U.S. Food and Drug Administration. Final determination regarding partially hydrogenated oils (removing *trans* fat). http://www.fda.gov/Food/IngredientsPackagingLabeling/Food AdditivesIngredients/ucm449162.htm. Last updated 7 October 2016.

57 Allain P, Berre S, Krari N, et al. Bromine and thyroid hormone activity. *J Clin Pathol*. 1993;46(5):456–58.

58 Aburto NJ, Abudou M, Candeias V, Wu T. *Effect and Safety of Salt Iodization to Prevent Iodine Deficiency Disorders: A Systematic Review with Meta-Analyses*. Geneva: World Health Organization, 2014.

59 Micha R, Wallace SK, Mozaffarian D. Red and processed meat consumption and risk of incident coronary heart disease, stroke, and diabetes mellitus: a systematic review and meta-analysis. *Circulation.* 2010;121:2271–83.
60 Sheweita SA, El-Bendery HA, Mostafa MH. Novel study on N-nitrosamines as risk factors of cardiovascular diseases. *BioMed Res Int.* 2014;2014:817019; Kim Y, Keogh J, Clifton P. A review of potential metabolic etiologies of the observed association between red meat consumption and development of type 2 diabetes mellitus. *Metabolism.* 2015;64:768–79.
61 Bondy SC. Low levels of aluminum can lead to behavioral and morphological changes associated with Alzheimer's disease and age-related neurodegeneration. *Neurotoxicology.* 2016;52:222–29.

CHAPTER TWO: THE BRAIN ON FAST FOOD

1 DeWall CN, Deckman T, Gailliot MT, et al. Sweetened blood cools hot tempers: physiological self-control and aggression. *Aggress Behav.* 2011;37(1):73–80.
2 DeWall CN, Pond RS, Bushman BJ. Sweet revenge: diabetic symptoms predict less forgiveness. *Personality and Individual Differences.* 2010;49(7):823–26.
3 Centers for Disease Control and Prevention. U.S. Diabetes Surveillance System. Division of Diabetes Translation. Diagnosed diabetes. http://gis.cdc.gov/grasp/diabetes/DiabetesAtlas.html.
4 Diabetes in Camden. Data from a Camden City Comprehensive Health Database (July 2002–June 2008). http://www.camconnect.org/datalogue/DiabetesSummary200806Data_300906Edits.pdf.
5 CamConnect. Know Your City: Camden City Crime Trends from 1989 to 2014. http://camconnect.org/datalogue/2015CrimeAnalysis.pdf.
6 U.S. Census Bureau. Welcome to QuickFacts: Camden City, New Jersey. http://www.census.gov/quickfacts/table/PST045215/3410000/accessible; QuickFacts: Cherry Hill Mall CDP, New Jersey. http://www.census.gov/quickfacts/table/SBO001212/3412385,34.
7 U.S. Department of Agriculture Economic Research Service. Food availability (per capita) data system. https://www.ers.usda.gov/data-products/food-availability-per-capita-data-system/. Last updated 23 November 2016.
8 Poll reported in Barford V. Why are Americans so angry? BBC News. 4 February 2016. http://www.bbc.com/news/magazine-35406324.
9 Kumar GP, Khanum F. Neuroprotective potential of phytochemicals. *Pharmacogn Rev.* 2012;6(12):81–90; Kennedy DO. Polyphenols and the human brain: Plant "secondary metabolite" ecologic roles and endogenous signaling functions drive benefits. *Adv Nutr.* 2014;5:515–33.
10 Akbaraly TN, Brunner EJ, Ferrie JE, et al. Dietary pattern and depressive symptoms in middle age. *Br J Psychiatry.* 2009;195(5):408–13.
11 Grosso G, Galvano F, Marventano S, et al. Omega-3 fatty acids and depression: scientific evidence and biological mechanisms. *Oxid Med Cell Longev.* 2014;2014:313570; Kennedy DO. B vitamins and the brain: mechanisms, dose and efficacy—a review. *Nutrients* 2016;8(2):68.
12 Sánchez-Villegas A, Toledo E, de Irala J, et al. Fast-food and commercial baked goods consumption and the risk of depression. *Public Health Nutrition.* 2011;15(3):424.
13 Gangwisch JE, Hale L, Garcia L, et al. High glycemic index diet as a risk factor for depression: analyses from the Women's Health Initiative. *Am J Clin Nutr.* 2015; doi:10.3945/ajcn.114.103846.
14 Kodl CT, Seaquist ER. Cognitive dysfunction and diabetes mellitus. *Endocr Rev.* 2008; 29:494–511; Sommerfield AJ, Deary IJ, Frier BM, et al. Acute hyperglycemia alters mood state and impairs cognitive performance in people with type 2 diabetes. *Diabetes Care.* 2004;27:2335–40.

15 Schopf V, Fischmeister FP, Windischberger C, et al. Effects of individual glucose levels on the neuronal correlates of emotions. *Front Hum Neurosci.* 2013;7:212.

16 Kodl CT, Seaquist ER. Cognitive dysfunction and diabetes mellitus. *Endocr Rev.* 2008;29:494–511; Starr VL, Convit A. Diabetes, sugar-coated but harmful to the brain. *Curr Opin Pharmacol.* 2007;7:638–42.

17 Suglia SF, Slonick S, Hemenway D. Soft drinks consumption is associated with behavior problems in 5-year-olds. *J Pediatr.* 2013;163(5):1323–28.

18 Wiles NJ, Northstone K, Emmett P, Lewis G. "Junk food" and childhood behavioural problems: results from the ALSPAC cohort. *Eur J Clin Nutr.* 2009;63(4):491–98.

19 Grosso G, Galvano F, Marventano S, et al. Omega-3 fatty acids and depression: scientific evidence and biological mechanisms. *Oxid Med Cell Longev* 2014;2014:313570.

20 Rahal A, Kumar A, Singh V. Oxidative stress, prooxidants, and antioxidants: the interplay. *BioMed Res Int.* 2014; 2014: 761264.

21 Grootveld M, Silwood CJL, Addis P, Claxson A. Health effects of oxidized heated oils. *FoodService Research International.* 2001;13:41–55.

22 DeMar JC, Jr., Ma K, Bell JM, et al. One generation of N-3 polyunsaturated fatty acid deprivation increases depression and aggression test scores in rats. *J Lipid Res.* 2006;47(1):172–80; Hibbeln JR, Ferguson TA, Blasbalg TL. Omega-3 fatty acid deficiencies in neurodevelopment, aggression and autonomic dysregulation: opportunities for intervention. *Int Rev Psychiatry.* 2006;18(2):107–18.

23 Higdon J, Drake VJ. Essential fatty acids. In: *An Evidence-Based Approach to Dietary Phytochemicals and Other Dietary Factors.* 2nd ed. New York: Thieme, 2013:183–208; Cole GM, Ma QL, Frautschy SA. Omega-3 fatty acids and dementia. *Prostaglandins Leukot Essent Fatty Acids.* 2009;81:213–21.

24 Simopoulos AP. The importance of the omega-6/omega-3 fatty acid ratio in cardiovascular disease and other chronic diseases. *Exp Biol Med.* 2008;233(6):674–88.

25 Wang DD, Li Y, Chiuve SE, et al. Association of specific dietary fats with total and all-cause mortality. *JAMA Int Med.* 2016;176(8):1134–45.

26 Chowdhury R, Warnakula S, Kunutsor S, et al. Association of dietary, circulating, and supplement fatty acids with coronary risk: a systematic review and meta-analysis. *Ann Intern Med.* 2014;160:398–406; Astrup A, Dyerberg J, Elwood P, et al. The role of reducing intakes of saturated fat in the prevention of cardiovascular disease: where does the evidence stand in 2010? *Am Clin Nutr.* 2011;93(4):684–88; Siri-Tarino PW, Sun Q, Hu FB, et al. Saturated fatty acids and risk of coronary heart disease: modulation by replacement nutrients. *Curr Atheroscler Rep.* 2010;12:384–90; Willett W, Sacks F, Stampfer M. Dietary fat and heart disease study is seriously misleading. Harvard School of Public Health, The Nutrition Source. 2014. https://www.hsph.harvard.edu/nutritionsource/2014/03/19/dietary-fat-and-heart-disease-study-is-seriously-misleading/.

27 Bittman, M. "Butter Is Back." *New York Times,* 25 March 2014. https://www.nytimes.com/2014/03/26/opinion/bittman-butter-is-back.html?_r=0.

28 Ramsden CE, Zamora D, Majchrzak-Hong S, et al. Re-evaluation of the traditional diet-heart hypothesis: analysis of recovered data from Minnesota Coronary Experiment (1968–73). *BMJ.* 2016;353:i1246.

29 Vogel RA, Corretti MC, Plotnick GD. The postprandial effect of components of the Mediterranean diet on endothelial function. *J Am Coll Cardiol.* 2000;36(5):1455–60.

30 Mattes RD, Dreher ML. Nuts and healthy body weight maintenance mechanisms. *Asia Pac J Clin Nutr.* 2010;19:137–41.

31 Depression: Patrick RP, Ames BN. Vitamin D and the omega-3 fatty acids control serotonin synthesis and action, part 2: relevance for ADHD, bipolar disorder, schizophrenia, and impulsive behavior. *FASEB J.* 2015;29:2207–22; Logan AC. Omega-3 fatty acids and major depression: a primer for the mental health professional. *Lipids Health Dis.* 2004;3:25; Osher Y,

Bemaker RH. Omega-3 fatty acids in depression: a review of three studies. *CNS Neurosci Ther.* 2009;15(2):128–33. Cognitive decline: Schaefer EJ, Bongard V, Beiser AS, et al. Plasma phosphatidylcholine docosahexaenoic acid content and risk of dementia in Alzheimer disease. *Arch Neurol.* 2006;63:1545–50; Beydoun MA, Kaufman JS, Satia JA, et al. Plasma n-3 fatty acids and the risk of cognitive decline in older adults: the Atherosclerosis Risk in Communities Study. *Am J Clin Nutr.* 2007;85:1103–11.

32 Schaefer EJ, Bongard V, Beiser AS, et al. Plasma phosphatidylcholine docosahexaenoic acid content and risk of dementia and Alzheimer disease: the Framingham Heart Study. Arch Neurol.2006;63(11):1545–50.

33 Shikany JM, Safford MM, Newby PK, et al. Southern dietary pattern is associated with hazard of acute coronary heart disease in the Reasons for Geographic and Racial Differences in Stroke (REGARDS) study. *Circulation.* 2015;132(9):804–14.

34 U.S. Department of Agriculture. *Agricultural Fact Book: Profiling Food Consumption in America.* Chapter 2, pp. 14–21. https://assets.documentcloud.org/documents/2461300/usda-chapter2.pdf.

35 Lewis MD, Hibbein JR, Johnson JE, et al. Suicide deaths of active duty U.S. military and omega-3 fatty acid status: a case control comparison. *J Clin Psychiatry.* 2011;72(12):1585–90.

36 Blasbalg TL, Hibbeln JR, Ramsden CE, et al. Changes in consumption of omega-3 and omega-6 fatty acids in the United States during the 20th century. *Am J Clin Nutr.* 2011;93(5):950–62.

37 Hibbeln JR, Nieminen LR, Lands WE. Increasing homicide rates and linoleic acid consumption among five Western countries, 1961–2000. *Lipids.* 2004;39(12):1207–13.

38 Patterson E, Wall R, Fitzgerald GF, et al. Health implications of high dietary omega-6 polyunsaturated fatty acids. *J Nutr Metab.* 2012;2012:539426, http://dx.doi.org/10.1155/2012/539426.

39 Patel B, Schutte R, Sporns P, et al. Potato glycoalkaloids adversely affect intestinal permeability and aggravate inflammatory bowel disease. *Inflamm Bowel Dis.* 2002;8(5):340–46.

40 Montgomery P, Burton JR, Sewell RP, et al. Low blood long chain omega-3 fatty acids in UK children are associated with poor cognitive performance and behavior: a cross-sectional analysis from the DOLAB study. *PloS One.* 2013;8(6):366697.

41 Hamazaki T, Hamazaki K. Fish oils and aggression or hostility. *Prog Lipid Res.* 2008;47(4): 221–32.

42 Grosso G, Galvano F, Marventano S, et al. Omega-3 fatty acids and depression: scientific evidence and biological mechanisms. *Oxid Med Cell Longev.* 2014;2014:313570.

43 Weiser MJ, Butt CM, Mohajeri MH. Docosahexaenoic acid and cognition throughout the lifespan. *Nutrients.* 2016;8(2):99.

44 Tan ZS, Harris WS, Beiser AS, et al. Red blood cell omega-3 fatty acid levels and markers of accelerated brain aging. *Neurology.* 2012;78:658–64; Pottala JV, Yaffe K, Robinson JG, et al. Higher RBC EPA + DHA corresponds with larger total brain and hippocampal volumes: WHIMS-MRI study. *Neurology.* 2014;82:435–42; Cole GM, Ma QL, Frautschy SA. Omega-3 fatty acids and dementia. *Prostaglandins Leukot Essent Fatty Acids.* 2009;81:213–21.

45 Hebert LE, Weuve J, Scherr PA, et al. Alzheimer disease in the United States (2010–2050) estimated using the 2010 census. *Neurology.* 2013;80(19):1778–83.

46 Eldho NV, Feller SE, Tristram-Nagle S, et al. Polyunsaturated docosahexaenoic Vs docosapentaenoic acid: differences in lipid matrix properties from the loss of one double bond. *J Am Chem Soc.* 2003;125(21):6409–21.

47 Milte CM, Sinn N, Street SJ, et al. Erythrocyte polyunsaturated fatty acid status, memory, cognition and mood in older adults with mild cognitive impairment and healthy controls. *Prostaglandins Leukot Essent Fatty Acids.* 2011;84:153–61.

48 Northstone K, Joinson C, Emmett P, et al. Are dietary patterns in childhood associated with IQ at 8 years of age?: a population-based cohort study. *J Epidemiol Community Health.*

2011;66(7):624–28; doi:10.1136/jech.2010.111955; Gale CR, Martyn CN, Marriott LD, et al. Dietary patterns in infancy and cognitive and neuropsychological function in childhood. *J Child Psychol Psychiatry.* 2009;50(7):816–23.

49 Oddy WH, Robinson M, Ambrosini GL, et al. The association between dietary patterns and mental health in early adolescence. *Preventive Med.* 2009;49(1):39–44; Wiles NJ, Northstone K, Emmett P, et al. "Junk Food" diet and childhood behavioural problems: results from the ALSPAC cohort. *Eur J Clin Nutr.* 2009;63(4):491–98.

50 Mujcic R, Oswald AJ. Evolution of well-being and happiness after increases in consumption of fruit and vegetables. *Am J Public Health.* 2016;106(8):1504–10.

51 Fruits and veggies give you that feel-good factor. Warwick News and Events. http://www2 .warwick.ac.uk/newsandevents/news/fruit_and_veg/. Last revised 8 July 2016.

52 Johnson PM, Kenny PJ. Dopamine D2 receptors in addiction-like reward dysfunction and compulsive eating in obese rats. *Nat Neurosci.* 2010;13(5):635–41.

53 Stranahan AM, Norman ED, Lee K, et al. Diet-induced insulin resistance impairs hippocampal synaptic plasticity and cognition in middle-aged rats. *Hippocampus.* 2008;18(11):1085–88.

54 Murphy C. Nutrition and chemosensory perception in the elderly. *Crit Rev Food Sci Nutr.* 1993;33(1):3–15.

55 Myers WC, Vondruska MA. Murder, minors, selective serotonin reuptake inhibitors, and the involuntary intoxication defense. *J Am Acad Psychiatry Law.* 1998;26(3):487–96; Patrick RP, Ames BN. Vitamin D and the omega-3 fatty acids control serotonin synthesis and action, part 2: relevance for ADHD, bipolar disorder, schizophrenia, and impulsive behavior. *FASEB J.* 2015;29(6):2207–22.

56 Williams E, Stewart-Knox B, Helander A, et al. Associations between whole-blood serotonin and subjective mood in healthy male volunteers. *Biol Psychol.* 2006;71(2):171–74.

57 Eppig C, Fincher CL, Thornhill R. Parasite prevalence and the worldwide distribution of cognitive ability. *Proc Biol Sci.* 2010;277(1701):3801–8.

58 Northstone K, Joinson C, Emmett P, et al. Are dietary patterns in childhood associated with IQ at 8 Years of Age?: a population-based cohort study. *J Epidemiol Community Health.* 2011;66(7):624–28; doi:10.1136/jech.2010.111955.

59 Wiles NJ, Northstone K, Emmett P, et al. "Junk food" diet and childhood behavioural problems: results from the ALSPAC cohort. *Eur J Clin Nutr.* 2009;63(4):491–98.

60 Rosales FJ, Reznick JS, Zeisel SH. Understanding the role of nutrition in the brain and behavioral development of toddlers and preschool children: identifying and addressing methodological barriers. *Nutr Neurosci.* 2009;12(5):190–202.

61 Jackson DB, Beaver KM. The role of adolescent nutrition and physical activity in the prediction of verbal intelligence during early adulthood: a genetically informed analysis of twin pairs. *Int J Environ Res Public Health.* 2015;12(1):385–401.

62 Purtell KM, Gershoff ET. Fast food consumption and academic growth in late childhood. *Clin Pediatr.* 2015;54(9):871–77.

63 Garcia-Lafuente A, Guillamon E, Villares A, et al. Flavonoids as anti-inflammatory agents: implications in cancer and cardiovascular disease. *Inflamm Res.* 2009;58(9):537–52.

64 Gale CR, Martyn CN, Marriott LD, et al. Dietary patterns in infancy and cognitive and neuropsychological function in childhood. *J Child Psychol Psychiatry.* 2009;50(7):816–23.

65 Thaler JP, Yi C-X, Schur EA, et al. Obesity is associated with hypothalamic injury in rodents and humans. *J Clin Invest.* 2012;122(1):153–62.

66 Zhang J, Hebert JR, Muldoon MF. Dietary fat intake is associated with psychosocial and cognitive functioning of school-aged children in the United States. *J Nutr.* 2005;135(8):1967–73.

67 Karlsson H, Ahlborg B, Dalman C, et al. Association between erythrocyte sedimentation rate and IQ in Swedish males aged 18–20. *Brain Behav Immun.* 2010;24(6):868–73.

68 Rijlaarsdam J, Cecil C, Walton E, et al. Prenatal unhealthy diet, insulin-like growth factor 2 gene (IGF-2) methylation, and attention deficit hyperactivity disorder symptoms in youth with early onset conduct problems. *J Child Psychol Psychiatry.* 2017;58(1):19–27; doi:10.1111 /jcpp.12589.

69 Hunchark M. Maternal intake of N-nitroso compounds from cured meat and the risk of pediatric brain tumors: a review. J Environ Pathol Toxicol Oncol. 2010;29(3):245–53. Kwan ML, Jensen CD, Maternal Diet and Risk of Childhood Acute Lymphoblastic Leukemia. Public Health Rep. 2009;124(4):503–514.

70 Li M, Fallin D, Riley A, Wang X. The association of maternal obesity and diabetes with autism and other developmental disabilities. *Pediatrics.* 2016;137(2):1–10; Dufault R, Lukiw WJ, Crider R, et al. A macroepigenetic approach to identify factors responsible for the autism epidemic in the United States. *Clin Epigenetics.* 2012;4(1):1.

71 Gesch CB. Influence of supplementary vitamins, minerals and essential fatty acids on the antisocial behaviour of young adult prisoners: randomised, placebo-controlled trial. *Brit J Psychiatry.* 2002;181(1):22–28.

72 Zaalberg A, Nijman H, Bulten E, et al. Effects of nutritional supplements on aggression, rule-breaking, and psychopathology among young adult prisoners. *Aggress Behav.* 2010;36(2):117–26.

73 Keeley J, Fields M. Case study: Appleton Central alternative charter high school's nutrition and wellness program. December 2004. http://www.sustainlv.org/wp-content/uploads /Appleton-school-food-study.pdf.

74 Bohannon J. The theory? Diet causes violence. The lab? Prison. *Science.* 2009;325:1614–16.

75 Moore SC, Carter LM, van Goozen S. Confectionery consumption in childhood and adult violence. *Br J Psychiatry.* 2009;195:366–67.

76 Ross LJ, Wilson M, Banks M, et al. Prevalence of malnutrition and nutritional risk factors in patients undergoing alcohol and drug treatment. *Nutrition.* 2012;28(7–8):738–43.

77 Grant LP, Haughton B, Sachan DS. Nutrition education is positively associated with substance abuse treatment program outcomes. *J Am Dietetic Assoc.* 2004;104(4):604–10.

78 Liester MB, Moore-Liester JD. Is sugar a gateway drug? *J Drug Abuse.* 2015;1(1):8.

79 Federal Bureau of Prisons. Statistics. https://www.bop.gov/about/statistics/statistics_inmate _offenses.jsp. Last updated 28 January 2017.

80 YouTube. Eric Clapton speaks about his drug and alcohol addiction. 1999 Interview with Ed Bradley. Posted June 2013. https://www.youtube.com/watch?v=kVPmfMDFS9A.

81 Fuchs E. Why the South is more violent than the rest of America. Business Insider. Law & Order. 18 September 2013. http://www.businessinsider.com/south-has-more-violent-crime -fbi-statistics-show-2013–9; Institute for Economics and Peace. *2012 United States Peace Index.* http://economicsandpeace.org/wp-content/uploads/2015/06/2012-United-States -Peace-Index-Report_1.pdf.

82 Nisbett RE. Violence and U.S. regional culture. *Am Psychol.* 1993;48(4),441–49.

83 *Diabetes Forecast,* Healthy Living Magazine. "The Diabetes Belt." http://www.diabetesforecast .org/2013/may/the-diabetes-belt.html.

84 CDC. Adults Meeting Fruit and Vegetable Intake Recommendations—United States, 2013 Weekly. MMWR 2015;64(26):709–713.

85 Martinson ML, Reichman NE. Socioeconomic inequalities in low birth weight in the United States, the United Kingdom, Canada, and Australia. *Am J Public Health.* 2016;106(4):748–54.

86 Hillemeier MM, Weisman CS, Chase GA, Dyer AM. Individual and community predictors of preterm birth and low birth weight along the rural–urban continuum in central Pennsylvania. *J Rural Health.* 2007;23(1):42–48.

CHAPTER THREE: LET FOOD BE THY MEDICINE

1 Werner H, Bruchim I. The insulin-like growth factor-I receptor as an oncogene. *Arch Physiol Biochem.* 2009;115:58–71; Levine ME, Suarez JA, Brandhorst S, et al. Low protein intake is associated with a major reduction in IGF-1, cancer, and overall mortality in the 65 and younger but not older population. *Cell Metab.* 2014;19:407–17; Key TJ, Appleby PN, Reeves GK, et al. Insulin-like growth factor 1 (IGF1), IGF binding protein 3 (IGFBP3), and breast cancer risk: pooled individual data analysis of 17 prospective studies. *Lancet Oncol.* 2010;11:530–42; Rowlands MA, Gunnell D, Harris R, et al. Circulating insulin-like growth factor peptides and prostate cancer risk: a systematic review and meta-analysis. *Int J Cancer.* 2009;124:2416–29.

2 Grant WR. A multicounty ecological study of cancer incidence rates in 2008 with respect to various risk-modifying factors. *Nutrients.* 2014;6:163–89.

3 Song M, Fung TT, Hu FB, et al. Association of animal and plant protein intake with all-cause and cause-specific mortality. *JAMA Intern Med.* 2016;176(10):1453–63; doi:10.1001/jama internmed.2016.4182.

4 Fung TT, Van Dam RM, Harkinson SE, et al. Low-carbohydrate diets and all-cause and cause-specific mortality: two cohort studies. *Ann Intern Med.* 2010;153:289–98.

5 Lagiou RP, Sandin S, Lof M, et al. Low carbohydrate, high protein diet and incidence of cardiovascular disease in Swedish women: prospective cohort study. *BMJ.* 2012;344:e4026.

6 Levine ME, Suarez JA, Brandhorst S, et al. Low protein intake is associated with a major reduction in IGF-1, cancer, and overall mortality in the 65 and younger but not older population. *Cell Metab.* 2014;19(3):407–7.

7 Wang X, Ouyang Y, Liu J, et al. Fruit and vegetable consumption and mortality from all causes, cardiovascular disease, and cancer: systematic review and dose-response meta-analysis of prospective cohort studies. *BMJ.* 2014;349:g4490.

8 Chuang YF, An Y, Bilgel M, et al. Midlife adiposity predicts earlier onset of Alzheimer's dementia, neuropathology and presymptomatic cerebral amyloid accumulation. *Mol Psychiatry.* 2015;21(7):910–15.

9 WHO Health Status Statistics: Mortality. Healthy Life Expectancy (HALE) http://www.who .int/healthinfo/statistics/indhale/en/.

10 Fuhrman J. Dietary protocols to maximize disease reversal and long term safety. *American Journal of Lifestyle Medicine.* 2015;9(5):343–53.

11 Fuhrman J, Singer M. Improved cardiovascular parameter with a nutrient-dense, plant-rich diet-style: a patient survey with illustrative cases. *American Journal of Lifestyle Medicine.* 7 July 2016; doi:10.1177/1559827615611024.

12 Dunaief DM, Fuhrman J, Dunaief JL, Ying G. Glycemic and cardiovascular parameters improved in type 2 diabetes with the high nutrient density (HND) diet. *Open Journal of Preventive Medicine.* 2012;2(3):364–71.

13 Buettner, D. *The Blue Zones: Lessons for Living Longer from the People Who've Lived the Longest,* 2nd ed. Washington, DC: National Geographic, 2012.

14 Lindeberg S, Berntorn E, Nilsson-Ehie P, et al. Age relations of cardiovascular risk factors in a traditional Melanesian society: the Kitava study. *Am J Clin Nutr.* 1997;66(4):845–52; Lindeberg S, Eliasson M, Lindhal B, Ahren D. Low serum insulin in traditional Pacific Islanders—the Kitava study. *Metabolism.* 1999;48(10):1216–19; Lindeberg S, Nilsson-Ehie P, Terent A, et al. Cardiovascular risk factors in a Melanesian population apparently free from stroke and ischaemic heart disease: the Kitava study. *J Intern Med.* 1994;236(3):331–40.

15 Higdon J, Delage B, Williams D, Dashwood R. Cruciferous vegetables and human cancer risk: epidemiologic evidence and mechanistic basis. *Pharmacol Res.* 2007;55:224–36.

16 Higdon J, Drake VJ. Cruciferous vegetables. In: *An Evidence-Based Approach to Phytochemicals*

and Other Dietary Factors. 2nd ed. New York: Thieme, 2013; Higdon J, Delage B, Williams D, Dashwood R. Cruciferous vegetables and human cancer risk: epidemiologic evidence and mechanistic basis. *Pharmacol Res.* 2007;55:224–36.

17 Yuan F, Chen DZ, Liu K, et al. Anti-estrogenic activities of indole-3-carbinol in cervical cells: implication for prevention of cervical cancer. *Anticancer Res.* 1999;19:1673–80; Meng Q, Yuan F, Goldberg ID, et al. Indole-3-carbinol is a negative regulator of estrogen receptor-alpha signaling in human tumor cells. *J Nutr.* 2000;130:2927–31; Ramirez MC, Singletary K. Regulation of estrogen receptor alpha expression in human breast cancer cells by sulforaphane. *J Nutr Biochem.* 2009;20:195–201.

18 Zhang CX, Ho SC, Chen YM, et al. Greater vegetable and fruit intake is associated with a lower risk of breast cancer among Chinese women. *Int J Cancer.* 2009;125:181–88.

19 Bosetti C, Filomeno M, Riso P, et al. Cruciferous vegetables and cancer risk in a network of case-control studies. *Ann Oncol.* 2012;23(8):2198–203.

20 Nechuta SJ, Lu W, Cai H, et al. Cruciferous vegetable intake after diagnosis of breast cancer and survival: a report from the Shanghai Breast Cancer Survival study. *Cancer Res.* 2012(suppl);72(8): abstract LB-322.

21 Cohen JH, Kristal AR, Stanford JL. Fruit and vegetable intakes and prostate cancer risk. *J Natl Cancer Inst.* 2000;92:61–68.

22 Larsson SC, Hakansson N, Naslund I, et al. Fruit and vegetable consumption in relation to pancreatic cancer risk: a prospective study. *Cancer Epidemiol Biomarkers Prev.* 2006;15:301–5.

23 Papanikolaou Y, Fulgoni VL III. Bean consumption is associated with greater nutrient intake, reduced systolic blood pressure, lower body weight, and a smaller waist circumference in adults: results from the National Health and Nutrition Examination Survey, 1999–2002. *J Am Coll Nutr.* 2008;27:569–76; Muir JG, O'Dea K. Measurement of resistant starch: factors affecting the amount of starch escaping digestion in vitro. *Am J Clin Nutr.* 1992;56:123–27.

24 Aune D, De Stefani E, Ronco A, et al. Legume intake and the risk of cancer: a multisite case-control study in Uruguay. *Cancer Causes Control.* 2009;20:1605–15; Singh PN, Fraser GE. Dietary risk factors for colon cancer in a low-risk population. *Am J Epidemiol.* 1998;148:761–74; O'Keefe SJ, Ou J, Aufreiter S, et al. Products of the colonic microbiota mediate the effects of diet on colon cancer risk. *J Nutr.* 2009;139:2044–48.

25 Bazzano LA, Thompson AM, Tees MT, et al. Non-soy legume consumption lowers cholesterol levels: a meta-analysis of randomized controlled trials. *Nutr Metab Cardiovasc Dis.* 2011;21:94–103.

26 Powolny A, Singh S. Multitargeted prevention and therapy of cancer by diallyl trisulfide and related Allium vegetable-derived organosulfur compounds. *Cancer Lett.* 2008;269:305–14; Ginter E, Simko V. Garlic (Allium sativum L.) and cardiovascular diseases. *Bratisl Lek Listy.* 2010;111:452–56; Taj Eldin IM, Ahmed EM, Elwahab HMA. Preliminary study of the clinical hypoglycemic effects of Allium cepa (red onion) in type 1 and type 2 diabetic patients. *Environ Health Insights.* 2010;4:71–77; Galeone C, Pelucchi C, Levi F, et al. Onion and garlic use and human cancer. *Am J Clin Nutr.* 2006;84:1027–32; Zhou Y, Zhuang W, Hu W, et al. Consumption of large amounts of Allium vegetables reduces risk for gastric cancer in a meta-analysis. *Gastroenterology.* 2011;141:80–89.

27 Cao QZ, Lin ZB. Antitumor and anti-angiogenic activity of Ganoderma lucidum polysaccharides peptide. *Acta Pharmacol Sin.* 2004;25:833–38.

28 Borchers AT, Krishnamurthy A, Keen CL, et al. The immunobiology of mushrooms. *Exp . Biol Med.* 2008;233:259–76; Yu L, Fernig DG, Smith JA, et al. Reversible inhibition of proliferation of epithelial cell lines by Agaricus bisporus (edible mushroom) lectin. *Cancer Res.* 1993;53:4627–32; Carrizo ME, Capaldi S, Perduca M, et al. The antineoplastic lectin of the common edible mushroom (Agaricus bisporus) has two binding sites, each specific for a different configuration at a single epimeric hydroxyl. *J Biol Chem.* 2005;280:10614–23; Fang N, Li Q, Yu S, et al. Inhibition of growth and induction of apoptosis in human cancer

cell lines by an ethyl acetate fraction from shiitake mushrooms. *J Altern Complement Med.* 2006;12:125–32; Ng ML, Yap AT. Inhibition of human colon carcinoma development by lentinan from shiitake mushrooms (Lentinus edodes). *J Altern Complement Med.* 2002;8:581–89; Adams LS, Phung S, Wu X, et al. White button mushroom (Agaricus bisporus) exhibits antiproliferative and proapoptotic properties and inhibits prostate tumor growth in athymic mice. *Nutr Cancer.* 2008;60:744–56; Lakshmi B, Ajith TA, Sheena N, et al. Antiperoxidative, anti-inflammatory, and antimutagenic activities of ethanol extract of the mycelium of Ganoderma lucidum occurring in South India. *Teratog Carcinog Mutagen.* 2003;Suppl 1:85–97; Lin ZB, Zhang HN. Anti-tumor and immunoregulatory activities of Ganoderma lucidum and its possible mechanisms. *Acta Pharmacol Sin.* 2004;25:1387–95; Patel S, Goyal A. Recent developments in mushrooms as anti-cancer therapeutics: a review. *3 Biotech.* 2012;2:1–15.

29 Grube BJ, Eng ET, Kao YC, et al. White button mushroom phytochemicals inhibit aromatase activity and breast cancer cell proliferation. *J Nutr.* 2001;131:3288–93; Chen S, Oh SR, Phung S, et al. Anti-aromatase activity of phytochemicals in white button mushrooms (Agaricus bisporus). *Cancer Res.* 2006;66(24):12026–34.

30 Zhang M, Huang J, Xie X, Holman CD, et al. Dietary intakes of mushrooms and green tea combine to reduce the risk of breast cancer in Chinese women. *Int J Cancer.* 2009;124:1404–8.

31 Schulzova V, Hajslova J, Peroutka R, et al. Influence of storage and household processing on the agaritine content of the cultivated Agaricus mushroom. *Food Addit Contam.* 2002;19:853–62.

32 Higdon J, Drake VJ. Flavonoids. In: *An Evidence-Based Approach to Dietary Phytochemicals and Other Dietary Factors.* 2d ed. New York: Thieme, 2012:83–108; Erdman JW, Jr., Balentine D, Arab L, et al. Flavonoids and heart health: proceedings of the ILSI North America Flavonoids Workshop, 31 May–1 June 2005, Washington, DC. *J Nutr.* 2007;137:718S–37S.

33 Bazzano LA, Li TY, Joshipura KJ, et al. Intake of fruit, vegetables, and fruit juices and risk of diabetes in women. *Diabetes Care.* 2008;31:1311–17; Cassidy A, O'Reilly EJ, Kay C, et al. Habitual intake of flavonoid subclasses and incident hypertension in adults. *Am J Clin Nutr.* 2011;93:338–47; Hannum SM. Potential impact of strawberries on human health: a review of the science. *Crit Rev Food Sci Nutr.* 2004;44:1–17; Joseph JA, Shukitt-Hale B, Willis LM. Grape juice, berries, and walnuts affect brain aging and behavior. *J Nutr.* 2009;139:1813S–17S; Roy S, Khanna S, Alessio HM, et al. Anti-angiogenic property of edible berries. *Free Radic Res.* 2002;36:1023–31; Stoner GD, Wang LS, Casto BC. Laboratory and clinical studies of cancer chemoprevention by antioxidants in berries. *Carcinogenesis.* 2008;29:1665–74; Bickford PC, Shukitt-Hale B, Joseph J. Effects of aging on cerebellar noradrenergic function and motor learning: nutritional interventions. *Mech Ageing Dev.* 1999;111:141–54; Krikorian R, Shidler MD, Nash TA, et al. Blueberry supplementation improves memory in older adults. *J Agric Food Chem.* 2010;58:3996–4000.

34 Huxley RR, Neil HA. The relation between dietary flavonol intake and coronary heart disease mortality: a meta-analysis of prospective cohort studies. *Eur J Clin Nutr.* 2003;57:904–8; Knekt P, Kumpulainen J, Jarvinen R, et al. Flavonoid intake and risk of chronic diseases. *Am J Clin Nutr.* 2002;76:560–68; Mursu J, Voutilainen S, Nurmi T, et al. Flavonoid intake and the risk of ischaemic stroke and CVD mortality in middle-aged Finnish men: the Kuopio Ischaemic Heart Disease Risk Factor study. *Br J Nutr.* 2008;100:890–95; Mink PJ, Scrafford CG, Barraj LM, et al. Flavonoid intake and cardiovascular disease mortality: a prospective study in postmenopausal women. *Am J Clin Nutr.* 2007;85:895–909.

35 Erdman JW, Jr., Balentine D, Arab L, et al. Flavonoids and heart health: proceedings of the ILSI North America Flavonoids Workshop, 31 May–1 June 2005, Washington, DC. *J Nutr.* 2007;137:718S–37S; Martin KR, Bopp J, Burrell L, et al. The effect of 100% tart cherry juice on serum uric acid levels, biomarkers of inflammation and cardiovascular disease risk factors. In: *Experimental Biology 2011.* Washington, DC: Federation of American Societies for Experimental Biology, 2011; Kelley DS, Rasooly R, Jacob RA, et al. Consumption of Bing sweet cherries

lowers circulating concentrations of inflammation markers in healthy men and women. *J Nutr.* 2006;136:981–86; Aviram M, Dornfeld L. Pomegranate juice consumption inhibits serum angiotensin converting enzyme activity and reduces systolic blood pressure. *Atherosclerosis.* 2001;158:195–98; Aviram M, Dornfeld L, Rosenblat M, et al. Pomegranate juice consumption reduces oxidative stress, atherogenic modifications to LDL, and platelet aggregation: studies in humans and in atherosclerotic apolipoprotein E-deficient mice. *Am J Clin Nutr.* 2000;71:1062– 76; Aviram M, Rosenblat M, Gaitini D, et al. Pomegranate juice consumption for 3 years by patients with carotid artery stenosis reduces common carotid intima-media thickness, blood pressure and LDL oxidation. *Clin Nutr.* 2004;23:423–33; Aviram M, Volkova N, Coleman R, et al. Pomegranate phenolics from the peels, arils, and flowers are antiatherogenic: studies in vivo in atherosclerotic apolipoprotein e-deficient (E 0) mice and in vitro in cultured macrophages and lipoproteins. *J Agric Food Chem.* 2008;56:1148–57.

36 Smart RC, Huang MT, Chang RL, et al. Disposition of the naturally occurring antimutagenic plant phenol, ellagic acid, and its synthetic derivatives, 3-O-decyllellagic acid and 3,3'-di-O-methylellagic acid in mice. *Carcinogenesis.* 1986;7:1663–67; Smart RC, Huang MT, Chang RL, et al. Effect of ellagic acid and 3-O-decyllellagic acid on the formation of benzo[a]-pyrene-derived DNA adducts in vivo and on the tumorigenicity of 3-methylcholanthrene in mice. *Carcinogenesis.* 1986;7:1669–75.

37 Stoner GD, Wang LS, Casto BC. Laboratory and clinical studies of cancer chemoprevention by antioxidants in berries. *Carcinogenesis.* 2008;29:1665–74.

38 Shukitt-Hale B. Blueberries and neuronal aging. *Gerontology.* 2012;58:518–23.

39 Krikorian R, Shidler MD, Nash TA, et al. Blueberry supplementation improves memory in older adults. *J Agric Food Chem.* 2010;58:3996–4000.

40 Brown MJ, Ferruzzi MG, Nguyen ML, et al. Carotenoid bioavailability is higher from salads ingested with full-fat than with fat-reduced salad dressings as measured with electrochemical detection. *Am J Clin Nutr.* 2004;80:396–403.

41 Nash SD, Nash DT. Nuts as part of a healthy cardiovascular diet. *Curr Atheroscler Rep.* 2008;10:529–35; Sabate J, Ang Y. Nuts and health outcomes: new epidemiologic evidence. *Am J Clin Nutr.* 2009;89:1643S–48S; Mattes RD, Dreher ML. Nuts and healthy body weight maintenance mechanisms. *Asia Pac J Clin Nutr.* 2010;19:137–41; Kendall CW, Josse AR, Esfahani A, et al. Nuts, metabolic syndrome and diabetes. *Br J Nutr.* 2010;104:465–73.

42 Saarinen NM, Warri A, Airio M, et al. Role of dietary lignans in the reduction of breast cancer risk. *Mol Nutr Food Res.* 2007;51:857–66; Coulman KD, Liu Z, Hum WQ, et al. Whole sesame seed is as rich a source of mammalian lignan precursors as whole flaxseed. *Nutr Cancer.* 2005;52:156–65.

43 Higdon J. Lignans. In: *An Evidence-Based Approach to Dietary Phytochemicals,* 2nd ed. New York: Thieme, 2006:155–61; Milder IE, Arts IC, van de Putte B, et al. Lignan contents of Dutch plant foods: a database including lariciresinol, pinoresinol, secoisolariciresinol and matairesinol. *Br J Nutr.* 2005;93:393–402; Coulman KD, Liu Z, Hum WQ, et al. Whole sesame seed is as rich a source of mammalian lignan precursors as whole flaxseed. *Nutr Cancer.* 2005;52:156–65.

44 Higdon J. Lignans. In: *An Evidence-Based Approach to Dietary Phytochemicals,* 2nd ed. New York: Thieme, 2006:155–61; Adlercreutz H. Lignans and human health. *Crit Rev Clin Lab Sci.* 2007;44:483–525.

45 Adlercreutz H, Bannwart C, Wahala K, et al. Inhibition of human aromatase by mammalian lignans and isoflavonoid phytoestrogens. *J Steroid Biochem Mol Biol.* 1993;44:147–53; Brooks JD, Thompson LU. Mammalian lignans and genistein decrease the activities of aromatase and 17beta-hydroxysteroid dehydrogenase in MCF-7 cells. *J Steroid Biochem Mol Biol.* 2005;94:461–67.

46 Adlercreutz H, Hockerstedt K, Bannwart C, et al. Effect of dietary components, including lignans and phytoestrogens, on enterohepatic circulation and liver metabolism of estrogens and on sex hormone binding globulin (SHBG). *J Steroid Biochem.* 1987;27:1135–44; Low YL, Dunning AM, Dowsett M, et al. Phytoestrogen exposure is associated with circulating sex hormone levels in postmenopausal women and interact with ESR1 and NR1I2 gene variants. *Cancer Epidemiol Biomarkers Prev.* 2007;16:1009–16.

47 Sturgeon SR, Heersink JL, Volpe SL, et al. Effect of dietary flaxseed on serum levels of estrogens and androgens in postmenopausal women. *Nutr Cancer.* 2008;60:612–18.

48 Thompson LU, Chen JM, Li T, et al. Dietary flaxseed alters tumor biological markers in postmenopausal breast cancer. *Clin Cancer Res.* 2005;11:3828–35.

49 Buck K, Vrieling A, Zaineddin AK, et al. Serum enterolactone and prognosis of postmenopausal breast cancer. *J Clin Oncol.* 2011;29:3730–38; Buck K, Zaineddin AK, Vrieling A, et al. Estimated enterolignans, lignan-rich foods, and fibre in relation to survival after postmenopausal breast cancer. *Br J Cancer.* 2011;105:1151–57.

50 McCann SE, Thompson LU, Nie J, et al. Dietary lignan intakes in relation to survival among women with breast cancer: the Western New York Exposures and Breast Cancer (WEB) study. *Breast Cancer Res Treat.* 2010;122:229–35.

51 Shardell MD, Alley DE, Hicks GE, et al. Low-serum carotenoid concentrations and carotenoid interactions predict mortality in US adults: the Third National Health and Nutrition Examination Survey. *Nutr Res.* 2011;31:178–89.

52 Krinsky NI, Johnson EJ. Carotenoid actions and their relation to health and disease. *Mol Aspects Med.* 2005;26:459–516.

53 Van Breemen RB, Pajkovic N. Multitargeted therapy of cancer by lycopene. *Cancer Lett.* 2008;269:339–51; Rizwan M, Rodriguez-Blanco I, Harbottle A, et al. Tomato paste rich in lycopene protects against cutaneous photodamage in humans in vivo. *Br J Dermatol.* 2011;164(1):154–62; Petyaev IM. Lycopene deficiency in ageing and cardiovascular disease. *Oxid Med Cell Longev.* 2016;2016:3218605.

54 Rissanen TH, Voutilainen S, Nyyssonen K, et al. Low serum lycopene concentration is associated with an excess incidence of acute coronary events and stroke: the Kuopio Ischaemic Heart Disease Risk Factor study. *Br J Nutr.* 2001;85:749–54; Rissanen T, Voutilainen S, Nyyssonen K, et al. Lycopene, atherosclerosis, and coronary heart disease. *Exp Biol Med (Maywood)* 2002;227:900–907; Rissanen TH, Voutilainen S, Nyyssonen K, et al. Serum lycopene concentrations and carotid atherosclerosis: the Kuopio Ischaemic Heart Disease Risk Factor study. *Am J Clin Nutr.* 2003;77:133–38.

55 Sesso HD, Buring JE, Norkus EP, et al. Plasma lycopene, other carotenoids, and retinol and the risk of cardiovascular disease in women. *Am J Clin Nutr.* 2004;79:47–53.

56 Hak AE, Ma J, Powell CB, et al. Prospective study of plasma carotenoids and tocopherols in relation to risk of ischemic stroke. *Stroke.* 2004;35:1584–88.

57 Canene-Adams K, Campbell JK, Zaripheh S, et al. The tomato as a functional food. *J Nutr.* 2005;135:1226–30.

58 Van het Hof KH, de Boer BC, Tijburg LB, et al. Carotenoid bioavailability in humans from tomatoes processed in different ways determined from the carotenoid response in the triglyceride-rich lipoprotein fraction of plasma after a single consumption and in plasma after four days of consumption. *J Nutr* 2000;130:1189–96; US Department of Agriculture, Agricultural Research Service, USDA Food Composition Databases. http://ndb.nal.usda.gov/ndb/search/list.

59 American Cancer Society, *Global Cancer Facts & Figures,* 2nd ed. Atlanta: American Cancer Society, 2011. http://www.cancer.org/acs/groups/content/@epidemiologysurveilance/documents/document/acspc-027766.pdf.

60 Kantor ED, Udumyan R, Signorello LB, et al. Adolescent body mass index and erythrocyte sedimentation rate in relation to colorectal cancer risk. *Gut*. 2016;65:1289–95; Pulgaron ER. Childhood obesity: a review of increased risk for physical and psychological comorbidities. *Clin Ther*. 2013;35:A18–32.

61 Steingraber S. The falling age of puberty in U.S. girls: what we know, what we need to know. Breast Cancer Fund: 2007; McDowell MA, Brody DJ, Hughes JP. Has age at menarche changed? Results from the National Health and Nutrition Examination Survey (NHANES), 1999–2004. *J Adolesc Health*. 2007;40:227–31; Anderson SE, Must A. Interpreting the continued decline in the average age at menarche: results from two nationally representative surveys of U.S. girls studied 10 years apart. *J Pediatr*. 2005;147:753–60.

62 Vandeloo MJ, Bruckers LM, Janssens JP. Effects of lifestyle on the onset of puberty as determinant for breast cancer. *Eur J Cancer Prev*. 2007;16:17–25; Leung AW, Mak J, Cheung PS, et al. Evidence for a programming effect of early menarche on the rise of breast cancer incidence in Hong Kong. *Cancer Detect Prev*. 2008;32:156–61; Pike MC, Pearce CL, Wu AH. Prevention of cancers of the breast, endometrium and ovary. *Oncogene*. 2004;23:6379–91.

63 Baanders AN, de Waard EL. Breast cancer in Europe and factors operating at an early age. *Eur J Cancer Prev*. 1993;2:1–89.

64 Berkey CS, Gardner JD, Frazier AL, Colditz GA. Relation of childhood diet and body size to menarche and adolescent growth in girls. *Am J Epidemiol*. 2000;152:446–52.

65 Rogers IS, Northstone K, Dunger DB, et al. Diet throughout childhood and age at menarche in a contemporary cohort of British girls. *Public Health Nutr*. 2010;13(12):2052–63; Berkey CS, Gardner JD, Frazier AL, Colditz GA. Relation of childhood diet and body size to menarche and adolescent growth in girls. *Am J Epidemiol*. 2000;152:446–52; Wiley AS. Milk intake and total dairy consumption: associations with early menarche in NHANES 1999–2004. *PloS One* 2011;6:e14685.

66 Dorgan JF, Hunsberger SA, McMahon RP, et al. Diet and sex hormones in girls: findings from a randomized controlled clinical trial. *J Natl Cancer Inst*. 2003;95(2):132–41.

67 Wolfswinkel EM, Lemaine V, Weathers WM, et al. Hyperplastic breast anomalies in the female adolescent breast. *Semin Plast Surg*. 2013;27(1):49–55.

68 Cho E, Spiegelman D, Hunter DJ, et al. Premenopausal fat intake and risk of breast cancer. *J Natl Cancer Inst*. 2003;95(14):1079–85.

69 Sutcliffe S, Colditz GA. Prostate cancer: is it time to expand the research focus to early-life exposures? *Nat Rev Cancer* 2013;13:208–518.

70 Liu RH. Potential synergy of phytochemicals in cancer prevention: mechanism of action. *J Nutr*. 2004;134(12 suppl):3479S–85S; Weiss JF, Landauer MR. Protection against ionizing radiation by antioxidant nutrients and phytochemicals. *Toxicology*. 2003;189 (1–2):1–20; Carratu B, Sanzini E. [Biologically-active phytochemicals in vegetable food.] *Ann 1st Super Sanita*. 2005;41(1):7–16; Liu RH. Health benefits of fruit and vegetables are from additive and synergistic combinations of phytochemicals. *Am J Clin Nutr* 2003;78:517S–520S; Davinelli S, Maes M, Corbi G, et al. Dietary phytochemicals and neuro-inflammaging: from mechanistic insights to translational challenges. *Immun Ageing* 2016;13:16; Banudevi S, Swaminathan S, Maheswari KU. Pleiotropic role of dietary phytochemicals in cancer: emerging perspectives for combinational therapy. *Nutr Cancer* 2015;67:1021–48.

71 Hanau C, Morre DJ, Morre DM. Cancer prevention trial of a synergistic mixture of green tea concentrate plus Capsicum (CAPSOL-T) in a random population of subjects ages 40–84. *Clin Proteomics*. 2014;11:2.

72 https://lifestylemedicine.org/What-is-Lifestyle-Medicine.

CHAPTER FOUR: THE LESSONS OF HISTORY

1 Stewart DO: *Impeached: The Trial of President Andrew Johnson and the Fight for Lincoln's Legacy*: Simon & Schuster; 2009. https://books.google.com/books?id=DHdhbBfNnlgC&dq=%22 Freedmen%27s+bureau%22+and+murders+and+texas+and+1865&q=44+murders#v =onepage&q=44%20murders&f=false.

2 Hegyl J, Schwartz RA, Hegyl V. Pellagra: dermatitis, dementia, and diarrhea. *Int J Dermatol.* 2004;43(1):1–5.

3 Savitt TL. *Medicine and Slavery: The Diseases and Health Care of Blacks in Antebellum Virginia*. Urbana: University of Illinois Press, 1978, 201.

4 Chambers DB. *Murder at Montpelier: Igbo Africans in Virginia*. Jackson: University Press of Mississippi, 2009.

5 Covey HC, Eisnach D. *What the Slaves Ate: Recollections of African American Foods and Foodways from the Slave Narratives*. Santa Barbara, CA: ABC-CLIO/Greenwood, 2009, 29.

6 Washington BT. *Frederick Douglass*. G. W. Jacobs, 1907, 252.

7 National Assessment of Adult Literacy. 120 years of Literary, Literacy from 1870 to 1979. National Center for Education Statistics. https://nces.ed.gov/naal/lit_history.asp.

8 Baker RS: Following the Color Line: An Account of Negro Citizenship in the American Democracy: Doubleday,1908, 53.

9 Baker RS: Following the Color Line: An Account of Negro Citizenship in the American Democracy: Doubleday, 1908, 248.

10 Washington BT: The Negro Problem: A Series of Articles by Representative American Negroes of Today: James Pott; 1903, 10. (Contains republished article "Industrial education for the Negro").

11 Washington BT. *Frederick Douglass*. G. W. Jacobs, 1907.

12 Litwack LF: Trouble in Mind: Black Southerners in the Age of Jim Crow: Knopf Doubleday Publishing Group; 1999. Page xiii.

13 Du Bois WEB: The Negro: Cosimo, Incorporated; 2007, 130.

14 Baker RS. *Following the Color Line: An Account of Negro Citizenship in the American Democracy*. New York: Doubleday, 1908, 247.

15 King ML, "Address at Conclusion of the Selma to Montgomery March" in Carson C, Shepard K, Young A: A Call to Conscience: The Landmark Speeches of Dr. Martin Luther King, Jr: Grand Central Publishing; 2001.

16 Frankenburg, FR. *Vitamin Discoveries and Disasters: History, Science & Controversies*. Santa Barbara, CA: Praeger/ABC-CLIO; The pellagra epidemic of the southern United States in the early 20th century. ActForLibraries.org. 2017. http://www.actforlibraries.org/the -pellagra-epidemic-of-the-southern-united-states-in-the-early-20th-century.

17 Harris HF. *Pellagra*. New York: Macmillan, 1919, 255.

18 Wheeler G. A note on the history of pellagra in the United States. *Public Health Rep.* 1931;46(6):2223.

19 National Association for the Study of Pellagra. *Transactions of the National Association for the Study of Pellagra*. R. L. Bryan: 1914, 391–92.

20 Ibid., 254.

21 Yarbrough JF. Pellagra: its etiology, symptomalogy, and treatment. *Medical Record.* 1917;92:893.

22 DeWall CN, Deckman T, Gailliot MT, et al. Sweetened blood cools hot tempers: physiological self-control and aggression. *Aggress Behav.* 2011;37(1):73–80.

23 Lytle LD, Messing RB, Fisher L, et al. Effects of long-term corn consumption on brain serotonin and the response to electric shock. *Science.* 1975;190(4215):692–94.

24 Patrick RP, Ames BN. Vitamin D and the omega-3 fatty acids control serotonin synthesis and action, part 2: relevance for ADHD, bipolar disorder, schizophrenia, and impulsive behavior. *FASEB J.* 2015;29(6):2207–22.

25 Birger M, Swartz M, Cohen D, et al. Aggression: the testosterone-serotonin link. *Isr Med Assoc.* 2003;5(9):653–58.

26 Wheeler G. A note on the history of pellagra in the United States. *Public Health Rep.* 1931(46):6.

27 Goldberger quoted in Etheridge EW. *The Butterfly Caste: A Social History of Pellagra in the South.* Greenwood, 1972, 77.

28 "South Resents Federal Alarm over Pellagra," *New York Times,* 27 July 1921.

29 Etheridge, EW. *The Butterfly Caste.*

30 New York Department of Mental Hygiene. *The Psychiatric Quarterly: Supplement.* State Hospitals Press, 1964, 207.

31 Kemble F. *Journal of a Residence on a Georgian Plantation in 1838–1839.* New York: Knopf, 1961; Cash WJ. *The Mind of the South.* New York: Knopf, 1941, 204.

32 Davenport CB. The hereditary factor in pellagra. *Arch Intern Med.* 1916;18(1):4–31.

33 Spencer HG, Paul DB. The failure of a scientific critique: David Heron, Karl Pearson and Mendelian eugenics. *Br J Hist Sci.* 1998;31(4):441–52.

34 Popenoe P, Johnson RH. *Applied Eugenics.* New York: Macmillan, 1918, 184.

35 Grant, M. *The Passing of the Great Race: Or, the Racial Basis of European History.* 4th rev ed. New York: Scribner's, 1922, 50–51.

36 Laughlin, HH, Deposition in Circuit Court Proceedings-Buck v. Bell 274 U.S. 200. Paragraph II.

37 Buck v. Bell, 274 U.S. 200 (May 7, 1927). Page 207. Opinion written by Oliver Wendell Holmes, Jr.

38 Kuhl S: The Nazi Connection: Eugenics, American Racism, and German National Socialism: Oxford University Press; 2002, 58.

39 Kuhl S: The Nazi Connection: Eugenics, American Racism, and German National Socialism: Oxford University Press; 2002, 37.

40 Proctor RN. Why did the Nazis have the world's most aggressive anti-cancer campaign? *Endeavour.* 1999;23(2):76–79.

41 Basil H. Preventive nutrition in Nazi Germany: a public health commentary. *Online Journal of Health Ethics.* 2013;9(1):10.

42 Shiva quoted in Pollan M. What's eating America. *Smithsonian.* July 2006. http://www.smithsonianmag.com/people-places/presence-jul06.html?c=y&story=fullstory.

43 Stark KD, Van Elswyk ME, Higgins MR, et al. Global survey of the omega-3 fatty acids, docosahexaenoic acid and eicosapentaenoic acid in the blood stream of healthy adults. *Prog Lipid Res.* 2016;63:132–52.

44 Daniel CR, Cross AJ, Koebnick C, Sinha R. Trends in meat consumption in the United States. Public Health Nutr. 2011;14(4):575–583.

45 Centers for Disease Control and Prevention. Long-Term Trends in Diabetes, April 2016.

46 World Health Organization. Lead poisoning and health. Fact sheet. Reviewed September 2016 http://www.who.int/mediacentre/factsheets/fs379/en/.

47 Nevin R. How lead exposure relates to temporal changes in IQ, violent crime, and unwed pregnancy. *Environ Res.* 2000;83(10):1–22.

48 Shy CM. Lead in petrol: the mistake of the XXth century. *World Health Stat Q.* 1989;43(3): 168–76.

49 Page IH, Allen EV, Chamberlain FL, et al. Dietary fat and its relation to heart attacks and strokes. *Circulation.* 1961;23(1):133–36.

50 Blasbalg TL, Hibbeln JR, Ramsden CE, et al. Changes in consumption of omega-3 and omega-6 fatty acids in the United States during the 20th century. *Am J Clin Nutr.* 2011;93(5):950–62.

51 Hibbeln JR, Nieminen LR, Lands WE. Increasing homicide rates and linoleic acid consumption among five Western countries, 1961–2000. *Lipids*. 2004;39(12):1207–13.

52 Iribarren C, Markovitz JH, Jacobs DR, Jr., et al. Dietary intake of N-3, N-6 fatty acids and fish: relationship with hostility in young adults—the CARDIA study. *Eur J Clin Nutr*. 2004;58(1):24–31.

53 Hibbeln JR. Seafood consumption and homicide mortality. In: *Fatty Acids and Lipids—New Findings*. Vol. 88. Basel: Karger, 2001, 41–46.

CHAPTER FIVE: DNA, SOCIAL ENERGY, AND FAST FOOD

1 Bygren LO, Kaati G, Edvinsson S. Longevity determined by paternal ancestors' nutrition during their slow growth period. *Acta Biotheoretica*. 2001;49(1):53–59.

2 O'Donoghue M, Boutin S, Krebs CJ, et al. Functional responses of coyotes and lynx to the snowshoe hare cycle. *Ecology*. 1998;79(4):1193–208.

3 Closs G, Watterson G, Donnelly P. Constant predator-prey ratios: an arithmetical artifact? *Ecology*. 1993;74(1):238–43.

4 Holzenberger M, Dupont J, Ducos B, et al. Igf-1 receptor regulates lifespan and resistance to oxidative stress in mice. *Nature*. 2003;421(6919):182–87. Altintas O, Park S, V. Lee S. The role of insulin/IGF-1 signaling in the longevity of model invertebrates, C. elegans *and* D. melanogaster. BMP Rep.2016;49(2):81–92.

5 Goldstein MS. Human paleopathology. *J Natl Med Assoc*. 1963;55(2):100–106.

6 Levine ME, Suarez JA, Brandhorst S, et al. Low protein intake is associated with a major reduction in IGF-1, cancer, and overall mortality in the 65 and younger but not older population. *Cell Metab*. 2014;19(3):407–17.

7 Fraser GE, Shavlik DJ. Ten years of life: is it a matter of choice? *Arch Intern Med*. 2001;161:1645–52; Song M, Fung TT, Hu FB, et al. Association of animal and plant protein intake with all-cause and cause-specific mortality. *JAMA Intern Med*. 2016;176(10):1453–63; Pan A, Sun Q, Bernstein AM, et al. Red meat consumption and mortality: results from 2 prospective cohort studies. *Arch Intern Med*. 2012;172(7):555–63; Sinha R, Cross AJ, Graubard BI, et al. Meat intake and mortality: a prospective study of over half a million people. *Arch Intern Med*. 2009;169:562–71; Rohrmann S, Overvad K, Bueno-de-Mesquita HB, et al. Meat consumption and mortality: results from the European Prospective Investigation into Cancer and Nutrition. *BMC Med*. 2013;11:63.

8 Zhang N. Epigenetic modulation of DNA methylation by nutrition and its mechanisms in animals. *ScienceDirect*. 2015;1(3):144–51; Bishop KS, Ferguson LR. The interaction between epigenetics, nutrition and the development of cancer. *Nutrients*. 2015;7(2):922–47.

9 Cacioppo S, Cacioppo JT. Decoding the invisible forces of social connections. *Front Integr Neurosci*. 2012;6:51.

10 Arce M, Michopoulos V, Shepard KN, et al. Diet choice, cortisol reactivity, and emotional feeding in socially housed rhesus monkeys. *Physiol Behav*. 2010;101(4):446–55.

11 Tung J, Barreiro LB, Johnson ZP, et al. Social environment is associated with gene regulatory variation in the rhesus macaque immune system. *Proc Natl Acad Sci*. 2012;109(17):6490–95.

12 Holt-Lunstad J, Smith TB, Layton JB. Social relationships and mortality risk: a meta-analytic review. *PLoS Med*. 2010;7(7):e1000316.

13 Giles LC, Glonek GFV, Luszcz MA, Andrews GR. Effect of social networks on 10 year survival in very old Australians: the Australian longitudinal study of aging. *J Epidemiol Commun Health* 2005;59:574–79.

14 Holt-Lunstad J, Smith TB, Layton JB. Social relationships and mortality risk: a meta-analytic review. *PLoS Med*. 2010;7(7):e1000316.

15 Murphy ML, Slavich GM, Rohleder N, et al. Targeted rejection triggers differential pro- and anti-inflammatory gene expression in adolescents as a function of social status. *Clin Psychol Sci.* 2013;1(1):30–40.

16 Gibson EL. Emotional influences on food choice: sensory, physiological and psychological pathways. *Physiol Behav.* 2006;89(1):53–61.

17 Fontana L. The scientific basis of caloric restriction leading to longer life. *Curr Opin Gastroenterol.* 2009;25:144–50; Canto C, Auwerx J. Caloric restriction, SIRT1 and longevity. *Trends Endocrinol Metab.* 2009;20:325–31.

18 Anton S. Leeuwenburgh C. Fasting or caloric restriction for healthy aging. *Exp Gerontol.* 2013;48(10):1003–5; Longo VD, Mattson MP. Fasting: molecular mechanisms and clinical applications. *Cell Metab.* 2014;19:181–92; Fontana L. The scientific basis of caloric restriction leading to longer life. *Curr Opin Gastroenterol.* 2009;25:144–50.

19 Slavich GM, Cole SW. The emerging field of human social genomics. *Clin Psychol Sci.* 2013;1(3):331–48.

20 Turrell G, Hewitt B, Patterson C, et al. Socioeconomic differences in food purchasing behaviour and suggested implications for diet-related health promotion. *J Hum Nutr Dietetics.* 2002;15(5):355–64.

21 Hosking DE, Nettelbeck T, Wilson C, Danthiir V. Retrospective lifetime dietary patterns predict cognitive performance in community-dwelling older Australians. *Br J Nutr.* 2014;112:228–37; Jones DE, Greenberg M, Crowley M. Early social-emotional functioning and public health: the relationship between kindergarten social competence and future wellness. *Am J Public Health.* 2015;105:2283–90.

22 Kandel ER. A new intellectual framework for psychiatry. *Am J Psychiatry.* 1998;155(4):457–69, see p. 461.

23 Kuhn TS, Hacking I. *The Structure of Scientific Revolutions.* 50th anniversary ed. Chicago: University of Chicago Press, 2012.

24 Cited in ibid.

25 Van den Bree MB, Przybeck TR, Cloninger CR. Diet and personality: associations in a population-based sample. *Appetite.* 2006;46(2):177–88.

26 Levinson CA, Rodebaugh TL. Social anxiety and eating disorder comorbidity: The role of negative social evaluation fears. Eat Behav 2012;13(1):27–35.

27 Padilla A, Hogan R, Kaiser RB. The toxic triangle: destructive leaders, susceptible followers, and conducive environments. *Leadership Quarterly.* 2007;18(3):176–94.

28 Nansel TR, Overpeck M, Pilla RS, et al. Bullying behaviors among US youth: prevalence and association with psychosocial adjustment. *JAMA.* 2001;285(16):2094–100.

29 Faris R, Felmlee D. Status struggles: network centrality and gender segregation in same- and cross-gender aggression. *Am Soc Rev.* 2011;76(1):48–73.

30 Warden D, Mackinnon S. Prosocial children, bullies and victims: an investigation of their sociometric status, empathy and social problem-solving strategies. *Br J Dev Psychol.* 2003;21(3):367–85.

31 Zahedi H, Kelishadi R, Heshmat R, et al. Association between junk food consumption and mental health in a national sample of Iranian children and adolescents: The Caspian-IV study. *Nutrition.* 2014;30(11–12):1391–97.

32 Fleming LC, Jacobsen KH. Bullying among middle-school students in low and middle income countries. *Health Promot Int.* 2009;25(1):73–84.

33 United Nations Office on Drugs and Crime. Intentional Homicide Count and Rate Per 100,000 Population, by Country/Territory (2000–2012). 2012. https://www.unodc.org/documents/data -and-analysis/statistics/GSH2013/2014_GLOBAL_HOMICIDE_BOOK_web.pdf

34 World Infozone. Tajikistan Information. http://worldinfozone.com/country php?country=Tajikistan.

35 FAO. Agriculture and Consumer Protection Department, Nutrition and Consumer Protection. Nutrition country profiles, Republic of Zambia. http://www.fao.org/ag/agn/nutrition/Zmb_en.stm.

36 Bee HL, Van Egeren LF, Pytkowicz Streissguth A, et al. Social class differences in maternal teaching strategies and speech patterns. *Dev Psychol.* 1969;1(6p1):726.

37 Neumark-Sztainer D, Wall M, Fulkerson JA, et al. Changes in the frequency of family meals from 1999 to 2010 in the homes of adolescents: trends by sociodemographic characteristics. *Journal Adolescent Health.* 2013;52(2):201–6.

38 Hammons AJ, Fiese BH. Is frequency of shared family meals related to the nutritional health of children and adolescents? *Pediatrics.* 2011;127(6):e1565–74.

39 Hunt G, Fazio A, MacKenzie K, et al. Food in the family: bringing young people back in. *Appetite.* 2011;56(2):394–402.

40 Muñiz EI, Silver EJ, Stein R. Family Routines and Social-Emotional School Readiness Among Preschool-Age Children. Journal of Developmental & Behavioral Pediatrics, 2014; 35 (2): 93.

41 Walker-Barnes CJ, Mason CA. Ethnic differences in the effect of parenting on gang involvement and gang delinquency: a longitudinal, hierarchical linear modeling perspective. *Child Dev.* 2001;72(6):1814–31.

42 Conklin AI, Forouhi NG, Surtees P, et al. Social relationships and healthful dietary behaviour: evidence from over-50s in the EPIC cohort, UK. *Social Sci Med.* 2014;100:167–75.

43 Cacioppo JT, Hawkley LC. Perceived social isolation and cognition. *Trends Cog Sci.* 2009;13(10):447–54.

44 Cortright J. City Report: Less in common. June 2015. http://cityobservatory.org/wp-content/uploads/2015/06/CityObservatory_Less_In_Common.pdf.

45 Rosenwald MS. "Can Gardening Transform Convicted Killers and Carjackers? Prison Officials Get Behind the Bloom." *Washington Post,* 7 June 2015.

46 Gesch CB. Influence of supplementary vitamins, minerals and essential fatty acids on the antisocial behaviour of young adult prisoners: randomised, placebo-controlled trial. *Br J Psychiatry.* 2002;181(1):22–28.

47 Zaalberg A, Nijman H, Bulten E, et al. Effects of nutritional supplements on aggression, rule-breaking, and psychopathology among young adult prisoners. *Aggress Behav.* 2010;36(2):117–26.

48 Frazee-Walker D. Vegan diet impacts recidivism. Zoukis Prisoner Resources. 20 May 2013. http://www.prisonlawblog.com/blog/vegan-diet-impacts-recidivism.

49 Nelson L, Lind D. The school to prison pipeline, explained. Justice Policy Institute. 24 February 2015. http://www.justicepolicy.org/news/8775.

50 Keeley J, Fields M. Case study: Appleton Central alternative charter high school's nutrition and wellness program. December 2004. http://www.sustainlv.org/wp-content/uploads/Appleton-school-food-study.pdf.

51 Ibid.

52 Boone-Heinonen J, Gordon-Larsen P, Kiefe CI, et al. Fast food restaurants and food stores: longitudinal associations with diet in young to middle-aged adults. The Cardia study. *Arch Intern Med.* 2011;171(13):1162–70.

CHAPTER SIX: MAKING DESERTS GREEN AGAIN

1 The State of Obesity. Food insecure children. http://stateofobesity.org/food-insecurity/.

2 Schmitz N, Nitka D, Gariepy G, et al. Association between neighborhood-level deprivation and disability in a community sample of people with diabetes. *Diabetes Care.* 2009;32(11):1998–2004.

3 Mari Gallagher Research and Consulting Group. Examining the impact of food deserts on public health in Chicago. 2006:6–7. http://www.marigallagher.com/site_media/dynamic/project_files/Chicago_Food_Desert_Report.pdf.

4 Gardner JW, Sanborn JS. Years of potential life lost (YPLL)—what does it measure? *Epidemiology.* 1990;1(4):322–29.

5 Brownlee S, Ohri-Vachaspati P, Lloyd K, et al. New Jersey Childhood Obesity Survey. Chartbook/Camden. Rutgers University Center for State Health Policy, 2010. http://www.cshp.rutgers.edu/downloads/8640.pdf.

6 The State of Obesity. Food insecure children. http://stateofobesity.org/food-insecurity/.

7 Drewnowski A, Darmon N. Food choices and diet costs: an economic analysis. *J Nutr.* 2005;135(4):900–904.

8 Semuels A. A potato-chip-shaped hole in ex-Detroiters' hearts. *LA Times* Oct 5 2014. http://www.latimes.com/nation/la-na-better-made-chips-20141005-story.html.

9 Lane SD, Keefe RH, Rubinstein R, et al. Structural violence, urban retail food markets, and low birth weight. *Health & Place.* 2008;14(3):415–23.

10 Levine TA, Grunau RE, McAuliffe FM, et al. Early childhood neurodevelopment after intrauterine growth restriction: a systematic review. *Pediatrics.* 2015;135(1):126–41.

11 Geva R, Eshel R, Leitner Y, Valevski AF, Harel S. Neuropsychological outcome of children with intrauterine growth restriction: a 9-year prospective study. *Pediatrics* 2006;118(1):91–100. doi:10.1542/peds.2005–2343; Poehlmann J, Schwichtenberg AJ, Shlafer RJ, et al. Emerging self-regulation in toddlers born preterm or low birth weight: differential susceptibility to parenting? *Dev Psychopathol.* 2011;23(1):177–93.

12 Rao S, Yajnik CS, Kanade A, et al. Intake of micronutrient-rich foods in rural Indian mothers is associated with the size of their babies at birth: Pune Maternal Nutrition Study. *J Nutr.* 2001;131(4):1217–24.

13 Lozoff B, Beard J, Connor J, et al. Long-lasting neural and behavioral effects of iron deficiency in infancy. *Nutr Rev.* 2006;64(suppl 2):S34–S43.

14 Andersson M, De Benoist B, Darnton-Hill I, et al. *Iodine Deficiency in Europe: A Continuing Public Health Problem.* Genva: World Health Organization Geneva, 2007.

15 Delange F. Iodine deficiency as a cause of brain damage. *Postgrad Med J.* 2001;77(906):217–20.

16 Lee S, Leung A, He X, et al. Iodine content in fast foods: comparison between two fast-food chains in the United States. *Endocr Pract.* 2010: 16(6):1071–72.

17 NEMO Study Group. Effect of a 12-mo micronutrient intervention on learning and memory in well-nourished and marginally nourished school-aged children: 2 parallel, randomized, placebo-controlled studies in Australia and Indonesia. *Am J Clin Nutr.* 2007;86(4):1082–93.

18 Sanger-Katz M. "The Decline in Big Soda." *New York Times,* 5 October 2015.

19 Campanile C. "Bloomberg Health Crusade Saved New Yorkers' Lives." *New York Post,* 11 May 2015, http://nypost.com/2015/05/11/new-yorkers-life-spans-improved-during-bloombergs-tenure-study/.

20 As of 2017; see "Food Retail Expansion to Support Health (FRESH)." NYCEDC, Financing and Incentives. https://www.nycedc.com/program/food-retail-expansion-support-health-fresh.

21 Decker H. "America's Most Obese State Passes 'Anti-Bloomberg Bill' to Ban Portion Control." National Memo, 13 March 2013. http://www.nationalmemo.com/americas-most-obese-state-passes-anti-bloomberg-bill-to-ban-portion-control/.

22 World Health Organization. *Global Status Report on Noncommunicable Diseases 2014.* Geneva: World Health Organization, 2014. http://apps.who.int/iris/bitstream/10665/148114/1/9789241564854_eng.pdf?ua=1.

23 "'Lifestyle' Diseases Linked to Unhealthy Habits Kill Millions of People Prematurely: WHO." Daily News, Lifestyle. 19 January 2015. http://www.nydailynews.com/life-style/health/lifestyle-diseases-kill-millions-prematurely-article-1.2083946.

24 Ibid.

25 Morland K, Wing S, Diez Roux A. The contextual effect of the local food environment on residents' diets: the atherosclerosis risk in communities study. *Am J Public Health.* 2002;92(11):1761–67.

26 Wrigley N, Warm D, Margetts B, Whelan A. Assessing the impact of improved retail access on diet in a "food desert:" a preliminary report. *Urban Studies.* 2002;39:2061–82.

27 American Heart Association. Food Access. https://www.heart.org/HEARTORG/Advocate/Voices-for-Healthy-Kids–Food-Access_UCM_460609_SubHomePage.jsp.

28 For more on these efforts, see the Voices for Healthy Kids 2016 progress report, *Building a Culture of Health for All Children.* http://voicesforhealthykids.org/2016progressreport/.

29 *A Review of Food Marketing to Children and Adolescents: Follow-Up Report.* Federal Trade Commission, 2012. https://www.ftc.gov/sites/default/files/documents/reports/review-food -marketing-children-and-adolescents-follow-report/121221foodmarketingreport.pdf.

30 Walsh B. "It's Not Just Genetics." *Time.* June 12, 2008. http://www.time.com/time/magazine /article/0,9171,1813984,00.html.

31 Stewart H, Hyman J, Carlson A, Frazao E. The cost of satisfying fruit and vegetable recommendations in the dietary guidelines. USDA Economic Research Service. Economic Brief # 27 Feb. 2016.

32 Eckel RH, Jakicic JM, Ard JD, et al. 2013 AHA/ACC guideline on lifestyle management to reduce cardiovascular risk. *Circulation.* 2014;129(25 Suppl 2):S76–99.

CHAPTER SEVEN: FOOD FOR THE HEART AND SOUL

1 Halberg O, Johansson O. Cancer trends during the 20th century. *J Aust Coll Nutr Environ Med.* 2002;21(1):3–8.

2 Nguyen B, Bauman A, Gale J, et al. Fruit and vegetable consumption and all-cause mortality: evidence from a large Australian cohort study. *Int J Behav Nutr Phys Act.* 2016;13:9; doi:10.1186/s12966–016–0334–5; Link LB, Potter JD. Raw versus cooked vegetables and cancer risk. *Cancer Epidemiol Biomarkers Prev.* 2004;13(9):1422–35; Oyebode O, Gordon-Dseagu V, Walker A, et al. Fruit and vegetable consumption and all-cause, cancer and CVD mortality: analysis of Health Survey for England data. *J Epidemiol Community Health.* 2014;68(9):856–62; doi:10.1136/jech-2013–203500.

3 World Cancer Research Fund International. Our cancer prevention recommendations. http://www.wcrf.org/int/research-we-fund/our-cancer-prevention-recommendations.

4 Orlich MJ, Singh PN, Sabaté J, et al. Vegetarian dietary patterns and mortality in Adventist Health Study 2. *AMA Intern Med.* 2013;173(13):1230–38; Li D. Effect of the vegetarian diet on non-communicable diseases. *J Sci Food Agric.* 2014;94(2):169–73.

5 Hightower JM, Moore D. Mercury levels in high-end consumers of fish. *Environ Health Perspect.* 2003;111(4):604–8; Mahaffey KR, Clickner RP, Bodurow CC. Blood organic mercury and dietary mercury intake: National Health and Nutrition Examination Survey 1999 and 2000. *Environ Health Perspect.* 112(5):562–70.

6 Stripp C, Overvad K, Christensen J, et al. Fish intake is positively associated with breast cancer incidence rate. *J Nutr.* 2003;133(11):3664–69.

7 Guillén MD, Uriarte PS. Aldehydes contained in edible oils of a very different nature after prolonged heating at frying temperature: presence of toxic oxygenated αβ unsaturated aldehydes. *Food Chem.* 2012;131(3):915; doi:10.1016/j.foodchem.2011.09.079; Marnett LJ. Oxy radicals, lipid peroxidation and DNA damage. *Toxicology.* 2002;181–182:219–22.

8 Linos E, Willet WC, Cho E, Frazier L. Adolescent diet in relation to breast cancer risk among premenopausal women. *Cancer Epidemiol Biomarkers Prev.* 2010;19(3):689–96.

9 Michels KB, Rosner BA, Chumlea WC, et al. Preschool diet and adult risk of breast cancer. *Int J Cancer.* 2006;118(3):749–54.

10 Alkaabi JM, Al-Dabbagh B, Ahmad S, et al. Glycemic indices of five varieties of dates in healthy and diabetic subjects. *Nutr J.* 2011;10:59.

CHAPTER NINE: FREQUENTLY ASKED QUESTIONS

1 Fortmann SP, Burda BU, Senger CA, et al. Vitamin and mineral supplements in the primary prevention of cardiovascular disease and cancer: an updated systematic evidence review for the U.S. Preventive Services Task Force. *Ann Intern Med.* 2013;159(120):824–34; Grodstein F, O'Brien J, Kang JH, et al. Long-term multivitamin supplementation and cognitive function in men: a randomized trial. *Ann Intern Med.* 2013;159(12):806–14.

2 Manshadi S, Ishiguro L, Sohn K, et al. Folic Acid Supplementation Promotes Mammary Tumor Progression in a Rat Model. *PLoS One.* January 21, 2014; http://dx.doi.org/10.1371/journal.pone.0084635.

3 Charles D, Ness AR, Campbell D, et al. Taking folate in pregnancy and the risk of maternal breast cancer. *BMJ.* 2004;329(7479):1375–76.

4 Larsson SC, Akesson A, Bergkvist L, et al. Multivitamin use and breast cancer incidence in a prospective cohort of Swedish women. *Am J Clin Nutr.* 2010;91:1268–72.

5 Stolzenberg-Solomon RZ, Chang SC, Leitzmann MF, et al. Folate intake, alcohol use, and postmenopausal breast cancer risk in the Prostate, Lung, Colorectal, and Ovarian Cancer Screening trial. *Am J Clin Nutr.* 2006;83:895–904.

6 Fife J, Raniga S, Hider PN, et al. Folic acid supplementation and colorectal cancer risk: a meta-analysis. *Colorectal Dis.* 2011;13(2):132–37; Baggott JE, Oster RA, Tamura T. Meta-analysis of cancer risk in folic acid supplementation trials. *Cancer Epidemiol.* 2012;36(1):78–81.

7 Figueiredo JC, Grau MV, Haile RW, et al. Folic acid and risk of prostate cancer: results from a randomized clinical trial. *J Natl Cancer Inst.* 2009;101:432–35.

8 Wien TN, Pike E, Wisloff T, et al. Cancer risk with folic acid supplements: a systemic review and meta-analysis. *BMJ Open.* 2012;2(1):e000653; doi:10.1136/bmjopen-2011–000653.

9 Haberg SE, London SJS, Stigum H, et al. Folic acid supplements in pregnancy and early childhood respiratory health. *Arch Dis Child.* 2009;94(3):180–84.

10 Raghaven R, Riley A, Caruso DM, et al. Maternal plasma folate, vitamin B12 levels and multivitamin supplement during pregnancy and the risk of autism spectrum disorder in the Boston Birth Cohort. Paper presented at the International Society of Autism Research meeting, Baltimore, 13 May 2016.

11 Pogoda JM, Preston-Martin S, Howe G, et al. An international case-control study of maternal diet during pregnancy and childhood brain tumor risk: a histology-specific analysis by food group. *Ann Epidemiol.* 2009;19:148–60; Kwan ML, Jensen CD, Block G, et al. Maternal diet and risk of childhood acute lymphoblastic leukemia. *Public Health Rep.* 2009;124:503–14; Petridou E, Ntouvelis E, Dessypris N, et al. Maternal diet and acute lymphoblastic leukemia in young children. *Cancer Epidemiol Biomarkers Prev.* 2005;14:1935–39; Jensen CD, Block G, Buffler P, et al. Maternal dietary risk factors in childhood acute lymphoblastic leukemia (United States). *Cancer Causes Control.* 2004;15:559–70.

12 Bjelkaovic G, Nikolava D, Gluud LL, et al. Mortality in randomized trials of antioxidant supplements for primary and secondary prevention. *JAMA.* 2007;297:842–57.

13 Melhus H, Michaelson K, Kindmark A, et al. Excessive dietary intake of vitamin A is associated with reduced bone mineral density and increased risk of hip fracture. *Ann Intern Med.* 1998;129(10):770–78.

14 Oregon State University, Linus Pauling Institute Micronutrient Information Center. Vitamin A. http://lpi.oregonstate.edu/infocenter/vitamins/vitaminA/. Last updated January 2015.

15 Bjelakovic G, Nikolova D, Gluud LL, et al. Antioxidant supplements for prevention of mortality in healthy participants and patients with various diseases. *Cochrane Database Syst Re.* 2012;3:CD007176; doi:10.1002/14651858.CD007176.pub2.

16 Barnett JB, Hamer DH, Meydani SN. Low zinc status: a new risk factor for pneumonia in the elderly? *Nutr Rev.* 2010;68:30–37; Meydani SN, Barnett JB, Dallal GE, et al. Serum zinc and pneumonia in nursing home elderly. *Am J Clin Nutr.* 2007;86:1167–73; Prasad AS, Beck FW, Bao B, et al. Zinc supplementation decreases incidence of infections in the elderly: effect of zinc on generation of cytokines and oxidative stress. *Am J Clin Nutr.* 2007;85:837–44; Barnett JB, Dao MC, Hamer DH, et al. Effect of zinc supplementation on serum zinc concentration and T cell proliferation in nursing home elderly: a randomized, double-blind, placebo-controlled trial. *Am J Clin Nutr.* 2016;103:942–51.

17 Bolland MJ, Grey A, Avenell A, et al. Calcium supplements with or without vitamin D and risk of cardiovascular events: reanalysis of the Women's Health Initiative limited access dataset and meta-analysis. *BMJ.* 2011:342:d2040; Bolland MJ, Avenell A, Baron JA, et al. Effect of calcium supplements on risk of myocardial infarction and cardiovascular events: meta-analysis. *BMJ.* 2010;341:c3691.

18 Reid IR, Bolland MJ, Grey A. Does calcium supplementation increase cardiovascular risk? *Clin Endocrinol (Oxf).* 2010;74(6):689–95.

19 Holick MF. Sunlight and vitamin D for bone health and prevention of autoimmune diseases, cancers, and cardiovascular disease. *Am J Clin Nutr.* 2004;80:1678S–88S; Bjelakovic G, Gluud LL, Nikolova D, et al. Vitamin D supplementation for prevention of mortality in adults. *Cochrane Database Syst Rev.* 2014;1:CD007470.

20 Rossini M, Gatti D, Viapiana O, et al. Short-term effects on bone turnover markers of a single high dose of oral vitamin D(3). *J Clin Endocrinol Metab.* 2012;97:E622–26; Zheng YT, Cui QQ, Hong YM, Yao WG. A meta-analysis of high dose, intermittent vitamin D supplementation among older adults. *PLoS One.* 2015;10:e0115850.

21 Foster M, Chu A, Petocz P, Samman S. Effect of vegetarian diets on zinc status: a systematic review and meta-analysis of studies in humans. *J Sci Food Agric.* 2013;93: 2362–71; Hunt JR. Bioavailability of iron, zinc, and other trace minerals from vegetarian diets. *Am J Clin Nutr.* 2003;78:633S–39S; Miller LV, Krebs NF, Hambidge KM. A mathematical model of zinc absorption in humans as a function of dietary zinc and phytate. *J Nutr.* 2007;137:135–41.

22 Prasad AS, Fitzgerald JT, Hess JW, et al. Zinc deficiency in elderly patients. *Nutrition.* 1993;9:218–24; Pepersack T, Rotsaert P, Benoit F, et al. Prevalence of zinc deficiency and its clinical relevance among hospitalised elderly. *Arch Gerontol Geriatr.* 2001;33:243–53.

23 Beulens JW, Booth SL, van den Heuvel EG, et al. The role of menaquinones (vitamin K(2)) in human health. *Br J Nutr.* 2013;110:1357–68; Cockayne S, Adamson J, Lanham-New S, et al. Vitamin K and the prevention of fractures: systematic review and meta-analysis of randomized controlled trials. *Arch Intern Med.* 2006;166:1256–61.

24 Sarter B, Kelsey KS, Schwartz TA, Harris WS. Blood docosahexaenoic acid and eicosapentaenoic acid in vegans: Associations with age and gender and effects of an algal -derived omega-3 fatty acid supplement. *Clinical Nutrition* 2015. http://www .clinicalnutritionjournal.com/issue/S0261-5614(15)X0003-3;34(2):212-18.

25 Pottala JV, Yaff K, Robinson JG, et al. Higher RBC EPA + DHA corresponds with larger total brain and hippocampal volumes. *Neurology.* 2014;82(5):435–42.

26 Pena-Rosas JP, De-Regil LM, Garcia-Casal MN, et al. Daily oral iron supplementation during pregnancy. *Cochrane Database Syst Rev.* 2015;12:CD004736; Scholl TO. Iron status during pregnancy: setting the stage for mother and infant. *Am J Clin Nutr.* 2005;81:1218S–22S; Song QY, Luo WP, Zhang CX. High serum iron level is associated with an increased risk of hypertensive disorders during pregnancy: a meta-analysis of observational studies. *Nutr Res.* 2015;35:1060–69.

27 Mei Z, Cogswell ME, Looker AC, et al. Assessment of iron status in US pregnant women from the National Health and Nutrition Examination Survey (NHANES), 1999–2006. *Am J Clin Nutr.* 2011;93:1312–20.

28 Murray-Kolb LE, Beard JL. Iron deficiency and child and maternal health. *Am J Clin Nutr.* 2009;89:946S–50S; Armony-Sivan R, Kaplan-Estrin M, Jacobson SW, et al. Iron-deficiency anemia in infancy and mother-infant interaction during feeding. *J Dev Behav Pediatr.* 2010;31:326–32; Lozoff B, Georgieff MK. Iron deficiency and brain development. *Semin Pediatr Neurol.* 2006;13:158–65; Gautam CS, Saha L, Sekhri K, et al. Iron deficiency in pregnancy and the rationality of iron supplements prescribed during pregnancy. *Medscape J Med.* 2008;10:283.

29 Jáuregui-Lobera I. Iron deficiency and cognitive functions. *J Neuropsychiatr Dis Treat.* 2014;10: 2087–95; Beard JL. Why iron deficiency is important in infant development. *J Nutr.* 2008;138:2534–36.

30 Waldmann A, Koschizke JW, Leitzmann C, et al. Dietary iron intake and iron status of German female vegans: results of the German vegan study. *Ann Nutr Metab.* 2004;48:103–8.

31 Stokowski LA. No amount of alcohol is safe. Medscape. 30 April 2014. http://www .medscape.com/viewarticle/824237.

32 See https://ntp.niehs.nih.gov/pubhealth/roc/index-1.html. Last updated 3 November 2016.

33 Nelson DE, Jarman DW, Rehm J, et al. Alcohol-attributable cancer deaths and years of potential life lost in the United States. *Am J Public Health.* 2013;103(4):641–48.

34 Bagnardi V, Rota M, Botteri E, et al. Alcohol consumption and site-specific cancer risk: a comprehensive dose-response meta-analysis. *Br J Cancer.* 2015;112:580–93.

35 Connor J. Alcohol consumption as a cause of cancer. *Addiction* 2016;112(2):222–28.

36 Hashibe M, Brennan P, Chuang SC, et al. Interaction between tobacco and alcohol use and the risk of head and neck cancer: pooled analysis in the International Head and Neck Cancer Epidemiology Consortium. *Cancer Epidemiol Biomarkers Prev.* 2009;18(2):541–50; Grewal P, Viswanathen VA. Liver cancer and alcohol. *Clin Liver Disease.* 2012;16(4):839–50; Fedirko V, Tramacere I, Bagnardi V, et al. Alcohol drinking and colorectal cancer risk: an overall and dose-response meta-analysis of published studies. *Annals Oncol.* 2011;22(9):1958–72; Bellocco R, Pasquali E, Rota M, et al. Alcohol drinking and risk of renal cell carcinoma: results of a meta-analysis. *Annals Oncol.* 2012;23(9):2235–44; Tramacere I, Pelucchi C, Bonifazi M, et al. A meta-analysis on alcohol drinking and the risk of Hodgkin lymphoma. *Eur J Cancer Prev.* 2012;21(3):268–73; Turati F, Garavello W, Tramacere I, et al. A meta-analysis of alcohol drinking and oral and pharyngeal cancers: results from subgroup analyses. *Alcohol Alcoholism.* 2013;48(1):107–18; Rehm J, Patra J, Popova S. Alcohol drinking cessation and its effect on esophageal and head and neck cancers: a pooled analysis. *Int J Cancer.* 2007;121(5):1132–37; Kanda J, Matsuo K, Suzuki T, et al. Impact of alcohol consumption with polymorphisms in alcohol-metabolizing enzymes on pancreatic cancer risk in Japanese. *Cancer Sci.* 2009;100(2):296–302; Yokoyama A, Omori T. Genetic polymorphisms of alcohol and aldehyde dehydrogenases and risk for esophageal and head and neck cancers. *Alcohol.* 2005;35(3):175–85.

37 Allen NE, Beral V, Casabonne D, et al. Moderate alcohol intake and cancer incidence in women. *J Natl Cancer Institute.* 2009;101(5):296–305; Hamajima N, Hirose K, Tajima K, et al. Alcohol, tobacco and breast cancer: collaborative reanalysis of individual data from 53 epidemiological studies, including 58,515 women with breast cancer and 95,067 women without the disease. *Br J Cancer.* 2002;87(11):1234–45; Chen WY, Rosner B, Hankinson SE, et al. Moderate alcohol consumption during adult life, drinking patterns, and breast cancer risk. *JAMA.* 2011;306:1884–90.

38 Stokowski LA. No amount of alcohol is safe. Medscape. 30 April 2014. http://www .medscape.com/viewarticle/824237.

39 Daniel S, Bereczki D. Alcohol as a risk factor for hemorrhagic stroke. *Ideggyogy Sz.* 2004;57:247–56.

40 George A, Figueredo VM. Alcohol and arrhythmias: a comprehensive review. *J Cardiovasc Med.* 2010;11:21–228; Klatsky AL. Alcohol and cardiovascular health. *Physiol Behav.* 2010;100:76–81.

41 Global status report on alcohol and health 2014. World Health Organization. http://apps
    .who.int/iris/bitstream/10665/112736/1/9789240692763_eng.pdf.

42 Athar M, Back JH, Tang X, et al. Resveratrol: a review of preclinical studies for human cancer
    prevention. *Toxicol Appl Pharmacol.* 2007;224(3):274–83; Patel KR, Scott E, Brown VA, et al.
    Clinical trials of resveratrol. *Ann NY Acad Sci.* 2011;1215:161–69.

43 Fuhrman J, Singer M. Improved cardiovascular parameter with a nutrient-dense, plant-rich
    diet-style: a patient survey with illustrative cases. *American Journal of Lifestyle Medicine.* 7 July
    2016; doi:10.1177/1559827615611024.

44 Dunaief DM, Fuhrman J, Dunaief JL, Ying G. Glycemic and cardiovascular parameters
    improved in type 2 diabetes with the high nutrient density (HND) diet. *Open J Prev Med.*
    2012;2(3):364–71.

45 Dickenson BD, Havas S. Reducing the population burden of cardiovascular disease by
    reducing sodium intake: a report of the Council on Science and Public Health. *Arch Intern
    Med.* 2007;167(14):1460–68.

46 Karppanen H, Mervaala E. Sodium intake and hypertension. *Prog Cardiovasc Dis.*
    2006;49(2):59–75; Cutler JA, Roccell E. Salt reduction for preventing hypertension and
    cardiovascular disease. *Hypertension.* 2006;48(5):818–19.

47 Cook N, Cutler J, Obarzanek E, et al. Long term effects of dietary sodium reduction on
    cardiovascular disease outcomes: observational follow-up of the trails of hypertension
    prevention (TOHP). *BMJ.* 2007;334:885.

48 Havas S, Roccella EJ, Lenfant C. Reducing the public health burden from elevated blood
    pressure levels in the United States by lowering intake of dietary sodium. *Am J Public Health.*
    2004;94(1):19–22.

49 Prospective Studies Collaboration. Age specific relevance of usual blood pressure to vascular
    mortality: a meta analysis of individual data for one million adults in 61 prospective studies.
    Lancet. 2002;360:1903–13.

50 Weinberger MH. Salt sensitivity is associated with an increased mortality in both normal and
    hypertensive humans. *J Clin Hypertens.* 2002;4(4):274–76.

51 Tuomilehto J, Jousilahti P, Rastenyte D, et al. Urinary sodium excretion and cardiovascular
    mortality in Finland: a prospective study. *Lancet.* 2001;357: 848–51.

52 Cook NR, Appel LJ, Whelton PK. Sodium intake and all-cause mortality over 20 years in the
    Trials of Hypertension Prevention. *J Am Coll Cardiol.* 2016;68(15):1609–17.

53 Luke R. President's address. *Trans Am Clin Climatol Assoc.* 2007;118: 1–22.

54 Freis E. The role of salt in hypertension. *Blood Pressure.* 1991;1:196–200.

55 National High Blood Pressure Education Program, National Heart, Lung and Blood Institute.
    National Institutes of Health. National High Blood Pressure Education Program Working
    Group report on primary prevention of hypertension. *Arch Intern Med.* 1993;153:186–208.

56 Sonnenberg A. Dietary salt and gastric ulcer. *Gut.* 1986;27(10):1138–42; Tsugane S, Sasazuki S.
    Diet and the risk of gastric cancer: review of epidemiological evidence. *Gastric Cancer.*
    2007;10(2):75–83.

57 De Wardener HE, MacGregor GA. Harmful effects of dietary salt in addition to hypertension.
    J Hum Hypertens. 2002;16(4):213–23.

58 Paddock C. CDC: 90 percent of Americans consume too much salt. Published Jan 8 2016
    Medical News Today. http://www.medicalnewstoday.com/articles/304833.php.
    Where's the sodium? CDC Vital Signs Feb 2012. https://www.cdc.gov/vitalsigns/sodium/.

59 McCann SE, Thompson LU, Nie J, et al. Dietary lignan intakes in relation to survival among
    women with breast cancer: the Western New York Exposures and Breast Cancer (WEB)
    study. *Breast Cancer Res Treat.* 2010;122:229–35.

INDEX

Page numbers in *italics* refer to illustrations.

ABOUT THE AUTHORS

JOEL FUHRMAN, M.D., specializes in preventing and reversing disease through nutritional and natural methods. Dr. Fuhrman is the president of the Nutritional Research Foundation. He is the author of several books, including the *New York Times* bestsellers *Eat to Live, Eat to Live Cookbook, Super Immunity, The End of Diabetes,* and *The End of Heart Disease.*

ROBERT B. PHILLIPS was a vice president at Merrill Lynch suffering with sarcoidosis, a serious health condition that affected his breathing. Six months after discovering Dr. Fuhrman's approach, his condition was completely reversed, and he quit his job at Merrill Lynch to help launch Dr. Fuhrman's member support website. Robert continues to write and conducts research at Drexel University in the field of social energy. He lives in New Jersey with his wife Marcia and two kids Joseph and Jacob. And he has two other grown kids Joey and Jennifer.